Herbal Medicine Handbook

Herbal Medicine Handbook

Editor: Melissa Gould

Callisto Reference

www.callistoreference.com

Callisto Reference,
118-35 Queens Blvd., Suite 400,
Forest Hills, NY 11375, USA

Visit us on the World Wide Web at:
www.callistoreference.com

ISBN: 978-1-64116-129-9 (Hardback)

Printed in China.

Cataloging-in-Publication Data

Herbal medicine handbook / edited by Melissa Gould.
p. cm.
Includes bibliographical references and index.
ISBN 978-1-64116-129-9
1. Herbs--Therapeutic use. 2. Traditional medicine.
3. Alternative medicine. I. Gould, Melissa.

RM666.H33 H47 2019
615.321--dc23

Table of Contents

Preface

The purpose of the book is to provide a glimpse into the dynamics and to present opinions and studies of some of the scientists engaged in the development of new ideas in the field from very different standpoints. This book will prove useful to students and researchers owing to its high content quality.

The study of botany that aims to use plants for medicinal purposes is known as herbalism. Some of the products of herbalism include herbal medicines, natural health products, herbal remedies, supplements, etc. Many herbs are applied to the skin in the form of essential oils. Herbalism is widely practiced throughout Africa and Asia. Traditional Chinese medicine and Ayurveda are examples of herbal medicine. This book presents researches and studies performed by experts across the globe. It covers in detail some existing theories and innovative concepts revolving around herbal medicine. For all those who are interested in this field, this book can prove to be an essential guide.

At the end, I would like to appreciate all the efforts made by the authors in completing their chapters professionally. I express my deepest gratitude to all of them for contributing to this book by sharing their valuable works. A special thanks to my family and friends for their constant support in this journey.

Editor

Phytochemical and antimicrobial activity of *Monechma ciliatum* (black mahlab) seed extracts

Oshi, M.A.M[*1], Abdelkareem, A.M[1], Eltohami, M.SH[2]

[1]*Department of Pharmaceutical Technology, Faculty of Pharmacy, Omdurman Islamic University, Omdurman, Sudan;*
Email:** ***oshipharm@hotmail.com

[2]*Department of Pharmacognosy, Faculty of Pharmacy, Omdurman Islamic University, Omdurman, Sudan;*

ARTICLE INFO

Topic: *Phytochemistry*

Key words:

Black mahlab

Monechma ciliatum

Antibacterial Activity

Antifungal Activity

Abbreviations:

Sa: *Staphylococcus aureus*;

Pa: *Pseudomonas aeruginosa*;

Kp: *Klebsiella pneumoniae*;

Ca: *Candida albicans*;

An: *Aspergillus niger*;

Af: *Aspergillus flavus*.

ABSTRACT

Background & Aim: The purpose of present study was to examine and validate the folk's claim of inhalation of *Monechma ciliatum* seeds powder by traditional African natives for cold and allergic conditions, so as to formulate a useful therapeutic agent to respiratory tract infections.

Experimental: Different extracts were bio-assayed *in vitro* for their bioactivity to inhibit the growth of pathogenic bacteria and fungi. Bacteria and fungi selected in the study were common pathogens for respiratory tract infections.

Results & Discussion: *Klebsiella pneumoniae* was highly sensitive to the hydroalcoholic extract (maceration by 70% ethanol and 30% water) and moderately sensitive to the extract (maceration by water). *Staphylococcus aureus* was found to be moderately sensitive to the hydroalcoholic extract (maceration by 70% ethanol 30% water). *Pseudomonas aeruginosa* was resistance to all extract used. In addition, all fungi used were found to be resistance to all extracts. Phytochemical screening test results of seeds of *Monechma ciliatum* to detect the major constituents showed the presence of flavonoids, tannins, triterpens, and anthraquinones. The findings of study support the traditional uses of the plant in the therapy of respiratory tract infections.

Recommended applications/industries: The extracts of black mahlab could be used in future direction as alternative therapeutic agents for the treatment of human's respiratory tract infectious diseases caused by *Klebsiella pneumoniae* and *Staphylococcus aureus*.

1. Introduction

According to World Health Organization (WHO), interest in traditional systems of medicine and, in particular, herbal medicines, has increased substantially in both developed and developing countries over the past two decades (WHO, 2003). A WHO survey indicates that about 70 - 80% of the world population, particularly in the developing countries; rely on non-conventional medicines mainly of herbal sources in their primary healthcare. WHO has described traditional medicine as one of the surest means to achieve total healthcare coverage of the world's population. In pursuance of its goal of providing accessible and culturally acceptable health care for the global population, WHO has encouraged the rational use of traditional plant based medicines by member states and has developed technical guidelines for the assessment of herbal medicine (Okunlola *et al.*, 2003).

Infection remains the main cause of morbidity and mortality in man, particularly in under-developed areas where it is associated with poverty and overcrowding. In the developed world increasing prosperity, universal immunization, and antibiotics have reduced the prevalence of infectious disease. However, antibiotic-resistant strains of bacteria as well as viruses and new diseases including Human Immunodeficiency Virus (HIV) infection and variant Creutzfeldt- Jackob Disease variant (vCJD) have emerged. The common respiratory tract infections are influenza (caused by *influenzae* virus, its main complications the secondary bacterial infection by *Staphylococcus aureus* having a mortality of up to 20%), Pneumonia (usually caused by bacteria *Staphylococcus aureus, Legionella pneumoniae, Coxiella burnentii, Pseudomonas aeruginosa, Pneumocystis carinii, Klebsiella pneumoniae*, and anaerobic organism) and Sinusitis infections are usually caused by *Streptococcus pneumoniae* and *Haemophilus influenzae* (Kumar & Clark, 2003). Deep fungus infections have increased rapidly in recent years. Most fungus infections are caused by candida germ, mainly *Candida albicans*. The death rate from these infections can reach to 30-60%. Unfortunately, few anti-fungus medicines are available for treating fungus infections, not to mention that most of them have serious side effects (Sheng *et al.*, 2012).

Monechma ciliatum is a plant distributed throughout tropical Africa, as wild and also cultivated in savanna (Fig.1). In Sudan, it is locally known as 'El-Mahlab El-Aswad', or 'El-Mehbab'. It grows in western and southwestern parts of Sudan, especially in the Nuba Mountains and Gabel Mara area. In Nigeria it is known as 'Bakin mata' in Hausa language. In Sudan the dried seeds (Fig. 2) are used as a scent preparation, also reported that in Sudan the entire dried plant is used for diarrhea and vomiting (Uguru & Evan, 2002). It is used as antispasmodic, and the aqueous extract used as laxative. The seeds are used as an effective laxative; it is further used in traditional Sudanese fragrances, lotions, and other cosmetics used for wedding preparation and childbirth rituals such as 'Dilka', 'Khumrra' (Mariod *et al.*, 2009).

Monechma ciliatum is a plant used in folk medicine by traditional midwives to induce labor and menses in the northern parts of Nigeria. It is reported that the dried leaves and seeds are powdered and burnt as an inhalation for treatment of cold. In Edo and Delta states of Nigeria, the plant is used as anthelmintic and anti-dysenteric (Uguru & Evan, 2002).

The seeds of plant contain hydrocarbons and fatty acids (Ayoub, 1981). Recently, the seeds were screened by Mariod et al. (2009); they found fatty acids (palmitic, stearic, linoleic, and others); tocopherols; protein; and elements (K, Ca, Mg, Al, Pb, Ni, Mn, Cu, Cr, Co, and Fe). The paucity of antimicrobial and chemical data of this herbal medicine prompted an investigation into its antimicrobial activity. Therefore, the present study was planned to find out the antimicrobial activity and their efficacy against different bacterial and fungal infections.

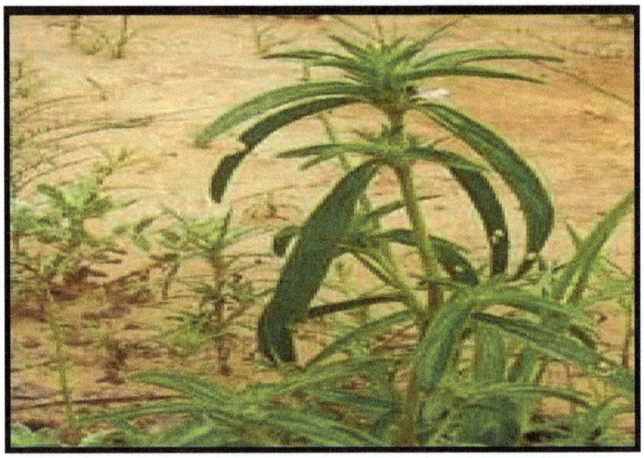

Fig. 1. *Monechma ciliatum* (A wild Sudanese medicinal plant)

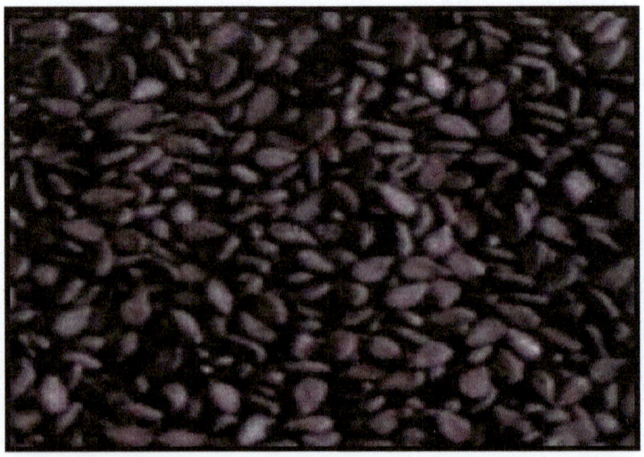

Fig. 2. Seeds of *Monechma ciliatum*

2. Materials and Methods

2.1. Plant materials and chemicals

The study was done at the Medicinal and Aromatic Plant Research Institute (MAPRI) of Khartoum, Sudan and Omdurman Islamic University, Omdurman, Sudan. Black mahlab seeds samples used in this study were collected from Nubia Mountains (South Kordofan state, Sudan). The seeds were identified in Department of pharmacognosy Alnaileen University-Sudan, and authenticated at the Medicinal and Aromatic Plant Research Institute (MAPRI) of Khartoum-Sudan. The seeds were collected between September and December (autumn), separated, and dried under shade. The dried seeds were stored in a covered bottle at room temperature until required for use.

Agar: HiMedia Laboratories Pvt. Ltd, India. Ampicillin: Bristol – Mayers Squibb, USA. Clotrimazole: General Medicine Co., Sudan. Ethanol: Scharlau Chemie S.A, Spain. Gentamicin: Roussel, UK. Methanol: BDH laboratory, UK. Nystatin: Sigma Medical Company, USA. Sabouraut agar: HiMedia Laboratories Pvt. Ltd, India. Standard bacteria and fungi: Three types of standard bacteria namely *Staphylococcus aureus* (ATCC 25923), *Klebsiella pneumoniae* (ATCC 53657) and *Pseudomonas aeruginosa* (ATCC 27853) were obtained from MAPRI. Three types of standard fungi namely *Aspergillus fumigates* (ATCC13073), *Aspergillus niger* (ATCC 9763) and *Candida albicans* (ATCC 7596) were obtained from MAPRI.

2.2. Preparation of the extracts

2.2.1. Maceration method by using water, methanol or ethanol as a solvent system. The dried seeds for *Monechma ciliatum* were reduced to a coarse powder by using mesh No. 35; 20 g of the coarse powder weighed, and transferred to flasks containing 400 mL of distilled water, methanol [30, 50, 70% (v/v)] or ethanol [30, 50, 70% (v/v)] separately. The flasks were allowed for 24h at room temperature, with occasional shaking. Then, the extract of each flask was passed through a cotton wool and the solid residue (marc) pressed (screw press). The strained and expressed liquid obtained was mixed, put for 12 h for clarification and filtrated. Finally, the filtrates were evaporated to reduce the solvent volume using rotary evaporator under reduced pressure at 40 °C and placed in a Petri dish, and left to dry to constant weight.

2.2.2. Infusion method. The dried seeds for *M. ciliatum* were reduced to a coarse powder by using mesh No. 35; 20 g of the coarse powder weighed, and transferred to flasks. 400 mL of cold and hot boiled water added to two flasks separately. The flasks were allowed for 24 h at room temperature, with occasional shaking. Then, the extract of each flask was passed through a cotton wool and the solid residue (marc) pressed (screw press). The strained and expressed liquid obtained was mixed, put for 12 h for clarification and filtrated. Finally, the filtrates were evaporated to reduce the solvent volume using rotary evaporator under reduced pressure at 40 °C and placed in a Petri dish, and left to dry to constant weight

2.2.3. Decoction method. The dried seeds for *M. ciliatum* were reduced to a coarse powder by using mesh No. 35; 20 g of the coarse powder weighed, and transferred to 4 flasks containing 200 mL of boiled water and allowed to stand for 5, 10, 15, and 20 min respectively. The flasks were allowed for 24 h at room temperature, with occasional shaking. Then, the extract of each flask was passed through a cotton wool and the solid residue (marc) pressed (screw press). The strained and expressed liquid obtained was mixed, put for 12 h for clarification and filtrated. Finally, the filtrates were evaporated to reduce the solvent volume using rotary evaporator under reduced pressure at 40 °C and placed in a Petri dish, and left to dry to constant weight.

2.2.4. Soxhlet extraction. The dried seeds for *M. ciliatum* were reduced to a coarse powder by using mesh No. 35; 20 g of the coarse powder weighed, and transferred to three Soxhlet containing 200 mL of methanol 70% (v/v), ethanol 70% (v/v) and chloroform separately, and allowed for 10 h. The flasks were allowed for 24 h at room temperature, with occasional shaking. Then, the extract of each flask was passed through a cotton wool and the solid residue (marc) pressed (screw press). The strained and expressed liquid obtained was mixed, put for 12 h for clarification and filtrated. Finally, the filtrates were evaporated to reduce the solvent volume using rotary evaporator under reduced pressure at 40 °C and placed in a Petri dish, and left to dry to constant weight.

2.5. Preparation of standard bacterial suspension

One milliliter aliquots of 24 h broth cultures of the standard organisms were aseptically distributed onto nutrient agar slopes and incubated at 37 °C for 24 h. The bacterial growth was harvested and washed off with sterile normal saline, to produce a suspension containing about 108 - 109 colony forming units per mL The suspension was stored in refrigerator at 4 °C until used (Kavanagh, 1972).

2.6. Preparation of standard fungal suspension

The fungal cultures were maintained on Sabouraut dextrose agar, incubated at 25 °C for three days. The fungal growth was harvested and washed with sterile normal saline, finally suspended in 100 mL of sterile normal saline, and the suspension was stored in the refrigerator until used (Kavanagh, 1972).

2.7. Antibacterial activity

Antibacterial activity was studied by an agar- diffusion method. Each of the incula of the tested organisms (1 mL) was poured into sterile Petri dish. A medium (at about 45 °C) was poured into each of the Petri dishes (20 mL). The medium was left to stand to allow it to set. Holes (disc shape) were made on the media with the aid of a sterile cork borer of 10 mm diameter and removal of the agar disc. The cups were marked, and different concentrations of the sterile extract were pipetted (0.1 mL) into the cups using sterile syringes. Plates were then incubated at 37 °C for 24 h. The sensitivities of the test organisms to the extracts were indicated by clear zones of growth inhibition around the cups containing the extracts and the diameter of the clear zone was taken as an index of the degree of sensitivity (Hassan *et al.*, 2010).

2.8. Antifungal activity

Antifungal activity was studied by an agar- diffusion method. Each of the incula of the tested organisms (1 mL) was poured into sterile Petri dish. A medium (about 45 °C) was poured into each of the Petri dishes (20 mL). The medium was left to stand to allow it to set. Holes (disc shape) were made on the media with the aid of a sterile cork borer of 10mm diameter and removal of the agar disc. The cups were marked, and different concentrations of the plant extracts were pipetted (0.1 mL) into the cups using sterile syringes. Plates were then incubated at 37 °C for 48 h. The sensitivities of the test organisms to the plant extracts were indicated by clear zones of growth inhibition around the cups containing the plant extracts and the diameter of the clear zone was taken as an index of the degree of sensitivity (Hassan *et al.*, 2010).

2.9. Phytochemical screening tests

Phytochemical screening was done for black mahlab seeds samples by using methods described by Sofowora (1993) and phytochemical analysis results were reported in Table 5.

2.10. Phytochemical screening

Ten gram of the powdered seeds was macerated in 100 mL of 70% (v/v) ethanol for 4h. The solution was filtered; enough 70% (v/v) ethanol added to complete the volume to 100 mL. This prepared extract (PE) was used for the various phytochemical tests.

2.10.1. Test for flavonoids. 17.5 mL of the PE was evaporated to dryness on a water bath, cooled, and the residue was defatted by several extractions with petroleum ether. The defatted residue was dissolved in 30 mL of 80% (v/v) ethanol, filtered, and the filtrate used for the following tests:

2.10.1.1. To 3 mL of the filtrate in a test tube, 1 mL of 1% of aluminum chloride in methanol solution was added. Formation of a yellow color immediately was taken as evidence of presence of flavonoids.

2.10.1.2. To 3 mL of the filtrate in a test tube, 1 mL of 1% potassium hydroxide solution was added. A dark yellow color indicates the presence of flavonoid.

2.10.2. Test for tannins. 7 mL of the PE was evaporated to dryness on a water bath. The residue was extracted several times with *n*- hexane and filtered. The insoluble residue was stirred with 10 mL of hot saline solution. The mixture was cooled, filtered, and the volume of filtrate adjusted to 10 mL normal saline.

2.10.2.1. Five milliliter portion of this solution was treated with few drops of gelatin salts reagent. Formation of immediate precipitate was taken as evidence for the presence of tannins in the sample.

2.10.2.2. To another portion of this solution, few drops of ferric chloride (test reagent) were added. Formation of blue, black or green color was taken as evidence for the presence of tannins in the sample.

2.10.3. Test for triterpens and unsaturated sterols. Ten milliliter of PE was evaporated to dryness on a water bath and the cooled residue stirred several times with chloroform to remove the most of coloring materials. The residue was then extracted with 20 mL of chloroform. The chloroform solution was dehydrated over anhydrous sodium sulphate. Five mL portion of the chloroform solution was mixed with 0.5 mL of acetic anhydride followed by 2drops of conc. sulfuric acid. The gradual appearance of green, blue, pink to purple color was taken as evidence of presence of sterols (green to purple) and triterpens (pink to purple) in the sample.

2.10.4. Test for alkaloids. 7.5 milliliter sample of the prepared extract was evaporated to dryness on water bath. 5 mL 2N hydrochloric acid was added, stirred while heating on a water bath for 10 min, cooled, and filtered. To test tube few drops of Mayer's reagent was added. Slightly turbidity or heavy precipitate was taken as evidence for the presence of alkaloids.

2.10.5. Test for saponins. One gram of the dried powdered seed was placed in a clean test tube. 10 mL of distilled water was added to test tube, stoppered, and vigorously shaken for about 30 s. The tube was then allowed to stand; the appearance of honey comb, persisted for at least an hour, was taken as evidence for the presence of saponins.

2.10.6. Test for cyanogenic glycosides. Three gram of the powdered seed was placed in flask and sufficient water added to moisten the sample, and followed by 1mL of chloroform. Apices of sodium picrate paper were carefully inserted between a split cork which used to stopper the flask. A change in color of the paper from yellow to various shaded red was taken as evidence for the presence of cyanogenic glycosides.

2.10.7. Test for anthraquinones. Ten gram of the powdered seed was boiled with 10 mL of 0.5 N KOH containing 1mL of 3% of hydrogen peroxide solution. The mixture was extracted by shaking with 10 mL of benzene. Five milliliter of the benzene solution was shaken with 3 mL of 10% ammonium hydroxide solution and the two layers allowed separating. The presence of anthraquinone was indicated by alkaline layer was found to have assumed pink or red color.

2.10.8. Test for coumarins. Three gram of the original powdered plant material boiled with 20 mL of distilled water in test tube and filter paper attached to the test tube. 0.5 N KOH was added, and then the filter paper inspected under UV light.

3. Results and Discussion

Extensive experimental work was done to select the most suitable extraction methods (maceration, infusion, decoction and Soxhlet) for antimicrobial activity tests against Gram positive bacteria, Gram negative bacteria and fungi, particularly those cause respiratory tract infections.

Maceration by water resulted in an extract with many limitations and drawbacks, as the high susceptibility to fermentation that took place after 24 h. It gave positive results against *Staphylococcus aureus* and *Klebsiella pneumoniae* as illustrated in Table 2.

Maceration by different concentrations of methanol and ethanol in water was found to be the best extraction method. Ethanol 70% (v/v) was selected for antimicrobial test, due to its high extraction yield (Table 1), and for economic factors (ethanol has low cost, more available and safer than methanol). Ethanol 70% (v/v) gave positive results against Gram negative bacterium *Klebsiella pneumoniae* and Gram positive bacterium *Staphylococcus aureus* (Table 2). In infusion method, the hot infusion gave high extraction yield than cold one (Table1). This method (hot infusion) did not give results as shown in Table 2. In decoction method, decoction for 20min gave high extraction yield than others (Table 1). It did not give positive results as shown in Table 2. In Soxhlet method, the extract by methanol was superior to its high extraction yield (Table 1). Soxhlet extract by methanol did not give results as shown in Table 2.

The negative antimicrobial results showed by infusion, decoction and Soxhlet extracts Table 2, may be attributed to thermolabile natures of active compounds of extract which decomposed by temperature more than 40 °C.

Pseudomonas aeruginosa and all fungi used were found to be insensitive to all extracts used as shown in Table 2. The resistance of *Pseudomonas aeruginosa* to extracts may be due to its permeability barrier afforded by its outer membrane lippolysaccharide and its tendency to colonize surfaces in the biofilm form makes the cells impervious to therapeutic concentrations of antibiotics (Omolola, 2011). The struggle of all fungi used in experiment to extracts may be due to its unique cell wall components glucans and chitin, make the diffusion of the extract difficult.

The phytochemical screening test results of seeds of *M. ciliatum* (Table 5), illustrated the presence of flavonoids, tannins and terpenoids which their antiallergic, anti- inflammatory, and antibacterial activities supporting the traditional uses of seeds for cold and allergic conditions. Medicinal plants have been used for centuries in folk medicines as remedies for human diseases, and many studies have been carried out in order to find out the scientific basis for their effectiveness. The main active antimicrobial agents isolated include alkaloids, phenolic acids, quinones, tannins, coumarins, flavonoids, and terpenoids (Ahmed *et al.*, 2006).

M. ciliatum seeds in this study exerted a high antibacterial activity against Gram positive bacteria *Staphylococcus aureus* and Gram negative bacteria *Klebsiella pneumoniae*. The study, therefore, provides the scientific basis for its traditional application as ethno-medicine for cold and allergic conditions. Therefore, this medicinal herb can be used for the treatment of respiratory tract infections caused by these two bacteria. The whole plant extract was chosen for the test due to the probability of synergistic action.

Table 1. The yield percentage and some organoleptic properties of extract

Extraction method	Yield % (± 0.5 %)	Color	Odor	Taste	Consistency
Maceration by water	9.05	yellow	aromatic	bitter	solid
Maceration by methanol 30%	5.15	brown	aromatic	bitter	semisolid
Maceration by methanol 50%	5.45	brown	aromatic	bitter	semisolid
Maceration by methanol 70%	7.40	brown	aromatic	bitter	semisolid
Maceration by ethanol 30%	2.45	brown	aromatic	bitter	semisolid
Maceration by ethanol 50%	5.00	brown	aromatic	bitter	semisolid
Maceration by ethanol 70%	5.15	brown	aromatic	bitter	semisolid
Infusion by cold water	6.50	yellow	aromatic	bitter	solid
Infusion by hot water	9.50	brown	aromatic	bitter	solid
Decoction by water 5min	7.15	brown	aromatic	bitter	solid
Decoction by water 10min	12.13	brown	aromatic	bitter	solid
Decoction by water 15min	12.60	brown	aromatic	bitter	solid
Decoction by water 20min	13.05	brown	aromatic	bitter	solid
Soxhlet by methanol	9.35	brown	aromatic	bitter	semisolid
Soxhlet by ethanol	6.00	brown	aromatic	bitter	semisolid
Soxhlet by chloroform	3.5	white	odorless	tasteless	liquid

Table 2. Comparative bioactivity of *Monechma ciliatum* seed extract against different standard bacteria and fungi

Extraction method	Solvent system	`Conc. (mg\mL)	Standard bacteria			Standard fungi		
			Sa	Pa	Kp	An	Ca	Af
Maceration (24 h)	water	25	11	-	-	-	-	-
		50	22	-	-	-	-	-
		100	26	-	-	-	-	-
		150	-	-	20	-	-	-
Maceration (24 h)	Ethanol (70%)	25	-	-	-	-	-	-
		50	11	-	16	-	-	-
		100	17	-	25	-	-	-
		150	11	-	33	-	-	-
Infusion (20 min)	water	25	-	-	-	-	-	-
		50	-	-	-	-	-	-
		100	-	-	-	-	-	-
		150	-	-	-	-	-	-
Soxhlet (10 h)	methanol (70%)	25	-	-	-	-	-	-
		50	-	-	-	-	-	-
		100	-	-	-	-	-	-
		150	-	-	-	-	-	-

Data are presented as mean diameter of growth inhibition zone (mm), average of three replicates, inhibition zone 15 mm: sensitive, 14-15 mm: intermediate, < 15 mm: resistant, - : no inhibition zone.

Table 3. Antibacterial activity of ampicillin and gentamicin

Drug	Conc. (mg/ml)	MDIZ(mm) Standard bacteria used		
		Sa	Pa	Kp
Ampicillin	0.04	30	-	-
	0.02	26	-	-
	0.01	22	-	-
	0.005	14	-	-
Gentamicin	0.04	18	22	16
	0.02	17	15	14
	0.01	14	12	-
	0.005	13	-	-

MDIZ: mean diameter of growth inhibition zone (mm), average of two replicates, inhibition zone ≥ 15 mm: sensitive, 14-15 mm: intermediate, < 15 mm: resistant, -: no inhibition zone

Table 4. Antifungal activity of nystatin and clotrimazole

Drug	Conc. (mg/ml)	MDIZ(mm) Standard fungi used		
		Ca	An	Af
Nystatin	0.05	28	17	-
	0.025	26	14	-
	0.0125	23	-	-
Clotrimazle	0.02	34	24	-
	0.01	30	29	-
	0.005	33	17	-

MDIZ: mean diameter of growth inhibition zone (mm), average of two replicates, inhibition zone ≥15mm: sensitive, 14-15mm: intermediate, < 15mm: resistant, -:no inhibition zone.

Table 5. The general phytochemical test results of *Monechma ciliatum* seeds

No.	Test	Result
1	Alkaloids	-ve
2	Anthraquinones	+ve
3	Coumarins	-ve
4	Cyanogenic glycosides	-ve
5	Flavonoids	+ve
6	Saponins	-ve
7	Tannins	+ve
8	Triterpenes and unsaturated sterols	+ve

As phytomedicines gain popularity, it is essential to educate the medical and scientific establishment that the pharmacological model of isolating constituents may not be the best methodology for the study of herbal medicines. The potentiation (or antagonism) provided by perturbation of multiple pharmacological targets converging in parallel biochemical pathways is often missed by standard laboratory searches for activity. If a chemical matrix is necessary for activity in phyto-medicines, then many remedies from the purification process from whole plant to isolated constituent may be overlooked. Ultimately, effective research into the mechanisms of actions of phyto-medicines will need to account for the possibility, indeed the probability, of synergistic activity between multiple constituents (Cseke *et al.*, 2006).

4. Conclusion

The high antibacterial activity of *Monechma ciliatum* seeds can be used to source antibiotic substances for drug development that can be used in the control of respiratory tract bacterial infections. Further investigations of its activity against a wider range of bacteria and fungi, identification and purification of its chemical constituents, and toxicological investigations of the plant extracts should be carried out with a view to developing novel drugs for human consumption.

Acknowledgment

The author is grateful to head of department of Pharmacognosy, Omdurman Islamic University, Omdurman-Sudan for providing lab facilities to do the research. In addition, he is thankful to Medicinal and Aromatic Plant Research Institute, Khartoum, Sudan for providing necessary facilities to do the research.

References

Ahmed, I., Agil, F. and Owais, M. 2006. *Modern Phytomedicine, Turning Medicinal Plants into Drugs*. Wieleyvch Verlag GmbH & Co. KGaA, Weinheim, pp. 200.

Ayoub, S. M. 1981. Component fatty acids from the oils from *Monechma ciliatum. Fitoterapia.*, 2: 251-253.

Cseke, L. J., Kirakosyan, A., Kaufman, P.B., Warber, S. L., Duke, J. A. and Brielmann, H. L. 2006. *Natural Products from Plants*, 2nd edition. The Synergy Principle at Work with Plants, Pathogens,

Insects, Herbivores and Humans. CRC Press Taylor & Francis Group, USA, pp: 494- 495.

Hassan, L. A., Sirat, H. M., Koko, W. S. and Abdelwahab, S. I. 2011. *In vitro* antimicrobial activities of chloroformic, hexane and ethanolic extracts of *Citrullus lanatus* var. *citroides* (Wild melon). *Journal of Medicinal Plants Research.*, 5(8): 1338-1344.

Kavanagh, F. 1972. *Analytical microbiology*. Academic press, New York, London.

Kumar, P. and Clark, M. 2002. *Basic Clinical Medicine*, 5th edition. W.B. Saunders, UK by path press Limited, pp.21.

Mariod, A. A., Aseel, K. M., Mustafa, A. A. and Ibrahim, S. 2009. Characterization of the Seed Oil and Meal from *Monechma ciliatum* and *Prunus mahaleb* Seeds. *Journal of the American* Oil *Chemists Society.*, 86: 749-755.

Okunlola, A., Adewoyin, B. A. and Odeku, O. A. 2007. Evaluation of Pharmaceutical and Microbial Qualities of Some Herbal Medicinal Products in South Western Nigeria. *Tropical Journal of Pharmaceutical Research.*, 6 (1): 661-670.

Omolola, O. 2011. The Isolation of *Pseudomonas aeruginosa* From Septic Sore Using Some Biological Tests. *Internet Journal of Food Safety.*, 13: 188-190.

Sheng, G. W., Hua, J. D., Hui, Y. M., Min, S. H. and Bo, L. I 2012. Mechanisms, clinically curative effects, and antifungal activities of cinnamon oil and pogostemon oil complex against three species of Candida. *Journal of Traditional Chinese Medicine.*, 32(1): 1-2.

Sofowora, A. 1993. *Medicinal Plants and Traditional Medicine in Africa*. 2nd edition. Spectrum Books Ltd., Sunshine House, Ibadan 81, pp.134-156.

Uguru, M. O. and Evan, F. 2002. Phytochemical and pharmacological studies on *Monechma ciliatum*. *Journal of Ethnopharmacology.*, 73: 289- 292.

WHO. 2003. *Guidelines on good agricultural and collection practices for medicinal plants*. Department of Essential Drugs and Medicines Policy, Geneva, Switzerland, pp. 1.

Nephroprotective activity of *Mammea africana* stem bark against paracetamol induced kidney injury

Jude Efiom Okokon*, and Bawo Michael

Department of Pharmacology and Toxicology Faculty of Pharmacy, University of Uyo, Uyo, Nigeria;
****Email:** judeefiom@yahoo.com*

ARTICLE INFO

***Topic:** Ethnopharmacology*

Key words:
- ✓ Mammea africana
- ✓ *Nephroprotective*
- ✓ *Antioxidant*
- ✓ *Kidney*

ABSTRACT

Background & Aim: *Mammea africana* sabine (Guttiferae) stembark commonly used traditionally to treat various diseases and ailments was evaluated for nephroprotective activity against paracetamol – induced kidney injury in rats to confirm its use in the treatment of kidney diseases.
Experimental: The nephroprotective effect of the extract was evaluated by the determination of some kidney function parameters such as serum urea and creatinine, electrolyes (K^+, Na^+, Cl^- and HCO^-_3), antioxidant enzymes (superoxide dismutase (SOD), catalase (CAT), reduced glutathione (GSH), malondialdehyde (MDA) and histopathological study of the liver.
Results & Discussion: The administration of the stembark extract caused significant dose-dependent reduction of high levels of serum creatinine and urea. The electrolytes levels were not affected. Histology of the kidney sections of extract and silymarin- treated animals showed reductions in the pathological features compared to the paracetamol- treated animals. The chemical pathological changes were consistent with histopathological observations suggesting marked nephroprotective effect of the stembark extract of *M. africana*
Recommended applications/industries: The results show that the stembark extract of *Mammea africana* has nephroprotective potential which may be due to its antioxidant effect activity.

1. Introduction

Mammea africana sabine (Guttiferae) (syn. *Ochrocarpus africana* Oliv.) is a large forest tree of 50 to 100 feet high with bark often yellow with pale scales and resinous yellow sap (Hutchison and Daziel, 1958). The plant is widely distributed in tropical Africa. The stem bark of the plant is used traditionally by the Ibibios of Niger Delta region of Nigeria in the treatment of malaria related fever, diabetes, microbial infections and mental disorders. The stembark is also used traditionally to treat stomach pains, rheumatispains, scabies,cough and hypertension (Raponda-Walter and Sillans, 1961; Adjanohoun *et al.*, 1996). The stembark extract have been reported to possess cytotoxic activity on cell culture (Chapuis *et al.*, 1988, Okokon *et al.*, 2012). Ouahouo et al. (2004) reported cytotoxic coumarins with antimicrobial activity against *Staphylococcus aureus* from the plant stembark. The stembark has been reported to posses antiplasmodial (Okokon *et al.*, 2006), cardioprotective (Okokon and Antia, 2007), antidiabetic and hypolipidaemic (Okokon *et al.,* 2007), vasorelaxant

(Dongmo *et al.*, 2007), antihypertensive (Nguelefack-Mbuyo *et al.,* 2008), anti-inflammatory and analgesic (Okokon *et al*., 2009), antioxidant (Nguelefack-Mbuyo *et al*., 2010), antidiarrheal and antiulcer (Okokon *et al*., 2010), immunomodulatory and anti-lesihmanial (Okokon *et al*., 2012), as well as depressant and anticonvulsant activities (Okokon *et al*., 2014). The stembark has been reported to contain 5,-7-dihydroxy-8-(12-methyl-butryl) –4- N - Pentyl coumarins (Carpenter *et al*., 1971; Crichton and Waterman, 1978; Carpenter *et al.,* 1970), 4-phenyl and 4-alkylcoumarins (Games, 1972), Mesuxanthone B (Carpenter *et al.,* 1971). Alkaloids have been reported to be absent in the entire plant parts (Gartlands *et al*., 1980).

We, therefore, report in this study the kidney protective activities of the stembark extract of *M. africana* from Nigeria.

2. Materials and Methods

2.1. Plants collection

The plant material *Mammea africana* (stembarks) were collected in a forest in Uruan area, Akwa Ibom State, Nigeria in April, 2013. The plant was identified and authenticated by Dr. Magaret Bassey of Department of Botany and Ecological Studies, University of Uyo, Uyo, Nigeria.

2.2. Extraction

The pieces of the stembark were washed and shade-dried for two weeks. The dried plants' materials were further chopped into smaller pieces and reduced to powder. The powdered material was soaked in 70% ethanol for 72 h. The liquid filtrates were concentrated and evaporated to dryness in vacuo 40°C using rotary evaporator.

2.3. Animals

Swiss albino rats of either sex (190 – 220 g) that were used for these experiments were obtained from University of Uyo animal house. The animals were housed in standard cages and were maintained on a standard pelleted feed (Guinea feed) and water *ad libitum*. Permission and approval for animal studies were obtained from College of Health Sciences Animal Ethics committee, University of Uyo.

2.4. Animal treatment

A total of 36 rats of both sexes were weighed and divided into six groups of 6 animals each and treated as follows: Groups A consisted of normal animals that were administered with distilled water (0.2 ml/kg), Group B was administered with vehicle control (distilled water, 0.2 ml/kg), while groups C, D and E were respectively administered p.o with 30, 60 and 90 mg/kg of *M. africana* stembark extract (MASBEX) daily for 8 days. Group F treated with silymarin (100 mg/kg) (standard drug) for the same period of time. Paracetamol, 2 g/kg, was administered to groups B – F on the eighth day. Twenty-four hours after paracetamol administration, the animals were sacrificed under light diethyl ether vapor. Blood were collected by cardiac puncture and used immediately.

2.5 The protective effect of the extract against Paracetamol-induced kidney injury on Biochemical parameters and hhistology of kidney of rats

The various serum samples collected after treatment of the animals were analyzed according to standard methods for effect of the extract on various biochemical parameters of rats such as uric acid, urea, and creatinine as well as some ions like sodium, potassium and chloride. This analysis were done at Department of Chemical Pathology, University of Uyo Teaching Hospital, (UUTH), Uyo using various diagnostic kits like Randox Laboratory kits, Dialab diagnostic kits, HUMAN diagnostic kits and TECO analytical kits. The kidneys of the animals fixed in 10% formaldehyde were processed, sectioned and stained with Heamatoxylin and eosin (H&E) according to standard procedures at Department of Chemical Pathology, University of Uyo Teaching Hospital, Uyo.

2.6. Preparation of renal homogenate

The kidneys were removed and dissected free from the surrounding fat and connective tissue. Each kidney was longitudinally sectioned, and renal cortex was separated and kept at −8°C. Subsequently, renal cortex was homogenized in cold potassium phosphate buffer (0.05 M, pH 7.4). The renal cortical homogenates were centrifuged at 5000rpm for 10 min at 4°C. The resulting supernatant was used for the determination of malondialdehyde (MDA) content (Wilbur *et al*., 1949; Esterbauer and Cheeseman, 1990), reduced glutathione (GSH) (Ellman,1959) and antioxidant enzyme levels such as superoxide dismutase (SOD) (Marklund *et al.,* 1974) and catalase (CAT) (Sinha, 1972) using colorimetric assay.

2.7. Statistical analysis and data evaluation

Data obtained from this work were analyzed statistically using Students't-test and ANOVA (One - way) followed by a post test (Tukey-Kramer multiple comparison test). Differences between means were considered significant at 1% and 5% level of significance i.e $p \leq 0.01$ and 0.05.

3. Results and discussion

In the present study the ethanolic stembark extract of *M. africana* was evaluated for nephroprotective activity against paracetamol-induced nephrotoxicity in rats. Biochemical markers of kidney function like blood urea, serum creatinine, electrolytes levels, tissue GSH, SOD, CAT, and lipid peroxidation were considered for assessing nephroprotective properties. Paracetamol administration exhibited a marked depletion of tissue GSH level with increased lipid peroxidation levels as shown by the increased MDA level. Kidney antioxidative enzymes like SOD and CAT activities were reduced. Significant elevation of serum markers like blood urea and serum creatinine were also observed. Various degrees of histological lesions were observed.

The kidney weights of rats treated with paracetamol were significantly ($p < 0.001$) increased when compared to that of the control group. However, animals in groups pre-treated with the stembark extract (30-90 mg/kg) and silymarin (100 mg/kg) had their kidney weights significantly ($p < 0.01 - 0.001$) reduced (Table 1). This results from the activity of the stembark extract against the damaging effect of paracetamol.

Paracetamol induces acute renal damage by elevating plasma creatinine and blood urea, while depleting glutathione levels with consequent induction of tubular necrosis (Abraham, 2005) as was observed histologically in this study. Blood urea nitrogen is found in the liver protein that is derived from diet or tissue sources and is normally excreted in the urine. In renal disease, the serum urea accumulates because the rate of serum urea production exceeds the rate of clearance. Elevation of urea and creatinine levels in the serum was taken as the index of nephrotoxicity.

Creatinine, on the other hand, is mostly derived from endogenous sources by tissue creatinine breakdown. Thus serum urea concentration is often considered a more reliable renal function predictor than serum creatinine (Palani *et al.,* 2009).

Table 1. Effect of *Mammea africana* stembark extract on Kidney weight in paracetamol-induced kidney injury in rats.

Parameters/Treatment	Kidney(g)
Normal control	1.42±0.06
PCM +Dist. water	$2.54{\pm}0.04^{c}$
MA. 30mg/kg + PCM	$1.52{\pm}0.08^{cd}$
MA. 60mg/kg+ PCM	$1.48{\pm}0.06^{f}$
MA. 90mg/kg+ PCM	$1.44{\pm}0.02^{f}$
Silymarin 100mg/kg + PCM	$1.53{\pm}0.06^{f}$

Data were expressed as mean ± SEM. significant at ap< 0.05, bp< 0.01, cp < 0.001 when compared to control. dp< 0.05, ep< 0.01, fp< 0.001 when compared to paracetamol. n = 6.

Treatment of rats with paracetamol (2g/kg) caused significant ($p < 0.001$) elevation of serum urea and creatinine levels when compared to normal control. These increased levels of serum urea and creatinine were significantly ($p<0.05$ - 0.001) reduced with the pretreatment of the rats with stembark extract of *M. africana* (30 – 90 mg/kg) in a dose dependent fashion. However, the administration of paracetamol did not affect the electrolytes (K^+, Na^+, Cl^- and HCO^-_3) levels of rats. Pretreatment of the rats did not also affect the levels of the electrolytes as there was no significant ($p>0.05$) different with that of the control rats. (Table 2). These findings further confirm the protective role of the extract.

Paracetamol treatment also caused significant ($p<0.001$) decreases in the activities of SOD, catalase and GSH levels and significant ($p<0.001$) increase in the concentration of MDA in kidney tissue when compared with control group (Table 3). Pre-treatment with stembark extract of *M. africana* (30 – 90 mg/kg) resulted in a significant ($p<0.05 – 0.001$) increase in the activities of SOD, catalase and GSH levels as well as significant ($p < 0.001$) decrease in the concentration of MDA. Silymarin treated animals also showed a significant ($p < 0.001$) increase in antioxidant enzymes; SOD, catalase and GSH levels with significant ($p < 0.001$) decrease in the level of MDA compared to paracetamol treated rats (Table 3).

Large quantities of oxidative free radicals such as superoxide anions and derivatives; especially the highly reactive and damaging hydroxyl radical which induces peroxidation of cell membrane lipids (Bhattacharya *et al.,* 1999), are generated in living cells Lipid peroxidation refers to the oxidative stress degradation of lipid in which malondialdehyde (MDA) is one of its end products (Asha *et al*., 2001). It mostly affects polyunsaturated fatty acids causing tissue damage (Khan *et al*., 2012) and the elevation in MDA levels in the kidney of paracetamol treated rats as observed in our results, which may be due to the enrichment of cell membrane with polyunsaturated highly oxidizable fatty acids (Cini *et al*., 1994). Lipid peroxidation (LP) has a relationship with the release of lysosomal enzymes. Hence, LP activates the phospholipases and removes the peroxidized lipid from the membrane (Kappus, 1985). The oxidation of unsaturated fatty acids in biological membranes by free radical leads to a decrease in membrane fluidity and disruption of membrane structure and function (Haragushi *et al*., 1997). In the present study, MDA level was significantly increased whereas catalase and SOD activities were decreased noticeably in paracetamol treated group as compared to control group. It has been proposed that oxidative stress may be responsible for tubular damage. It is well known that the production of ROS causes cell damage due to cytotoxic action of oxygen and nitrogen derived free radical species.

Natural antioxidant systems are inactivated by lipid peroxidation and reactive oxygen species (ROS) (Halliwell and Gutteridge, 1984). Antioxidants act as cell's defense against free radicals. Enzymatic antioxidants such as SOD, CAT and GPx are the first line of defense against oxidative injury. SOD is the first antioxidant enzyme to deal with oxyradicals by accelerating the dismutation of superoxide radicals (O_2) to hydrogen peroxide (H_2O_2). In the present study, significant decreases in SOD and CAT activities in the tissues of paracetamol treated rats were observed. These decreases could have resulted from ineffective scavenging of ROS and possibly, oxidative inactivation of enzymes (Pigeolet *et al.,* 1999). CAT acts as a preventive antioxidant and plays an important role in protecting against the deleterious effects of lipid peroxidation. A significant decrease in catalase activity during paracetamol ingestion indicates inefficient scavenging of H_2O_2 (Mallikarjuna *et al.,* 2008; Husain and Somani, 1997). The results of this study corroborate the above reports. Thus paracetamol consumption suppresses the activities of these enzymatic antioxidants and renders the cells more susceptible to free radical induced injury. Besides, non-enzymatic antioxidants play significant role in protecting the cells from oxidative damage. Non enzymatic antioxidant systems such as GSH, Vitamin C and E are considered as the second line of defense against free radicals. GSH a major non-protein thiol, considered as an important endogenous defense against peroxidative destruction of cellular membranes. Glutathione reacts directly with ROS and electrophilic metabolites, protects essential thiol groups from oxidation and serves as a substrate for several enzymes including GPx. In this study, the concentration of GSH was significantly reduced in paracetamol treated rats, which corroborates other reports (Fernandez and Videla, 1981; Jaya *et al.,* 1993). The reduced form of GSH therefore becomes readily oxidized to GSSG on interacting with free radicals (Frenandez-Checa *et al.,* 1997). Other antioxidants such as naturally occurring free radical scavengers like vitamin C and E (Yu *et al.,* 1994), also play great role in preventing lipid peroxidation under experimental conditions. Vitamin C (ascorbic acid) is an important H_2O soluble antioxidant in biological fluids and an essential micronutrient required for normal metabolic functioning of the body.

Histopathological study revealed the normal renal architecture in control group showing normal tubular brush borders and intact glomeruli and Bowman's capsule (Figure 6 A). Paracetamol treated rats showed severe damage in the kidney cells observed as variable size and atrophic cellular glomeruli, marked cloudy swelling in tubules, narrow lumens, cortical vascular dilation and congestion, chronic inflammation and destruction of glomeruli, focal cortical degeneration, and chronic inflammatory exudates in the cortex around glomeruli (Figure 6B) Pretreatment with stembark extract of *M. africana* (30 – 90 mg/kg) and standard drug, Silymarin (100 mg/kg) helped in decreasing the cellular damage induced by Paracetamol. Cellular appearance showed mostly nearly normal glomeruli with few variable size atrophic glomeruli, mild tubular degeneration, glomerular inflammation, necrosis and cloudy swelling (Figure 6 C – F).

Table 2. Effect of ethanolic stembark extract of *Mammea africana* on some kidney function parameters of rat.

Parameters/Treatment	Na^+(mmol/l)	K^+(mmol/l)	CL(mmol/l)	HCO(mmol/l)	UREA(mmol/l)	Creatinine(mmol/l)
Normal control	136.8±0.73	7.06±0.37	105.8±2.30	25.46±1.25	4.40±0.53	63.46±3.34
PCM +Dist. water	136.0±1.64	7.92±0.59	111.6±2.37	26.10±0.96	12.02±0.95^C	95.48 ±3.11^C
MA. 30mg/kg + PCM	136.2±1.06	8.64±0.93	107.8±2.95	27.04± 1.21	6.76±0.67^f	75.38±6.36^d
MA. 60mg/kg+ PCM	131.6 ± 3.72	7.98±0.85	106.4±2.65	25.57± 0.97	5.96±0.95^f	69.68±4.51^e
MA. 90mg/kg+ PCM	138.2 ± 1.77	7.28±0.41	109.8±3.21	27.45± 0.65	5.36±0.47^f	68.40±2.98^f
Silymarin 100 mg/kg + PCM	136.8±1.59	7.66±0.49	108.6±1.16	27.72± 0.75	5.92±0.95^f	69.54±2.36^f

Data were expressed as mean ± SEM. significant at ap< 0.05, bp< 0.01, cp< 0.001 when compared to control. dp< 0.05, ep< 0.01, fp< 0.001 when compared to paracetamol. n = 6.

Table 3. Effect of *Mammea africana* stembark extract on kidney antioxidant enzymes in paracetamol-induced kidney injury in rats.

Parameters/Treatment	SOD(U/mg of protein)	CAT(U/mg of protein)	MDA(U/mg of protein)	GSH(µg/mg of protein)
Normal control	20.26 ±0.86	45.38±1.86	46.42±3.66	0.30±0.01
PCM +Dist. water	7.33 ± 0.22^c	23.20±1.64^c	84.34±4.42^c	0.10±0.01^c
MA. 30mg/kg + PCM	10.18±0.16^{cd}	32.02±1.38^{cd}	62.12±4.54^c	0.16±0.02^{ce}
MA. 60mg/kg+ PCM	15.26 ±0. 28^{bf}	35.11±1.41^f	54.86±2.25^{cf}	0.20±0.02^{bf}
MA. 90mg/kg+ PCM	17.78± 0.19^{cf}	41.12±1.22^f	48.24±1.65^{bf}	0.22±0.01^{af}
Silymarin 100mg/kg + PCM	19.45 ±0.28^{cf}	53.25± 1.33^f	48.86±1.14^f	0.25±0.01^f

Data were expressed as mean ± SEM. significant at ap< 0.05, bp< 0.01, cp< 0.001 when compared to control. dp< 0.05, ep< 0.01, fp< 0.001 when compared to paracetamol. n = 6.

Table 4. Effect of treatment with ethanolic extract of *Mammea africana* on the blood hematological parameters, in rats with paracetamol -induced nephrotoxicity.

Parameters Treatment Dose (mg/kg)	RBC ($X 10^{12}$/l)	PCV(%)	Hb(g/dl)	WBC ($X 10^9$/l)	Neutrophils. (%)	Lymphocytes (%)	Monocytes (%)	Eosinophils (%)	Basophils (%)
Normal control	3.82±0.32	44.2±10.37	14.8±0.12	11.4±1.85	20.2±1.42	73.8±1.06	2.00±0.05	4.0±0.37	2.20±0.40
PCM +Dist. water	3.08±0.34	44.4±1.80	14.82±0.52	10.74±1.80	41.60±1.23^c	54.4±2.39^c	1.0±0.02^c	2.80±0.96^a	0.2±0.20^c
MA. 30mg/kg + PCM	3.98±0.52	46.2±1.24	15.4±0.34	9.92±1.28	36.9±1.65^c	62.6±2.47^b	1.0±0.01^c	0.00±0.00^{c,e}	0.00±0.00^c
MA. 60mg/kg+ PCM	4.13±0.26	43.5±2.63	14.62±0.63	9.80±1.34	43.2±2.02^c	56.6±2.30^c	0.4±0.04^{c,f}	0.2±0.20^{c,e}	0.00±0.00^c
MA. 90mg/kg+ PCM	4.18±0.60	44.8±1.15	14.62±0.34	11.36±1.24	35.8±2.66^c	61.2±1.57^b	0.8±0.02^{c,e}	2.00±0.14^a	0.00±0.00^c
Silymarin 100mg/kg+ PCM	4.05±0.12	43.2±1.56	14.8±0.12	9.66±2.34	30.4±1.47^{b,f}	68.2±2.57^c	1.0±0.04^c	0.4±0.40^{c,e}	0.00±0.00^c

Data were expressed as mean ± SEM. significant at ap< 0.05, bp< 0.01, cp< 0.001 when compared to control. dp< 0.05, ep< 0.01, fp< 0.001 when compared to paracetamol . n = 6.

GROUP - A

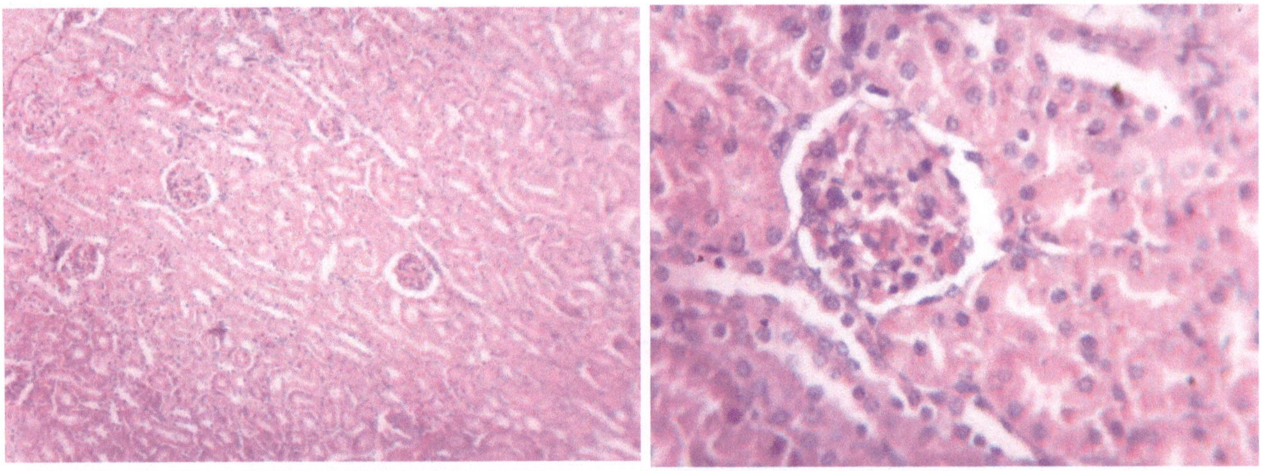

***Keys: RC** –Renal corpuscle, **PCT**- proximal convoluted tubules, DCT- Distal convoluted tubules, G- glomerulus, SEL – Squamous epithelial lining, **C** – Cortex and **M** – Medulla, **LH**- loop of Henles, **CT**- Collecting ducts*

Figure 1 - A(X100) and B(X400) of Kidney tissue without treatment revealed normal cellular pattern with area of distal and proximal convoluted tubules, renal corpuscle, collecting tubules and loop of Henles, no abnormality seen.

GROUP - B

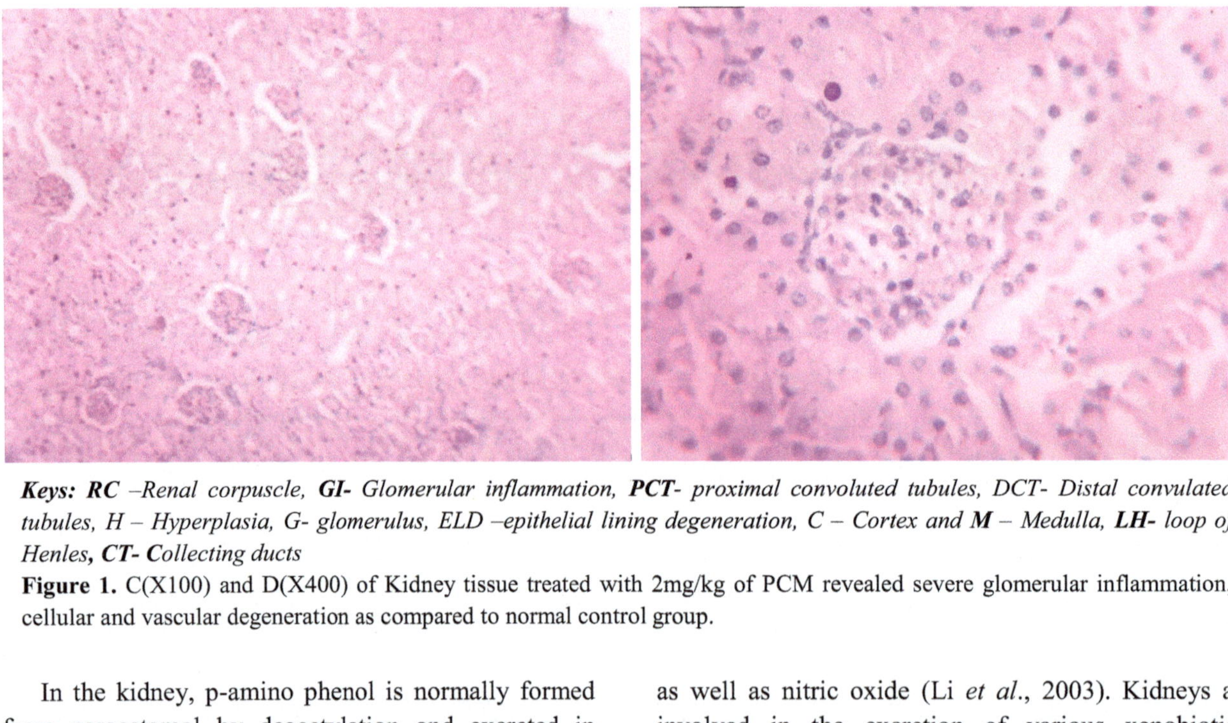

***Keys: RC** –Renal corpuscle, **GI**- Glomerular inflammation, **PCT**- proximal convoluted tubules, DCT- Distal convulated tubules, H – Hyperplasia, G- glomerulus, ELD –epithelial lining degeneration, C – Cortex and **M** – Medulla, **LH**- loop of Henles, **CT**- Collecting ducts*

Figure 1. C(X100) and D(X400) of Kidney tissue treated with 2mg/kg of PCM revealed severe glomerular inflammation, cellular and vascular degeneration as compared to normal control group.

In the kidney, p-amino phenol is normally formed from paracetamol by deacetylation and excreted in urine. This exposes the kidney to damage by p-amino phenol as it plays a major role in the pathogenesis of paracetamol induced renal damage (Carpenter and Mudge, 1981; Mugford and Tarlolf, 1997). Hepatically derived glutathione conjugates are also involved in paracetamol induced renal injury (Trumper *et al.*, 1996) as well as nitric oxide (Li *et al.*, 2003). Kidneys are involved in the excretion of various xenobiotics, pollutants, toxins and are exposed to high quantities of free radicals which contribute to high oxidative stress. This is responsible for the pathogenesis of kidney damage. Since the paracetamol induced nephrotoxicity was reported to be via NAPQI radical.

GROUP - C

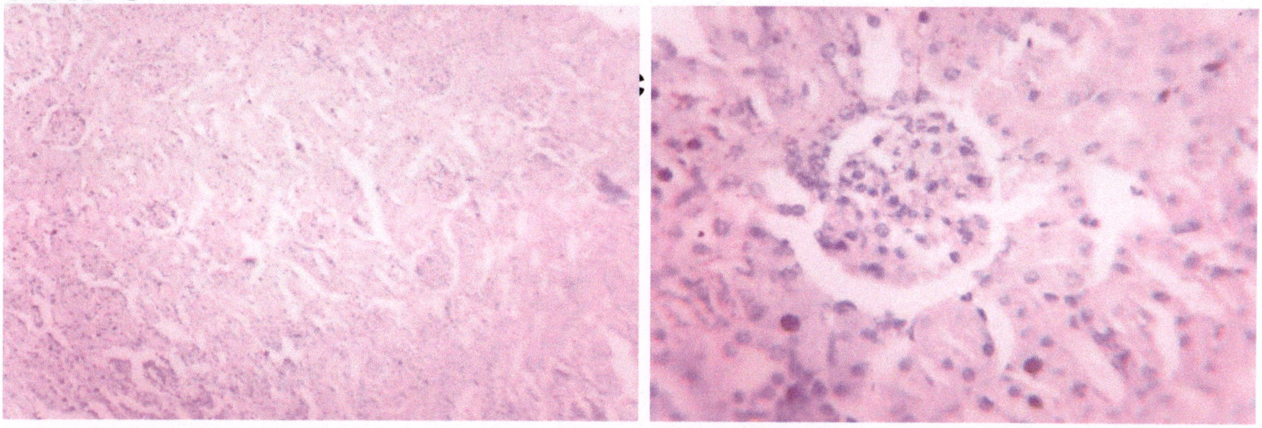

__Keys: RC__ –Renal corpuscle, __GI-__ Glomerular inflammation, __PCT-__ proximal convoluted tubules, DCT- Distal convulated tubules, H – Hyperplasia, G- glomerulus, __ELD__ –epithelial lining degeneration, __C__ – Cortex and __M__ – Medulla, __LH-__ loop of Henles, __CT- C__ollecting ducts

Figure 1 - E(X100) and F(X400) of Kidney tissue treated with 30 mg/kg of *Mammea africana* revealed glomerular inflammation as compared to normal control group.

GROUP - D

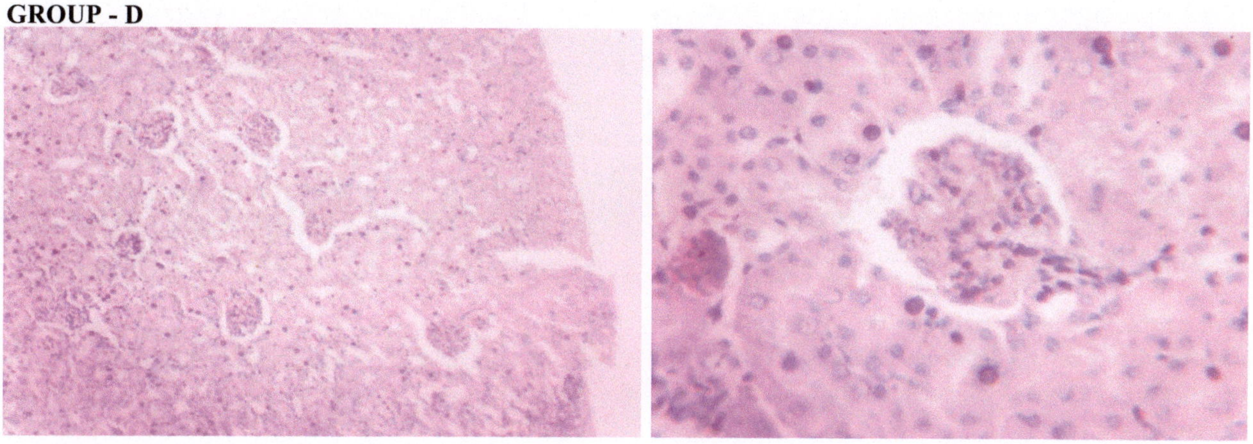

__Keys: RC__ –Renal corpuscle, __GI-__ Glomerular inflammation, __PCT-__ proximal convoluted tubules, DCT- Distal convulated tubules, H – Hyperplasia, G- glomerulus, __ELD__ –epithelial lining degeneration, __C__ – Cortex and __M__ – Medulla, __LH-__ loop of Henles, __CT- C__ollecting ducts

Figure 1 - G(X100) and H(X400) of Kidney tissue treated with 60 mg/kg of *Mammea africana* revealed mild glomerular inflammation as compared to normal control group

GROUP - D

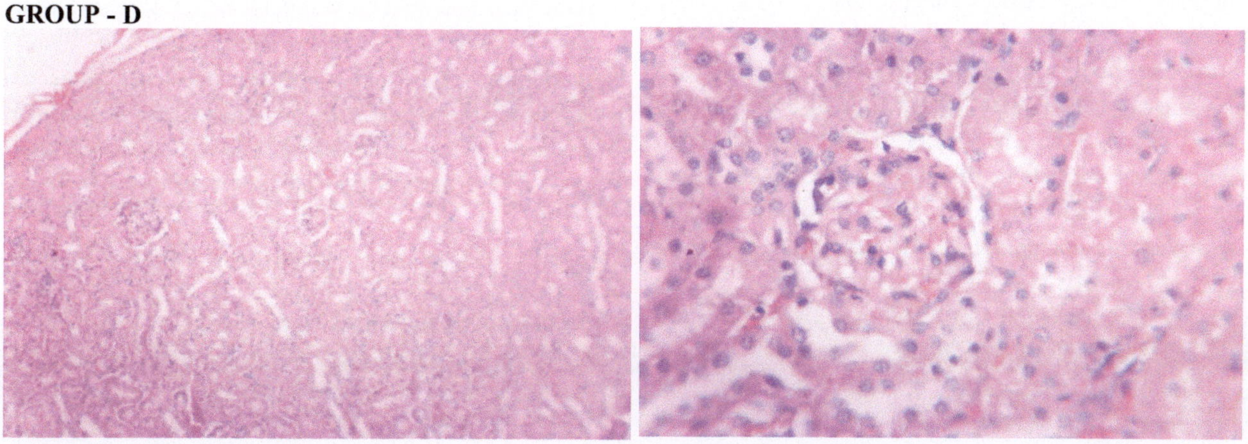

Keys: ***RC*** *–Renal corpuscle,* ***PCT****- proximal convoluted tubules, DCT- Distal convulated tubules, G- glomerulus, SEL –Squamous epithelial lining, C – Cortex and* ***M*** *– Medulla,* ***LH****- loop of Henles,* ***CT****- Collecting ducts.*

Figure 1 - I(X100) and J(X400) of Kidney tissue treated with 90 mg/kg of *Mammea africana* revealed mild glomerular

GROUP - F

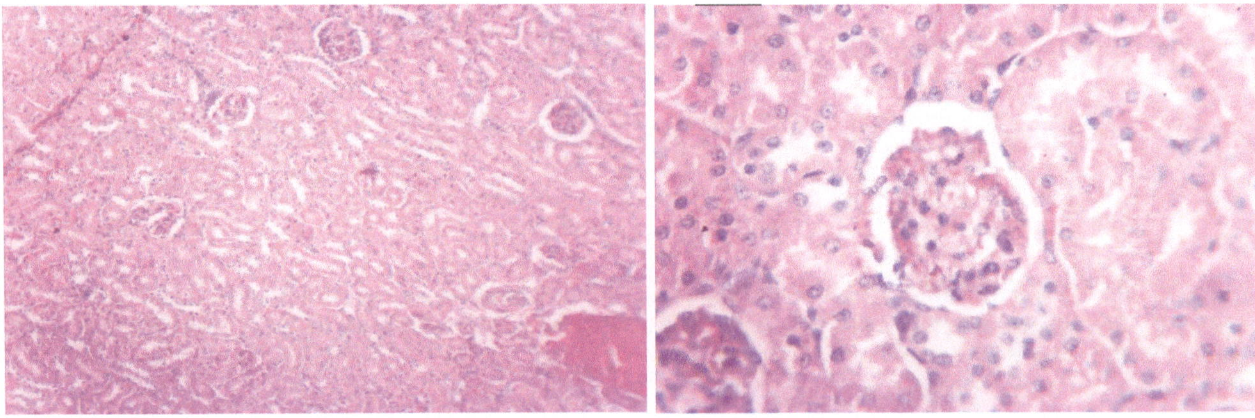

Keys: ***RC*** *–Renal corpuscle,* ***GI-*** *Glomerular inflammation,* ***PCT****- proximal convoluted tubules, DCT- Distal convulated tubules, G- glomerulus,* ***ELD*** *–epithelial lining degeneration,* ***C*** *– Cortex and* ***M*** *– Medulla,* ***LH-*** *loop of Henles,* ***CT-*** *Collecting ducts*

Figure 1 - K(X100) and L(X400) of Kidney tissue treated with Sylamrin revealed mild glomerular inflammation as compared to normal control group.

Co-administration of test extract normalized tissue lipid peroxidation level and prevented the reduction of tissue GSH level as well as activities of antioxidant enzymes. The nephro protective property of the extract is further confirmed by significant improvement of the kidney architecture by reversing the glomerular congestion, interstium with inflammatory cells, tubular necrosis, peritubular necrosis and basement degeneration over paracetamol administered group.

The stembark extract and fractions have been reported to exhibit strong cellular antioxidant activity in whole blood, neutrophils (extracellular and intracellular) and macrophages (Okokon *et al.,* 2013). Similarly, the cytotoxic coumarins isolated from the stembark have also been reported to exert strong antioxidant activity (Nguelefack-Mbuyo *et al.*, 2010). This activity demonstrate the potential of the extract to inhibit reactive oxygen species (ROS) and scavenge free radicals; superoxide, hydrogen peroxide, etc which can be attributable to the presence of coumarins and other phenolic compounds in the stembark as reported earlier (Carpenter *et al.,* 1970; Carpenter *et al.*, 1971; Games, 1972; Crichton and Waterman, 1978; Ouahouo *et al.*, 2004; Okokon *et al.*, 2013).

The strong antioxidant activities of antioxidant counteract the redox state precipitated intracellular and hence ensure nephroprotection against paracetamol -induced kidney injury. The antioxidant activity of this extract may as well explain the mechanism of action of the observed hepatoprotective activity of *Mammea africana*. Besides, *M. africana* stem bark extract has been reported to possess renal protective activity on L-NAME hypertensive rats as well as caused transcient diuretic effect at high doses (Nguelefack-Mbuyo *et al.*, 2010).

4. Conclusion

The findings of this study further support the renal protective potential of stembark of *M. africana* which can be attributed to its antioxidant and diuretic properties which are important in renal protective activities of medicinal plants. Hence, the stembark of *Mammea africana* possess nephroprotective active against paracetamol induced kidney injury.

5. Acknowledgement

The authors are grateful to Mr Adewale Adebisi of Department of Anatomy, University of Uyo, for his Technical assistance

6. References

Abraham, P. 2005. Oxidative stress in paracetamol induced pathogenesis: (I) renal damage. *Indian Journal of Biochemistry and Biophysics.,* 42: 59-62.

Adjanohoun, J.E., Aboubakar, N., Dramane, K., Ebot, M. E., Ekpere, J.A., Enoworock, E.G., Foncho, D., Gbile, Z. O., Kamanyi, A., Kamoukom, J., Keeta, A., Mbenkum, T., Mbi, C.M., Mbielle, A.L., Mbome, I.L., Mubiru, N.K., Naney, W.L., Nkongmeneck, B., Satabie, B., Sofowora, A., Tanze, V. and Wirmum, C. K. 1996. *Traditional Medicine and Pharmacopeia-Contribution to Ethnobotanical and Floristic Studies in Cameroon.* Porto-Novo, Benin: CNPMS, p. 15.

Asha, V.V. 2001. Preliminary studies on hepatoprotective activities of *Momordica sabangulata* and *Naragama alat. Indian Journal of Pharmacology.,* 33: 276-279.

Bhattacharya, A., Chatterjee, A., Ghosal, S. and Bhattacharya, S. K. 1999. Antioxidant activity of active tannoid principles of *Emblica officinalis* (amla). *Indian Journal of Experimental Biology*., 37: 676–680.

Carpenter, H.M. and Mudge, G.H. 1981. Acetaminophen nephrotoxicity: studies on renal acetylation and deacetylation. *Journal of Pharmacology and Experimental Therapeutics.,* 218: 161-167.

Carpenter I, Mc Garry EJ. and Scheimann F. 1970. The neoflavonoids and 4-alkylcoumarins from *Mammea africana* G. Don. *Tetrahedron Letters*., 46: 3983 - 3986.

Carpenter, I., Mc Garry, E. J. and Scheimann, F. 1971. Extractives from Guttiferae. Part XXI. The isolation and structure of nine coumarins from the bark of *Mammea africana* G. Don. *Journal of Chemical Society*., 22: 3783 - 3789.

Chapius, J. C., Sordat, B., Hostettman, K. 1988. Screening for cytotoxic activities of Plants used in traditional Medicine. *Journal of Ethnopharmacology*., 2322 (2/3): 273 - 284.

Cini, M., Fariello, R.Y., Bianchettei, A. and Morettei, A. 1994. Studies on lipid peroxidation in the rat brain. *Neurochemical Research.,* 19:283.

Crichton, E.G. and Waterman, P. G. 1978. Dihydromammea c/ob: A New Coumarin from the seed of *Mammea africana. Phytochemistry* 17: 1783 - 1786. Dongmo, A.B., Azebaze, A. and Nguelefack, T.B. 2007. Vasodilator effect of the extracts and some coumarins from the stem bark of *Mammea africana* (Guttiferae). *Journal of Ethnopharmacology.,* 111:329 - 334.

Ellman, G. L. 1959. Tissue sulfhydryl groups. *Archieves of Biochemistry and Biophysics*., 82, 70-77.

Esterbauer, H. and Cheeseman, K.H. 1990 Determination of aldehydic lipid peroxidation products: malonaldehyde and 4-hydroxynonenal. *Methods in Enzymology*., 186: 407–421.

Fernandez, V. and Videla, I. A. 1981. Effect of acute and chronic ethanol ingestion on the content of reduced glutathione on various tissues of the rat. *Experientia*., 37:392-394.

Fernández-Checa, J.C., Kaplowitz, N., García-Ruiz, C., Colell, A., Miranda, M., Marí, M., Ardite, E. and Morales, A. 1997. GSH transport in mitochondria: defense against TNF-induced oxidative stress and alcohol induced defect. *American Journal of Physiology*., 273:7-17.

Games, D. E. 1972. Identification of 4-phenyl and 4-alkylcoumarins in *Mammea Americana, Mammea africana* and *Calophyllum ionophyllum* by gas chromatography – mass spectrometry. *Tetrahedron.,* 31: 3187 - 3190.

Gartlans, J. S., Key, D. B,, Waterman, P. G., Mbi, C. N. and Struhsaker, T. T.1980. Comparative study of the Phytochemistry of two African rain forests. *Biochemical Systematics and Ecology.,* 8: 401- 422.

Halliwell, B. and Gutteridge, J. M. 1984. Oxygen toxicity, oxygen radicals, transition metals and disease. *Biochemical Journal*., 219: 1–14.

Haragushi, H., Ishikawa, H. and Kubo, I. 1997. Antioxidant action of diterpenoids from *Prodocarpas nagi*, *Planta Medica*., 63: 213-215.

Husain, K., Somani, S. M. 1997. Interaction of exercise and ethanol and hepatic and plasma antioxidant system in rat. *Pathophysiology*., 4:60-74.

Hutchinson, L. J. and Daziel, J.M. 1958. *Flora of West Tropical Africa*, revised by R. W. J. Keay.Vol.1, part 2, 2nd edition. White Press, London.

Jaya, D.S., Augustine, J., Menon, V. P. 1993. Role of lipid peroxides, glutathione and antiperoxidative enzymes in alcohol and drug toxicity. *Indian Journal of Experimental Biology*., 31:453-459.

Kappus, H.1985. Oxidative stress Academic Press, London, 273.

Khan, R.A., Khan, M.R., Sahreen, S. and Ahmed, M. 2012. Evaluation of phenolic contents and antioxidant activity of various solvent extracts of *Sonchus asper* (L.) Hill. *Chemistry Central Journal.*, 6: 12.

Li, C., Lui, J., Saaedra, J.E., Keefer, L.K. and Waalkes, M.P. 2003. The Nitric oxide donor, V-PYRRO/NO, protects against acetaminophen-induced nephrotoxicity in mice.*Toxicology.*, 189: 173-80.

Mallikarjuna, K., Sahitya, P., Sathyavelu, K. and Rajendra, W. 2008. Ethanol toxicity: Rehabilitation of hepatic antioxidant defense system with dietary ginger. *Fitoterapia.,* 79: 174-178.

Marklund, S., Marklund, G. 1974. Involvement of superoxide anion radical in the autooxidation of pyrogallol and a convenient assay for superoxide dismutase. *European Journal Biochemistry.,* 47: 469-474.

Mingatto, F. E., dos Santos, A. C., Rodrigues, T., Pigoso, A. A., Uyemura, S. A. and Curti, C. 2000. Effects of nimesulide and its reduced metabolite on mitochondria. *British Journal of Pharmacology.*, 131: 1154–1160.

Mitchell, J.R., Jollow, D. J., Potter, W. Z., Davis, D. C., Gillette, J. R. and Brodie, B. B. 1973. Acetaminophen-induced hepatic necrosis. 1. Role of drug metabolism. *Journal of Pharmacology and Experimental Therapeutics.,* 187: 185-194.

Mugford, C.A. and Tarlolf, J.B. 1997. The contribution of oxidation and deacetylation to acetaminophen nephrotoxicity in female Sprague-Dawley rats. *Toxicological Letter.*, 93: 15-18.

Nguelefack-Mbuyo, E.P., Dimo, T., Nguelefack, T.B., Azebaze, A.G., Dongmo, A.B., Kamtchouing, P. and Kamanyi, A. 2010. In vitro antioxidant activity of extracts and coumarins from the stem bark of *Mammea africana* Sabine. *Journal of Complementary and Integrative Medicine.*, 7(1): 1-11.

Nguelefack-Mbuyo, P. E., Nguelefack, T. B. and Dongmo, A. B. 2008. Anti- hypertensive effects of the methanol/methylene chloride stem bark extract of *Mammea africana* in L-NAME- induced hypertensive rats. *Journal of Ethnopharmacology.,* 117: 446 – 450.

Okokon, J.E., Dar, A. and Choudhary, M. I. 2012. Immunostimulatory, Anticancer, and antileishmanial activities of *Mammea africana* from Nigeria. *Journal of Natural Pharmaceuticals.*, 3(2): 105 - 109.

Okokon, J. E. and Antia, B. S. 2007. Hypolipidaemic and Cardioprotective activity of *Mammea africana. Research Journal Medicinal Plants.*, 1(4): 154 – 157.

Okokon, J. E., Antia, B. S., Osuji, L., Udia, P. M. 2007. Antidiabetic and Hypolipidaemic activity of ethanolic stembark extract of *Mammea africana. Journal of Pharmacology and Toxicology.*, 2: 278 - 283.

Okokon, J.E and Davies, K. 2014. Psychopharmacological studies of *Mammea africana* stembark extract. *The Journal of Phytopharmacology.*, 4 (3): (In Press)

Okokon, J. E., Udokpoh, A. E. and Essiet, G. A. 2006. Antimalarial Activity of *Mammea africana. African Journal of Traditional, Complementary and Alternative Medicine.,* 3: 43 – 49.

Okokon, J. E., Umoh, E. and Umoh, U. 2009. Antiinflammatory and antinociceptive effects of ethanolic stembark extract of *Mammea africana. Journal of Biomedical Research.,* 12(2): 135 – 139.

Okokon, JE., Umoh, U. F., Umoh, E. E. and Etim E. I. 2010. Antiulcer and antidiarrhoeal activity of *Mammea africana. Iranian Journal of Pharmacology and Therapeutics.,* 9(2): 96-101.

Ouahouo, B. M. W., Asebaze, A. G. B., Meyer, M., Bodo, B., Fomum, Z.T. and Ngengfack, A. E. 2004. Cytotoxic and antimicrobial coumarins from *Mammea africana. Annal of Tropical Medicine and Parasitology.*, 98: 737 – 739.

Palani, S., Raja, S., Rajalingam, D., Praveen Kumar, R. and Senthil Kumar B. 2009. Therapeutic efficacy of *Pimpinella tirupatiensis* (Apiaceae) on acetaminophen induced nephrotoxicity and oxidative stress in male albino rats, *International Journal of PharmTech Research.*, 1(3): 925-934

Pigeolet, E., Corbisier, P., Houbion, A., Lambrt, D., Michiels, C. and Raes, M. 1999. Antioxidant and oxidative stress in exercise. *Experimental Biology and Medicine.*, 22: 283-292.

Raponda-Walker, A. and Sillans, R. 1961. Les plantes utiles du Gabon. Paris: Paul Leechevalier.

Sinha, A. K. 1972. Colorimetric assay of catalase. *Analytical Biochemistry.,* 47: 389-94.

Trumper, L., Mansterolo, L.A. and Elias, M. M.1996. Nephrotoxicity of acetaminophen in male Wistar rats: role of hepatically derived metabolites. *Journal of Pharmacology and Experimental Therapeutics*., 279: 548 - 554

Wilbur, K. M., Bernhein, F. and Shapiro, O.W.1949. Determination of lipid peroxidation. *Archieves of Biochemistry*., 24: 305-310.

Yu, B.P. 1994. Cellular defenses against damage from reactive oxygen species. *Physiological Reviews.,* 74: 139-162.

Comparison of the antibacterial, antiplaque and anti-gingivitis activity of herbal mouthwash with chlorhexidine in dog

Saadat Moshkelani[1], Mohamad Javaheri-Koupaei[2], Hassan Momtaz[3*]

[1]*Department of Surgery, Faculty of Specialized Veterinary Sciences, Tehran Science and Research Branch, Islamic Azad University, Tehran, Iran;*

[2]*Young Researchers and Elite Club, Shahrekord Branch, Islamic Azad University, Shahrekord, Iran;*

[3]*Faculty of Veterinary Medicine, Shahrekord Branch, Islamic Azad University, Shahrekord, Iran;*
Email: *hamomtaz@iaushk.ac.ir

ARTICLE INFO

Topic: *Ethnoveterinary*

Key words:

- ✓ *Antibacterial*
- ✓ *Anti-gingivitis*
- ✓ *Antiplaque*
- ✓ *Green tea*
- ✓ *Dog*

ABSTRACT

Background & Aim: Oral diseases including gingivitis and periodontal diseases are most common diseases in pets, especially dogs. The aim of this study was to evaluate the potency of herbal composition containing green tea extract as a mouthwash on preventing plaque formation and oral diseases in dogs.
Experimental: In order to achieve this goal, 20 male dogs selected and were divided randomly in to two groups including control (Chlorhexidine 0.1%) and treatment (herbal mouthwash) groups. total microbial cunt was performed in swab samples were taken from each dog-oral cavity. In addition, Silness-Loe Plaque Index System was used to evaluate the Improvement of dental plaque and gingivitis.
Results: Percentage of colonies reduction on the last day of the study compared with the first day in control and treatment groups are 84.90% and 73.41%, respectively. In addition, Silness-Loe Plaque Index for control and treatment groups is 0.71 and 0.75, respectively. Results of the present study indicate a favorable effect of herbal mouthwash to prevention and reduce plaque and bacteria in the mouth of pet animals.
Recommended applications/industries: The herbal mouthwash could reduce the aerobic mouth bacterial load and may prevent plaque formation on teeth and come over halitosis due to infection of the bacteria.

1. Introduction

Inflammation and recession of perialveolar gum margins are common findings in dogs and cats. These lesions are initially caused by excessive accumulation of dental plaque resulting from deposition of by-products from breakdown of food and saliva by normal resident microflora (Crossley and Penman, 1995). Plaque is an organic matrix of salivary glycoproteins and polysaccharides adhering to the tooth surface that provides sites for oral bacteria to proliferate. Adjunctive management methods such as providing hard diets, regular tooth brushing, and oral hygiene chews have been shown to reduce the incidence of calculus accumulation (Emily and Penman, 1990;

Nelson and Couto, 2014). Treatment includes the extraction of severely affected teeth, debriding necrotic or proliferative gum margins, root planning with curettes, and scaling calculi from the remaining involved supragingival and subgingival dental surfaces by manual or ultrasonic means. In addition, flushing dental surfaces once daily with antibacterial material like 0.1% to 0.2% chlorhexidine or alternate-day brushing may delay accumulation of calculi. Unfortunately, chlorhexidine may stain teeth light blue and also leads to the re-accumulation of plaque (Greene, 2013).

Herbal extracts have been widely used in topical and oral applications for disease treatment in both animals and human. Green tea (*Camellia sinensis*), which is not fermented at all during the drying process, has numerous medicinal benefits mainly due to its antibacterial and antioxidant properties (LaGow, 2004). A short list of phenolic phytochemicals with promising properties to benefit human and animal's health includes a group of polyphenol compounds called Catechins which are found in green tea. Animals and humans that have tea compounds in their drinking water develop fewer dental caries and less plaque formation than those drinking plain water (Moghbel and Abbaspour, 2010; Wynn and Fougere, 2007). Therefore, the aim of this study was to evaluate the potency of herbal composition containing Iranian green tea extract as a mouthwash on mouth microbial load and then approving its effect on preventing plaque formation in dogs.

2. Materials and Methods

2.1. Herbal formula

Poly-herbal mouthwash (Camodex) used in this study was blended in Zist Dam Sepahan Co., Esfahan, Iran for the first time. The major component of Camodex is Iranian green tea extract and this product was standardized to contain 2.5% polyphenols.

2.2. Animals and Study design

The experiment was conducted on 20 male Persian shepherd dogs (with gingivitis and dental plaque) aging one to two years with 20-25 kg average body weights that were divided in two groups (n=10). The test group consisted of treatment and control group as follows: (*i*) control group were used chlorhexidine 0.1% spray; (*ii*) treatment group were used Poly-herbal spray (Camodex). They have to use it twice daily each time three puffs in their mouth for 56 days.

2.3. Samples and microbial analysis

To evaluate the oral flora in the days 0, 14, 28, 42, and 56 swab samples were taken from each dog oral cavity. All samples were cultured on nutrition agar medium and then were incubated in 37 °C for 24 h. To investigate the bacterial load, all of the colonies on each plate were counted under loop.

2.4. Plaque Index

In order to evaluate the Improvement of dental plaque and gingivitis complete examination of the mouth was conducted in the days 0 and 56. The modified Silness-Loe Plaque Index System was used to compare the results of dental plaque and gingivitis (Fischman, 1986).

2.5 Statistical analysis

Data of this research were analyzed using Chi-Square by SPSS version 20.0 software by means of $p < 0.05$.

3. Results and discussion

To the best of our knowledge, the present study is the first report about effect of a mouthwash containing Green tea on gingivitis, plaque and microbial load of oral cavity in pet animals. The results showed that average colonies (Mean ± SD) formed on the culture medium on days 0, 14, 28, 42, and 56 in the control group were 675.30 ±306.52, 354±153.23, 220.6±117.86, 142.7±93.99, and 99.80±76.85, respectively. In addition, average colonies in same days in treatment group were 957.60±485.11, 661.8±314.73, 481.80±190.37, 315.60±139.60, and 228±113.55, respectively. The results indicated that significant difference ($p < 0.05$) between treatment and control groups (Table 1).

Averages of colonies reduction on the last day of the study compared with the first day in control and treatment groups are 84.90±9.21 and 73.41±10.36, respectively (Table 2). The modified Silness-Loe Plaque Index System was used to compare the results of dental plaque and gingivitis in the study population (Table 3). Although, the results of Silness-Loe index showed no significant differences between treatment and control groups, but the positive effects of herbal mouthwash in preventing plaque formation were observed.

Table 1. Average colonies (Mean ± SD) formed on the culture medium during the investigation

Groups	0	14	28	42	56
Control	675±306	354±153	220±117	142±93	99±76
Treatment	957±485	661±314	481±190	315±139	228±113
P value	0.14	0.012*	0.002**	0.004**	0.008**

Systemic antimicrobials such as tetracycline, metronidazole, and tinidazole and topical chlorhexidine have been evaluated for treatment of periodontitis in experimentally affected dogs (Green, 2013). The uses of antibiotics and chemicals materials have irreversible effects on the health of the animals and humans. For this reason, several researches conducted for evaluation of herbal mouthwash in human. Effect of green tea on prevention of mouth bacterial infection, halitosis, and plaque formation on teeth were evaluated in human. A total of 25 volunteer female students, aged 20-25 years, were selected and then evaluated by green tea extract and mouthwashes containing 0.2, 0.5, and 1% tannin, as the most effective antibacterial complex in green tea.

Table 2. Averages of colonies reduction (Mean ± SD) during the investigation

Groups	14	28	42	56
Control	47±14	67±12	78±11	84±9
Treatment	26±16	44±14	62±18	73±10
P value	0.008*	0.002**	0.023**	0.017**

Table 3. Silness-Loe Plaque Index (Mean ± SD) during the investigation.

Groups	0	56
Control	1.27±0.57	0.71±0.38
Treatment	1.28±0.46	0.75±0.30
Pvalue	0.97	0.80

The result indicated that green tea mouthwash containing 1% tannin was more effective than other concentrations and there were no meaningful differences between the green tea mouthwashes containing 10% alcohol and alcohol free, as well as the herbal and chemical chlorhexidine 0.2% (Moghbel *et al.*, 2011). Other study aimed to determine the effect of green tea mouthwash on oral malodor, plaque, and gingival inflammation. After using for four weeks, green tea mouthwash could significantly reduce volatile sulfur compounds (VSC) level in gingivitis subjects without causing remarkable side effects (Rassameemasmaung *et al.*, 2013). The results of the present study indicate that daily application of Camodex was effective in reducing recurrence of dental plaque and gingivitis in dogs.

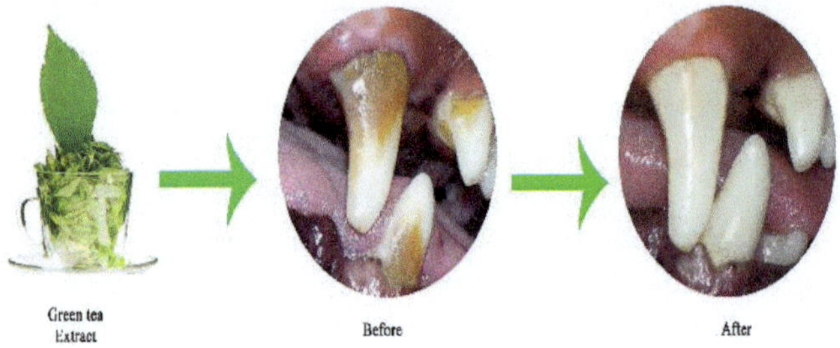

4. Conclusion

The herbal green tea mouthwash could reduce the aerobic mouth bacterial load and may prevent plaque formation on teeth and come over halitosis due to infection of the bacteria.

5. References

Crossley, D. A. and Penman, S. 1995. *Manual of small animal dentistry*. British Small Animal Veterinary Association.

Emily, P. and Penman, S. 1990. *Handbook of small animal dentistry*. Pergamon Press plc.

Fischman, S. L. 1986. Current status of indices of plaque. *Journal of Clinical Periodontology.*, 13: 371-374.

Greene, C. E. 2013. *Infectious diseases of the dog and cat*. Elsevier Health Sciences.

LaGow, B. 2004. *PDR for herbal medicines*. Thomson PDR.

Moghbel, A. and Abbaspour, H. 2010. A study on the factors affecting the compressibility of green tea leaves powder to make a herbal tablet. *Scientific Medical Journal.*, 8:463-478.

Moghbel, A., Farjzadeh, A., Aghel, N., Agheli, H., Raisi, N. 2011. The Effect of Green Tea on Prevention of Mouth Bacterial Infection, Halitosis, and Plaque Formation on Teeth. *Iranian Journal of Toxicology.*, 5: 502-515.

Nelson, R. W. and Couto, C. G. 2014. *Small animal internal medicine.* Elsevier Health Sciences.

Rassameemasmaung, S., Phusudsawang, P. and Sangalungkarn, V. 2013. Effect of Green Tea Mouthwash on Oral Malodor. *Hindawi Publishing Corporation.*, 1-6.

Wynn, S. G. and Fougère, B. 2007. *Veterinary herbal medicine.* Elsevier Health Sciences.

Evaluation of chemical composition, anti-inflammatory and anti-nociceptive effects of *Eugenia caryophyllata* buds essential oil

Emad Khalilzadeh*, **Reza Hazrati, Gholamreza Vafaei Saiah**

Division of Physiology, Department of Basic Science, Faculty of Veterinary Medicine, University of Tabriz, Tabriz, Iran;

***Email:** e.khalilzadeh@gmail.com

ARTICLE INFO

Topic: *Medicinal Plants*

Key words:
- ✓ *Clove essential oil*
- ✓ *Ketoprofen*
- ✓ *Morphine*
- ✓ *Naloxone*
- ✓ *Orofacial pain*
- ✓ *Tail immersion*

ABSTRACT

Background & Aim: *Eugenia caryophyllata* well known as Clove is a tree from Myrtaceae family that several parts of this plant traditionally used in dental care as an analgesic. This study aimed to assess the chemical composition, anti-inflammatory and anti-nociceptive activities of the essential oil extracted from Clove buds.

Experimental: The essential oil of Clove buds (EOC) was extracted by Clevenger type apparatus and its chemical composition determined by gas chromatography-mass spectrometry (GC-MS). Analgesic activities of EOC were measured by formalin-induced orofacial pain and tail immersion test in rat. Also anti-inflammatory effect of the EOC was evaluated by using xylene induced ear edema test in mice.

Results: EOC (100, 200 mg/kg, SC) and ketoprofen (80 and 160 mg/kg, IP) inhibit only the second phase of orofacial pain. Morphine (5 mg/kg) as a positive control significantly ($p <0.05$) reduced pain response in the both phases of pain. Pre-treatment of animals with naloxone did not prevent the EOC (200 mg/kg) analgesic activity. Co-administration of sub-analgesic doses of EOC (50 mg/kg) and ketoprofen (40 mg/kg) significantly ($p <0.05$) reduced nociceptive behavior in second phase. Also EOC (100 and 200 mg/kg) failed to increase nociceptive response latency in the tail immersion test. Meanwhile, EOC (100 and 200 mg/kg) and ketoprofen (80 mg/kg) significantly ($p <0.001$) attenuated xylene-induced ear edema in mice. Also according to GC-MS results the major components of the EOC were eugenol (54.86%), β-Caryophyllene (20.19%), α-Humulene (7.11%), eugenol acetat (4.85%) and Chavibetol (2.23%).

Recommended applications/industries: These data showed that EOC possessed potent anti-inflammatory activity and produced non-opioid mediated analgesia in the second phase of orofacial pain without any effect on tail immersion response.

1. Introduction

Eugenia caryophyllata well known as Clove is a tree from Myrtaceae family with a height ranging from 10 to 20 meters that widely cultivated in Indonesia, Sri Lanka, Madagascar, Tanzania and Brazil (Arung *et al.,* 2011). Clove buds and leaves are used in cooking and food industries as a food flavoring agent, pharmaceutical company, perfumery and cosmetic products (Daniel *et al.*, 2009). Clove oil and its essential oil traditionally used in aromatherapy (Schiller and Schiller, 2008), relief of headaches, joint pain, toothaches and also as an oral antiseptic (Shelef, 1983; Soto and Burhanuddin, 1995; Chaieb *et al.,* 2007) Eugenol, as major component of clove essential oil has many of biological activities including antifungal, (Pinto *et al.*, 2009) antiallergic, (Kim *et al.,* 1998) antioxidant (Gülçin *et al.*, 2012) and insecticidal (Park *et al.,* 2000) properties. Essential oil of Eugenia caryophyllata has been recognized as an effective, safe and inexpensive anesthetic for fishes and amphibians (Kildea *et al.,* 2004). It was reported that clove essential oil has cytotoxic and anti-cancerogenic properties (Kouidhi *et al.,* 2010). Also, analgesic effect of eugenol in different models of pain has been well documented (Park *et al.,* 2011; Lionnet *et al.,* 2010; Kurian *et al.,* 2006; Peana *et al.,* 2004; Okhubo and Shibata, 1997). It has also been reported that, eugenol activates calcium channels and inhibits of Na^+ currents in rat dorsal root ganglion cells (Okhubo and Kitamura, 1997; Cho *et al.,* 2008) blocks calcium and potassium channels in guinea pig cardiac muscles (Sensch *et al.,* 2000). Topical application of eugenol in small quantities to dental cavity could produce anti-inflammatory and local analgesic effects (Markowitz *et al.*, 1992).

The orofacial region is one of the most densely innervated (by trigeminal nerves) areas of the body, which wide range of conditions like trigeminal neuralgia, post-herpetic neuralgia, temporomandibular joint disorders, periodontal inflammation and pathological states of the teeth produce acute and chronic painful sensation in this region (Raboisson and Dallel, 2004). Because of the lack of recognition and understanding of orofacial pain mechanisms, there are many difficulties in management of this kind of pain (Miranda *et al.*, 2009; Belmonte *et al.*, 2004) Natural therapies, because of less adverse effects and also more beneficial effects have a great advantage over common pain killers like opioids and non-steroidal anti-inflammatory drugs when side effects are taken into account (Petrović *et al.*, 2008; Zdunić *et al.*, 2009).

Therefore, we investigated the effects of EOC in two models of nociception (tail immersion test and formalin induced orofacial pain) as well as xylene induced ear edema as a model of inflammation to determine its possible anti-nociceptive and anti-inflammatory activities. Naloxone pretreatment was performed to clarify the involvement of opioidergic system in EOC-induced analgesia in the orofacial test. The possible contribution of cyclooxygenase system was assessed using ketoprofen (as positive control with peripheral analgesic and anti-inflammatory actions) with and without EOC.

2. Materials and Methods

2.1. Plant material and essential oil extraction

The buds of *Eugenia caryophyllata* was purchased from local market in Tabriz and were subsequently authenticated by Dr A. Ebrahimi, a botanist at the Herbarium of Faculty of Pharmacy (Tbz-Fph), Medical University of Tabriz, Tabriz, Iran. The buds were ground into a fine powder. The essential oil of Eugenia caryophyllata buds were extracted from powdered plant by hydro-distillation in a Clevenger type apparatus for 3 h and produced 8% (v/w) yield. Obtained EO was dried over anhydrous sodium sulfate until the last traces of water were removed, and then stored in dark glass bottles at 4 °C.

2.2. Animals

Adult male Wistar rats, weighing 270–300 g and adult male mice, weighing 32-36 g were used in this study. They were randomly housed in polyethylene cages with *ad libitum* access to food and water in a room with controlled temperature (22±1 °C) and under a 12 h light-dark cycle (lights on from 07:00 a.m.) Six rats were used in each group of orofacial formalin test and tail immersion test. All experiments were performed between 11:00 h and 15:00 h. All research and animal care procedures were approved by the Veterinary Ethics Committee of the Faculty of Veterinary Medicine, University of Tabriz and were performed in accordance with the current guidelines for the care of laboratory animals and the ethical guidelines for investigations of experimental pain in conscious animals (Zimmermann, 1983).

2.3. Drugs and chemicals

Morphine sulfate was purchased from Toliddarou Co (Tehran, Iran). Atropine sulfate and naloxone hydrochloride, Tween 80 and ketoprofen were purchased from Sigma Chemical Co (St. Louis, MO, USA) and formalin solution 37% and NaCl from Merck chemicals (Darmstadt, Germany). Xylene was purchased from Dr. Mojalali Chemical Co (Tehran, Iran). All drugs and chemicals were dissolved in physiological saline. Xylene is used in pure form in the xylene-induced ear edema test. An emulsion of essential oil was prepared using Tween 80 and saline (0.5%, v/v) as solvent.

2.4. Essential oil GC-MS analyze

The essential oil was analyzed by gas chromatography – mass spectrometry (GC-MS). The chromatograph instrument (Agilent 6890 UK) was equipped with an HP-5MS capillary column (30 × 0.25 mm ID × 0.25 mm film thickness) and the data were taken under the following conditions: initial temperature 50°C, temperature ramp 5°C/min, 240°C/min to 300°C (holding for 3 min), and injector temperature at 290°C. The carrier gas was helium and the split ratio was 0.8 mL-1/min. For confirmation of analysis results, EOs were also analyzed by gas chromatography–mass spectrometry (Agilent 6890 gas chromatograph equipped with an Agilent 5973 mass-selective detector; Agilent UK) and the same capillary column and analytical conditions as above. The MS was run in electron-ionization mode with ionization energy of 70 eV.

2.5. Xylene-induced ear edema in mice

Ear edema was induced by topical application of pure xylene (20 µl) to inner and outer surfaces of the left ear of each mouse and right ear was considered as control. Mice were divided into four groups (n=5/group). Group 1 served as control administered with Tween 0.5% (100 µl, s.c.). Group 2 served as positive control and was dosed with 80 mg/kg, IP ketoprofen 30 min before induction of ear edema. Groups 3 and 4 were treated with 100 and 200 mg/kg, SC of EOC 30 min prior to induction of ear edema. Mice were sacrificed by cervical dislocation 1 h after xylene application. The plug (7mm in diameter) was removed with a stainless steel punch from both xylene treated ear and untreated ear then weighted by a sensitive digital balance (Zhang *et al.*, 2008). The ear edema percent was calculated according to the following formula:

Ear edema percent =100 × (left ear punch weight - right ear punch weight) / (right ear punch weight).

2.6. Orofacial formalin test

For reduction of possible effects of stress during the test, on two successive days prior to the orofacial formalin test, animals were placed 30 minute inside a Plexiglas observation chamber (30×30×25 cm) that equipped with a mirror angled at 45° below the chamber. In the test day after 30-min adaptation period, formaldehyde solution (1.5% in saline; 50µl) was injected subcutaneously into the left side of the upper lip (narrow area between upper lip and vibrissal pad) just lateral to the nose using a 31-gauge injection needle (insulin syringe 0.5 ml, BD® USA) (Raboisson and Dallel, 2004).

Following formalin injection, the rat was immediately put back in the observation chamber. The time spent in face rubbing with the forepaws determined as a nociceptive behavior and it was recorded in uninterrupted 3-min blocks over a period of 45 min (Erfanparast *et al.,* 2010). The first 3 min measured as the first phase (phasic pain, neurogenic phase) while the period between 18 - 36 min was considered as the second phase (inflammatory pain). Vehicle (Tween 80, 0.5% in saline; 1ml/kg, SC), EOC (50, 100 and 200 mg/kg), morphine sulphate (5 mg/kg, IP) and ketoprofen (40, 80, 160 mg/kg; IP) were administered 30 min prior to formalin injection. Naloxone (1 mg/kg, IP) was administered 40 min before formalin injection. In combination treatment, 50 mg/kg EOC was co-administered with 40 mg/kg ketoprofen.

2.7. Tail Immersion Test

The tail of rats was immersed (on 5 cm) in a water bath at noxious temperature of 55± 0.5 C until the tail was withdrawn or when the whole body was recoiled. The cut-off time was fixed at 15 seconds to prevent any tissue damage to the tail (Le Bars *et al.,* 2001). Reaction latencies at the 0, 15, 30, 45 and 60 min after chemicals administration were used as a parameter reflecting of the pain experienced.

2.8. Statistics

To evaluate significant differences among treated groups in the orofacial pain test as well as xylene-induced ear edema test, one-way analysis of variance

(ANOVA) were applied followed by Tukey HSD test. Also two way ANOVA with repeated measure and Bonferroni post hoc were used to assess the effects of time and drug in tail immersion test using IBM® SPSS® software version 19 (IBM company, USA). In figures, all values are expressed as Mean±SEM. A value of P <0.05 was considered statistically significant.

3. Results and discussion

3.1. GC-MS Analysis

The chemical composition of EOC was determined by GC-MS, which identified 9 compounds, representing 93.66% of total oil compounds. According to these results, the major components of the oil were Eugenol (54.86%), β-Caryophyllene (20.19%), α-Humulene (7.11%), eugenol acetat (4.85%) and Chavibetol (2.23%). The main percentage compositions of EOC are represented in table1.

3.2. Orofacial pain

The SC injection of formalin into the upper lip region in the normal saline and vehicle (Tween 80, 0.5% 200µl) treated animals without any significant differences produced pain responses in the first and 6th – 12th three min blocks. Therefore, formalin produced a biphasic pattern (first phase: 0-3 min and second phase: 18-36 min) of pain response in orofacial region (Figure 1).

The results are presented in Figure 2 showed that essential oil of *Eugenia caryophyllata* at dose of 50 mg/kg did not produce any significant effects in the both first and second phases of pain. The SC injection of EOC at doses of 100 and 200 mg/kg induced significant (p<0.05) anti-nociceptive activities only in the second phase when compared to control group. Morphine (5 mg/kg) significantly (p<0.05) inhibited behavioral responses in the both phases of the orofacial formalin test (Figure 2).

The IP injection of ketoprofen at doses of 80 and 160 mg/kg but not 40 mg/kg induced significant (p<0.05) antinociceptive activities only in the second phase of orofacial formalin test when compared to the control group in a dose dependent manner (Figure 3).

Naloxone (1 mg/kg) alone had no any significant effect. Pre-treatment of animals with naloxone did not prevent the EOC (200 mg/kg) analgesic activity (p<0.05) (Figure 4).

Co-administration of sub-analgesic doses of EOC (50 mg/kg) and ketoprofen (40 mg/kg) significantly (p<0.05) reduced nociceptive behavior in the second phase of formalin induced pain when compared with control group (Figure 5).

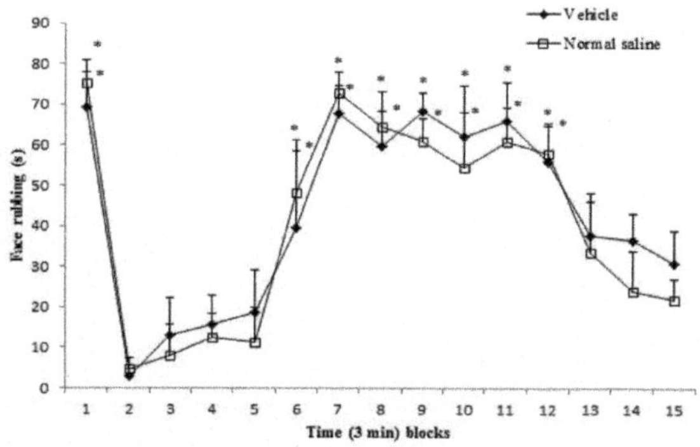

Fig. 1. Three-min blocks of face rubbing induced by injection of formalin into the upper lip in normal saline and Tween 80 0.5% treated groups. Values are expressed as the mean ± SEM (n=6/group). * p < 0.05 compared with other 3-min blocks (Two way ANOVA followed by Bonferroni post hoc test).

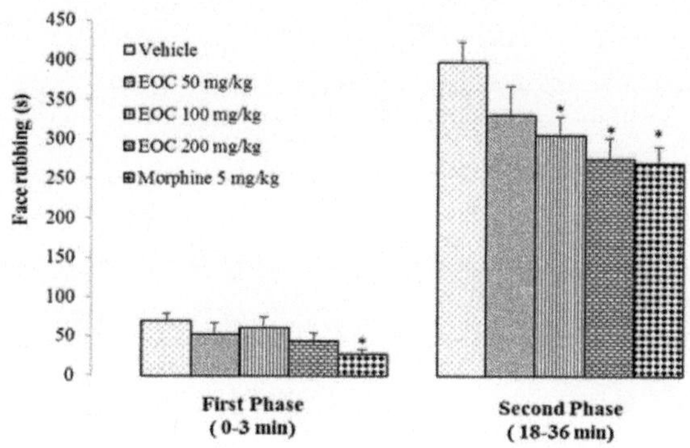

Fig. 2. Effects of P injection of essential oil of *Eugenia caryophyllata* (EOC) and Morphine on formalin-induced orofacial pain. Values are expressed as the mean ± SEM (n = 6/group). * p < 0.05 compared with vehicle (Tween 80 0.5%) group (One way ANOVA followed by Tukey HSD post hoc test).

3.3. Tail immersion test

As is shown in Figure 6, morphine (5 mg/kg) analgesic activity was started 30 min after IP injection (p<0.0001) and last until the end of observation period (60 min). SC injection of EOC at doses of 100 and 200 mg/kg failed to prolong withdrawal latency during the observation period.

3.4. Xylene-induced ear edema

Subcutaneous injection of EOC at doses of 100 and 200 mg/kg as well as ketoprofen at dose of (80 mg/kg) significantly ($p<0.01$, $p<0.001$ and $p<0.001$ respectively) attenuated xylene-induced ear edema in mice (Figure 7).

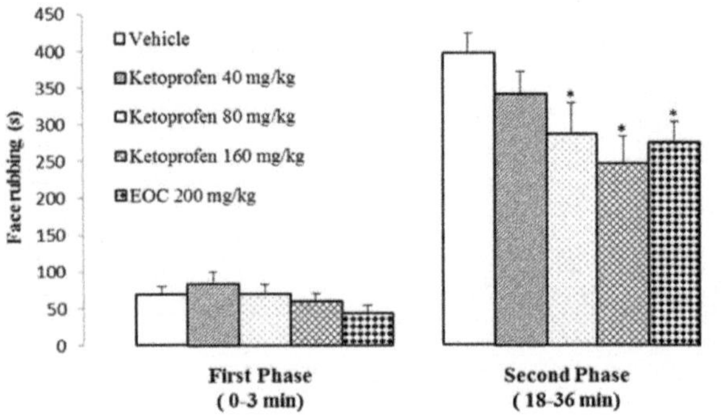

Fig. 3. Effects of IP injection of Ketoprofen on formalin-induced orofacial pain. Values are expressed as the mean ± SEM (n = 6/group). * $p < 0.05$ compared with vehicle (Tween 80 0.5%) group (One way ANOVA followed by Tukey HSD post hoc test).

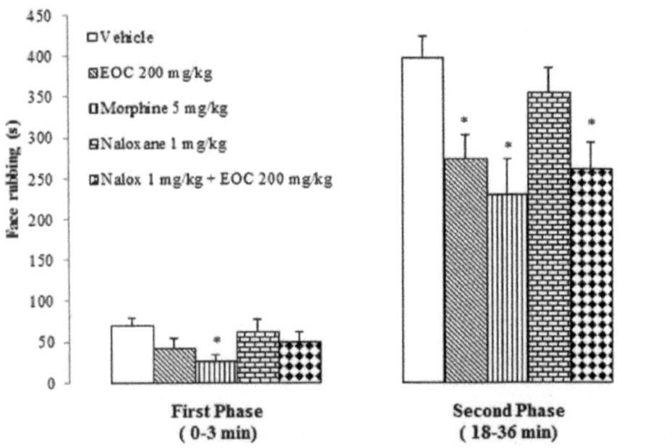

Fig. 4. Effects of IP injection of naloxone alone and before essential oil of *Eugenia caryophyllata* on on formalin-induced orofacial pain. Values are the means ± SEM (n = 6/group). * $p < 0.05$ compared with vehicle (Tween 80 0.5%) group (One way ANOVA followed by Tukey HSD post hoc test). EOC: Essential oil of *Eugenia caryophyllata*, Nalox: Naloxone.

Topical administration of Clove essential oil widely and traditionally used for relief of tooth pain and also it is well known in the dentistry because of its local analgesic and local anesthetic effects (Daniel *et al.*, 2009). Nonetheless, there aren't any published data about its systemic effects and mechanisms of action in the different kinds of pain arise from orofacial region and trigeminal nerve territory.

In this experiment chemical composition of EOC was analyzed by GC-MS, which identified 9 compounds, representing 93.66% of total oil compounds. The major components of the oil were Eugenol (54.86%), β-Caryophyllene (20.19%), α-Humulene (7.11%), Eugenol acetat (4.85%) and Chavibetol (2.23%).

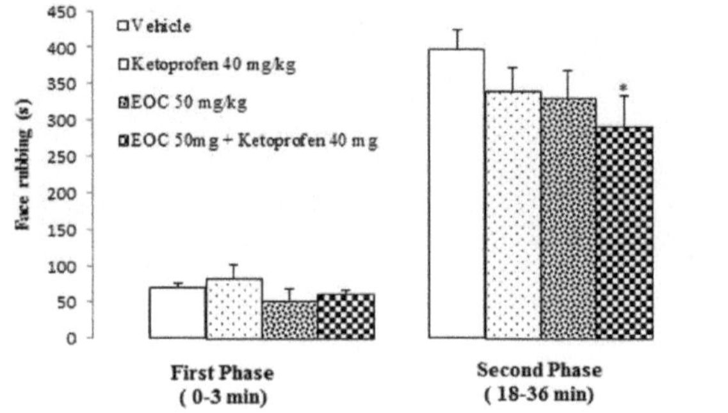

Fig. 5. Effects of combination treatments with sub-analgesic dose of essential oil of *Eugenia caryophyllata* (EOC) with Ketoprofen on formalin-induced orofacial pain. Values are expressed as the mean ± SEM (n = 6/group). * $p < 0.05$ compared with vehicle (Tween 80 0.5%) group (One way ANOVA followed by Tukey HSD post hoc test).

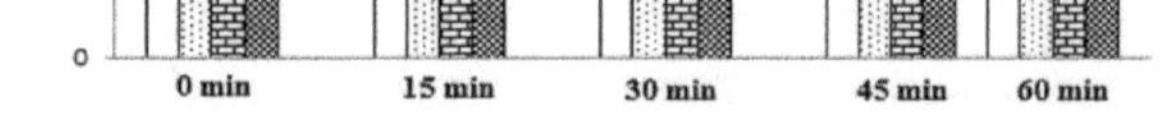

Fig. 6. The effects of essential oil of *Eugenia caryophyllata (EOC)* and morphine on tail immersion test response. * $p < 0.0001$ compared with other time points of vehicle. (n=6/group). (Two way ANOVA with repeated measure followed by Bonferroni post hoc test) EOC: Essential oil of *Eugenia caryophyllata*.

We identified high concentration of Eugenol and β-Caryophyllene in the extracted essential oil. Eugenol is a phenylpropene derivative, well known as local anesthetic (Park *et al.*, 2009), analgesic (Okhubo and Kitamura, 1997; Park *et al.*, 2006) and anti-inflammatory agent (Hashimoto et al., 1988) that widely used in dentistry. The analgesic effects of eugenol may be modulated by its inhibitory effect on voltage-gated Na^+ channels (Park *et al.,* 2006) and on high voltage-activated $Ca2^+$ channels (Lee *et al.,* 2005). β-Caryophyllene is another component exists in the Eugenia caryophyllata essential oil, this sesquiterpene has a functional non-psychoactive CB_2 cannabinoid receptor agonistic activity (Gertsch *et al.,* 2008). Cannabinoid receptor CB_2 and its selective agonist accepted as a new pharmacological target for treatment of pain (Anand *et al.*, 2009).

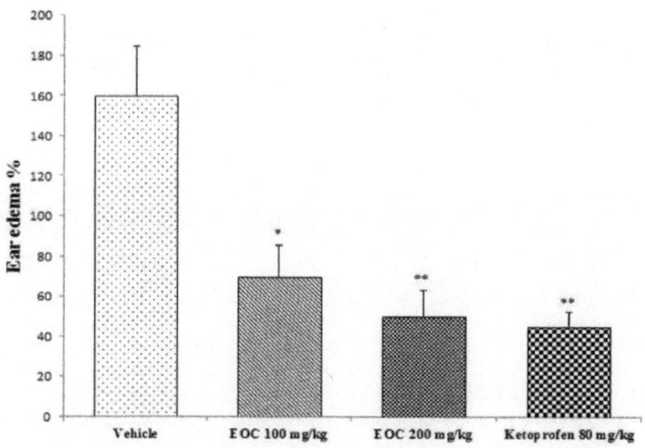

Fig. 7. Effect of essential oil of *Eugenia caryophyllata* (EOC) and ketoprofen on xylene induced ear edema in mice. Values are expressed as the mean ± SEM (n = 5/group). * $p < 0.01$ and **$p < 0.001$ compared with vehicle (Tween 80, 0.5%) group (One way ANOVA followed by Tukey HSD post hoc test).

Table1. The main components (%) of the *Eugenia caryophyllata* buds essential oil.

NO	Compound	RT[1]	%
1	Eugenol	12.99	54.86
2	β- Caryophyllene	14.00	20.19
3	α -Humulene	14.54	7.11
4	Iso-eugenol	13.49	1.23
5	Chavibetol	13.61	2.23
6	O- egunol	14.17	1.70
7	cis- Ocimene	15.51	1.41
8	Eugenol acetat	16.08	4.85
9	Caryophyllene oxide	17.29	0.08

[1]Retention Time.

Topical application of xylene to ear leads to an acute inflammatory response and is known to cause severe vasodilation and oedematous changes of skin (Kim *et al.*, 2007). This method is used for the evaluation of anti-inflammatory steroids as well as non-steroidal antiphlogistic agents especially those inhibiting phospholipase A_2 (Zaninir *et al.*, 1992).

Our data obtained from ear edema test revealed that EOC and ketoprofen can modulate inflammatory response induced by xylene which suggests it might peripherally reduce the release of inflammatory mediators.

Our results in the present study indicate antinociceptive effects of clove essential oil in the formalin induced orofacial nociception in rats, and also provide some evidence for determination of possible mechanisms of antinociceptive action in this model of pain.

In the orofacial formalin test, morphine (5 mg/kg) reduced pain response in both phases of orofacial pain. Also the results (Fig.2 and Fig. 4) showed that the essential oil of clove at doses of 100 and 200 mg/kg considerably inhibited second phase (inflammatory phase) of formalin induce orofacial pain response but this analgesic effect was not antagonized with non-selective opioid receptors antagonist, naloxone. Moreover high dose of EOC (200 mg/kg) reduced pain response in the first phase of formalin induce orofacial pain but this effect was not statistically significant. These findings suggest that analgesic effect of EOC is not mediated through opioidergic mechanisms and it's containing active analgesic properties acting predominantly with peripheral mechanisms (anti-inflammatory action) in this model of nociception. In addition, ketoprofen (non-selective cyclooxygenase and lipoxygenase inhibitor) at doses of 80 and 160 mg/kg significantly reduced pain response only in the second phase of orofacial pain and co-administration of sub-analgesic doses of EOC (50 mg/kg) and ketoprofen (40 mg/kg) significantly ($p<0.05$) reduced nociceptive behavior only in the second phase when compared with control group (Fig. 3 and 5). This potentiated analgesic effect may indicates that EOC can inhibits cyclooxygenase pathway and reduce inflammatory mediators of pain in the second phase of this test.

Two different phases of orofacial formalin test have different properties and are very useful tools, not only for assessing the potency of analgesics, but also for elucidating the mechanisms of pain and analgesia (Chen *et al.,* 1995). Analgesic drugs that inhibit both phases of formalin pain like morphine primarily act centrally but peripherally acting drugs such as anti-inflammatory drugs as the cyclooxygenase inhibitors only inhibit the second phase of formalin-induced nociception (Chen *et al.,* 1995).

In the tail immersion test SC injection of EOC failed to prolong withdrawal latency during the observation period. The tail immersion test well known as a proper method to evaluate the central mechanisms of pain relief as observed in the case of opioids like morphine (Halder *et al.,* 2009).

Our results in formalin induced orofacial pain as well as tail immersion test revealed that EOC has a relatively more potent peripheral action than central action in causing pain relief.

4. Conclusion

In conclusion, the results of present study indicated that EOC possesses potent anti-inflammatory activity in xylene induced ear edema and also EOC and ketoprofen exhibited antinociceptive activities only in the inflammatory phase of formalin induced orofacial pain and opioidergic system may not be involved in the antinociceptive activity of Clove essential oil in this model of nociception.

5. Acknowledgments

This work was financially supported by University of Tabriz grant. We thank the Vice Chancellor of Research and technology of University of Tabriz for financially support.

6. Conflicts of interest

The authors declare that they have no conflict of interest.

7. References

Anand, P., Whiteside, G., Fowler, C.J., and Hohmann, A.G. 2009. Targeting CB2 receptors and the endocannabinoid system for the treatment of pain. *Brain Res Rev*, 60: 255-266.

Arung, E.T., Matsubara, E., Kusuma, I.W., Sukaton, E., Shimizu, K., and Kondo, R. 2011. Inhibitory components from the buds of clove (Syzygium aromaticum) on melanin formation in B16 melanoma cells. *Fitoterapia*, 82: 198-202.

Belmonte, C., Acosta, M.C., and Gallar, J. 2004. Neural basis of sensation in intact and injured corneas. *Exp Eye Res*, 78: 513-525.

Chaieb, K., Hajlaoui, H., Zmantar, T., Kahla-Nakbi, A.B., Mahmoud, R., Mahdouani, K., and Bakhrouf, A. 2007. The chemical composition and biological activity of clove essential oil, Eugenia caryophyllata (Syzigium aromaticum L. Myrtaceae): a short review. *Phytother Res*, 21: 501-506.

Chen, Y.F., Tsai, H.Y., and Wu, T.S. 1995. Anti-inflammatory and analgesic activities from root of Angelica pubescens. *Planta Med*, 61: 2-8.

Cho, J.S., Kim, T.H., Lim, J.M., Song, J.H. 2008. Effects of eugenol on Na^+ currents in rat dorsal root ganglion neurons. *Brain Res*, 1243: 53-62.

Daniel, A.N., Sartoretto, S.M., Schmidt, G., Caparroz-Assef, S.M., Bersani-Amado, C.A., and Cuman, R.K.N. 2009. Anti- inflammatory and antinociceptive activities A of eugenol essential oil in experimental animal models. *Rev Bras Farmacogn*, 19: 212-217.

Erfanparast, A., Tamaddonfard, E., Farshid, A.A., and Khalilzadeh, E. 2010. Effect of microinjection of histamine into the dorsal hippocampus on the orofacial formalin-induced pain in rats. *Eur j Pharmacol*, 627:119-123.

Gertsch, J., Leonti, M., Raduner, S., Racz, I., Chen, J.Z., Xie, X.Q., Altmann, K.H., Karsak, M., and Zimmer, A. 2008. Beta-caryophyllene is a dietary cannabinoid. *Proc Natl Acad Sci USA*, 26: 9099-9104.

Gülçin, I., Elmastas, M., and Aboul-Enein, H.Y. 2012. Antioxidant activity of clove oil – A powerful antioxidant source. *Arabian J Chem*, 5: 489-499.

Halder, S., Bharal, N., Mediratta, P.K., Kaur, I., and Sharma, K.K. 2009. Antiinflammatory, immunomodulatory and antinociceptive activity of Terminalia arjuna Roxb bark powder in mice and rats. *Indian J Exp Biol*, 47: 577-583.

Hashimoto, S., Uchiyama, K., Maeda, M., Ishitsuka, K., Furumoto, K., and Nakamura, Y. 1988. In vivo and in vitro effects of zinc oxide-eugenol (ZOE) on biosynthesis of cyclooxygenase products in rat dental pulp. *J Dent Res*, 67: 1092-1096.

Kildea, M.A., Allanb, G.L., and Kearney, R.E. 2004. Accumulation and clearance of the anaesthetics clove oil and AQUI-S from the edible tissue of silver perch (Bidyanus bidyanus). *Aquaculture*, 232: 265-277.

Kim, H.M., Lee, E.H., Hong, S.H., Song, H.J., Shin, M.K., Kim, S.H., and Shin, T.Y. 1998. Effect of Syzygium aromaticum extract on immediate hypersensitivity in rats. *J Ethnopharmacol*, 60: 125-131.

Kim, H.D., Cho, H.R., Moon, S.B., Shin, H.D., Yang, K.J., Park, B.R., Jang, H.J., Kim, L.S., Lee, H.S., and Ku, S.K. 2007. Effects of beta-glucan from Aureobasidium pullulans on acute inflammation in mice. *Arch Pharmacal Res*, 30: 323-328.

Kouidhi, B., Zmantar, T., and Bakhrouf, A. 2010. Anticariogenic and cytotoxic activity of clove essential oil (Eugenia caryophyllata) against a large number of oral pathogens. *Ann Microbiol*, 60: 599-604.

Kurian, R., Arulmozhi, D.K., Veeranjaneyulu, A., and Bodhankar, S.L. 2006. Effect of eugenol on animal models of nociception. *Indian J Pharmacol*, 38: 341-345.

Le Bars, D., Gozariu, M., and Cadden, S.W. 2001. Animal models of nociception. *Pharmacol Rev*, 53: 597-652.

Lee, M.H., Yeon, K.Y., Park, C.K., Li, H.Y., Fang, Z., Kim, M.S., Choi, S.Y., Lee, S.J., Lee, S., Park, K., Lee, J.H., Kim, J.S, and Oh, S.B. 2005. Eugenol inhibits calcium currents in dental afferent neurons. *J Dent Res*, 84: 848-51.

Lionnet, L., Beaudry, F., and Vachon, P. 2010. Intrathecal eugenol administration alleviates neuropathic pain in male Sprague-Dawley rats. *Phytother Res*, 24: 1645-1653.

Markowitz, K., Moynihan, M., Liu, M., and Kim, S. 1992. Biologic properties of eugenol and zinc oxide-eugenol. A clinically oriented review. *Oral Surg Oral Med Oral Pathol*, 73: 729-737.

Miranda, H.F., Sierralta, F., and Prieto, J.C. 2009. Synergism between NSAIDs in the orofacial formalin test in mice. *Pharmacol Biochem Be*, 92: 314–318.

Okhubo, T., Kitamura, K. 1997. Eugenol activates $Ca2^+$-permeable currents in rat dorsal root ganglion cells. *J Dent Res*, 76: 1737-1744.

Okhubo, T., Shibata, M. 1997. The selective capsaicin antagonist capsazepine abolishes the antinociceptive action of eugenol and guaiacol. *J Dent Res*, 76: 848-851.

Park, C.K., Li, H.Y., Yeon, K.Y., Jung, S.J., Choi, S.Y., Lee, S.J., Lee, S., Park, K., Kim, J.S., and Oh, S.B. 2006. Eugenol inhibits sodium currents in dental afferent neurons. *J Dent Res*, 85: 900-904

Park, C.K., Kim, K., Jung, S.J., Kim, M.J., Ahn, D.K., Hong, S.D., Kim, J.S., and Oh, S.B. 2009. Molecular mechanism for local anesthetic action of eugenol in the rat trigeminal system. *Pain*, 144: 84-94.

Park, I.K., Lee, H.S., Lee, S.G., Park, J.D., and Ahn, Y.J. 2000. Insecticidal and fumigant activities of Cinnamomum cassia bark-derived material against Mechoris ursulus (Coleoptera Attelabidae). *J Agric Food Chem*, 48: 2528-2531.

Park, S.H., Sim, Y.B., Lee, J.K., Kim, S.M., Kang, Y.J., Jung, J.S., and Suh, H.W. 2011. The analgesic effects and mechanisms of orally administered eugenol. *Arch Pharm Res*, 34(3): 501-507.

Peana. A.T., Chessa, G., Carta, G., Delogu, G., and Fabbri, D. 2004. Eugenol, bis-eugenol and synthesized related-dimer compounds produce antinociception in the acetic acid-induced-writhing responses. *Curr Top Phytochem*, 6: 137-143.

Petrović, S., Dobrić, S., Mimica-Dukić, N., and Simin, N. 2008. The antiinflammatory, gastroprotective and antioxidant activities of Hieracium gymnocephalum extract. *Phytother Res*, 22: 1548–1551.

Pinto, E., Vale-Silva, L., Cavaleiro, C., and Salgueiro. L. 2009. Antifungal activity of the clove essential oil from Syzygium aromaticum on Candida, Aspergillus and dermatophyte species. *J Med Microbiol*, 58: 1454-1462.

Raboisson, P., Dallel, R. 2004. The orofacial formalin test. *Neurosci Biobehav Rev*, 28: 219-226.

Schiller, C., Schiller, D. 2008. *The Aromatherapy Encyclopedia: A concise guide to 385 Essential Plant Oils*. Basic Health Publications, Inc.

Sensch, O., Vierling, W., Brandt, W., and Reiter, W. 2000. Effects of inhibition of calcium and potassium currents in guinea-pig cardiac contraction: comparison of beta-caryophyllene oxide, eugenol, and nifedipine. *Br J Pharmacol*, 131: 1089-1096.

Shelef, L.A. 1983. Antimicrobial effects of spices. *J Food Saf*, 6: 29-44.

Soto, C.G., Burhanuddin, C.G. 1995. Clove oil as a fish anaesthetic for measuring length and weight of rabbit fish (Siganus lineatus). *Aquaculture,* 136: 149-152.

Zaninir, J.C., Medeiros, Y.S., Cruz, A.B., Yunes, R.R.A., and Calixto, J.B. 1992. Action of compounds from Mandevilla velutina on croton oil induced ear oedema in mice: a comparative study with steroidal and non-steroidal anti-inflammatory drugs. *Phytother Res*, 6: 1-5.

Zdunić, G., Godevac, D., Milenković, M., Vucićević, D., Savikin, K., Menković, N., and Petrović, S. 2009. Evaluation of Hypericum perforatum oil extracts for an antiinflammatory and gastroprotective activity in rats. *Phytother Res*, 23: 1554-1564.

Zhang, G.Q., Huang, X.D., Wang, H., Leung, A.K., Chan, C.L., Fong, D.W., and Yu. Z.L. 2008. Anti-inflammatory and analgesic effects of the ethanol extract of Rosa multiflora Thunb. hips. *J Ethnopharmacol*, 118:290-294.

Zimmermann, M. 1983. Ethical guidelines for investigations of experimental pain in conscious animals. *Pain*, 16: 109-110.

Antioxidant activity of Sage (Salvia officinalis), Red Cabbage (Brassica oleracea), Walnut Leaf (Juglans regia L.), Yellow Sweet Clover (Melilotus officinalis) and Hawthorn (Crataegus oxyacantha) at different temperatures

Mohammad Momen Heravi, Shahla Daneshmehr*, Ali Morsali

Department of Chemistry, Mashhad Branch, Islamic Azad University, Mashhad, Iran;

***Email:** *daneshmehr@mshdiau.ac.ir*

ARTICLE INFO

Topic: *Medicinal Plants*

Key words:

- ✓ *Cancer*
- ✓ *Free Radical*
- ✓ *Scavenging Activity*
- ✓ *Medicinal Plant*

ABSTRACT

Background & Aim: Medicinal plants can be a good replacement for common cancer treatment including chemotherapy, radiation therapy and surgery because they don't have many side effects. The aim of this study was to investigate the effect of temperature on the free radical scavenging in the presence of medicinal plants.
Experimental: For determination of free radical scavenging activity by using the stable 2,2-diphenyl-1-picrylhydrazyl (DPPH) assay at different temperatures, two investigations were carried out: first ethanolic extracts of Sage (Salvia officinalis), Red Cabbage (Brassica oleracea), Walnut Leaf (Juglans regia L.), Yellow Sweet Clover (Melilotus officinalis) and Hawthorn (Crataegus oxyacantha) one by one and then the mixtures of each pair of plants in order to determine plant-plant interactions.
Results: Because of Herb-Herb interactions, the most free radical scavenging percentages are related to plants in single forms not mixtures. The results demonstrated that with increasing temperature free radical scavenging increased in the presence of Sage, while it decreased in the presence of Hawthorn. The highest free radical scavenging percentages at temperatures ranging from ambient to body and fever are related to Sage at 25°C, then Walnut Leaf at 37°C and finally, Hawthorn at 40°C.
Recommended applications/industries: The results indicated that for preventing herb-herb interactions, medicinal plants as tea, food and fruit are used alone.

1. Introduction

Cancer has existed for all of human history (Hajdu *et al.*, 2011). It is a disease in which abnormal cells divide and to be multiply in a malignant tumor. In a healthy organism, always between the rate of cell division and cell death is a balance (Munari *et al.*, 2014; Markert 1968). Reactive oxygen species (ROS) are a byproduct of normal metabolism. Additionally, ROS are produced in cells as a response to several factors, including oxidative and thermal stresses, ultraviolet light, chemical agents, and ionizing radiation. Oxidative stress can cause DNA damage, cell functions inhibition, lipid and protein peroxidation, and disturbance of glutathione levels (Yoo *et al.*, 2008). In addition, ROS contribute to the development of cancer, diabetes, atherosclerosis, inflammatory diseases, and ageing (Beal, 1995; Harman, 1956 & 1992; Lee *et al.*, 2005). ROS are divided into free radical species, such as superoxide anion radical, hydroxyl radical, and non-free radical that are involved in oxidative reactions, such as singlet oxygen (Esmaeili *et al.*, 2010). ROS free radicals contain unpaired electrons, which usually show a high degree of reactivity with biological macromolecules such as proteins, lipids, and DNA (Halliwell & Gutteridge, 1999). Free radicals can oxidize DNA bases (especially guanine), leading to mutations (Harman, 1956 & 1992). Oxidative damages can be reduced through enzymatic mechanisms such as superoxide dismutase (SOD) and catalase (CAT) or by antioxidants presented as natural products (Boo *et al.*, 2012). The antioxidants realize the balance of formation and destroying the free radicals. They are able to trap or to block, to scavenge, to remove free radicals by substitution, addition or electron transfer reactions (Popescu *et al.*, 2011; Rizea *et al.*, 2012). As part of a healthy lifestyle and a well-balanced, wholesome diet, antioxidant supplementation is now being recognized as an important means of improving free radical protection (Rock *et al.*, 2012). Many synthetic drugs protect against oxidative damage, but some have adverse side effects (Munari *et al.*, 2014). An alternative solution to overcome ROS is to consume natural antioxidants from food, beverages, and traditional medicines containing natural antioxidants such as L-ascorbic acid, tocopherol, and polyphenols (Van Wyk & Wink, 2004 & 2008; Yazdanparast & Ardestani, 2007; Wink & Abbas, 2013). The use of medicinal plants is perhaps the oldest method of coping with illnesses throughout the world and physicians and patients have looked for the natural drugs, nontoxic remedy and suitable to the organism. Because of the quality of medicinal plants and some research results, many people have the mistaken notion that, being natural, all herbs and foods are safe. Especially in the last decade, with more intensive studies devoted to natural therapies (Dejica, 2000; Feher *et al.*, 1988). Medicinal plants are commonly rich in phenolic compounds, such as flavonoids, phenolic acids, stilbenes, tannins, coumarins, lignans and lignins (Van Wyk & Wink, 2004;, Atanassova *et al.*, 2011; Jeong *et al.*, 2004; Hamdy Roby *et al.*, 2013; Packer *et al.*, 1999; Daffodil *et al.*, 2014; Ali *et al.*, 2008; Velioglu *et al.*, 1998; Amarowicza *et al.*, 2004). These compounds in various plant products (such as fruits, leaves, seeds, and oils) have multiple biological effects including antioxidant activity and radical scavenging in the last several years (Lugasi *et al.*, 1998; Kähkönen *et al.*, 1999; Mensor *et al.*, 2001; Singh *et al.*, 2002; Parejo *et al.*, 2002). Sage (Salvia officinalis), Red Cabbage (Brassica oleracea), Walnut Leaf (Juglans regia L.), Yellow Sweet Clover (Melilotus officinalis) and Hawthorn (Crataegus oxyacantha) are medicinal plants , are economically and nutritionally important vegetable consumed widely around the globe and they are good source of health-promoting compounds that show preventive effect against cancer, atherosclerosis, nephritis and diabetes mellitus (Singh *et al.*, 2009; Taveira *et al.*, 2009; Jaiswal *et al.*, 2012; Miliauskas *et al.*, 2004).

DPPH (2, 2-diphenyl-1-picrylhydrazyl) radical scavenging assay is mostly applied to rapidly examine the antioxidant capacity of samples. This method is widely used, as its reliability on giving information about the main property of antioxidant potential for many medicinal plants (Kedare & Singh, 2011; Huang *et al.*, 2009; Fu *et al.*, 2010).

DPPH can accept an electron or hydrogen radical to become a stable and diamagnetic molecule. It can be oxidized difficulty, and then irreversibly. When DPPH reacts with antioxidant compounds, it can donate hydrogen, so it is reduced. Fig 1. Many studies investigated interaction between herb-drug, food-drug, herb-herb, nutrient-drug and drug-drug (Sørensen, 2002; San Miguel *et al.*, 2005; Williamson, 2003 & 2005; Evans & McLeod, 2003; Tarirai *et al.*, 2010; Cheng *et al.*, 2010; Manek *et al.*, 2011; Fasinu *et al.*, 2012; Zeping *et al.*, 2005; *Izzo & Ernst, 2001;* Zhou *et al.*, 2010) and other

research results showed that the radical scavenging activities of all the plants extracts increased with increasing concentration (Ghasemi *et al.*, 2011; Heo *et al.*, 2014; Anissi *et al.*, 2014; Zhang *et al.*, 2014; Krishnaiah *et al.*, 2011; Turkmen *et al.*, 2006). Therefore, this work investigates the effects of temperature on free radical scavenging percentage with same concentration at temperatures ranging from ambient to body and fever.

2. Materials and Methods

2.1. Chemical and reagent

The reagent 2,2-Diphenyl-1-picrylhydrazyl (DPPH) was supplied by Sigma (St. Louis, USA). All other reagents (acetonitrile, Hydrochloric acid and ethanol) were purchased from Merck.

2.2. Plant materials and preparation of extracts

Fresh plants including: sage (Salvia officinalis), hawthorn (Crataegus oxyacantha), walnut leaf (Juglans regia L.), red Cabbage (*Brassica oleracea*), yellow sweet clover (Melilotus officinalis) were collected from Azerbaijan mountains located at northwest of Iran. The gathered samples were dried at ambient temperature and under sunlight for 5 days. Dried plants were milled with sample mill (300 Waufn S2, Germany) and in turn extracted with two solvents: HCl (1.5M) and ethanol (95%). A 2gr of each samples were extracted by dissolving in 85mL ethanol and 15mL HCl. Flasks were kept in a shaking incubator (Boekel Jitterbug Microplate, Cole-Parmer, USA) at 1000 rpm and 40°C for 1 h. The extracts were concentrated at 40°C for 15 min. The infusions were filtered through Whatman filter paper twice, until a clear extract was obtained.

2.3. Instrumentation

All spectrophotometric data were acquired using Perkin Elmer Lambda 25 UV-Vis spectrophotometer. Glass cuvettes (1 cm × 1 cm × 4.5 cm) were used for UV-Vis absorbance measurements. The temperature in the cell was controlled by using JULABO Heating Immersion Circulator.

2.4. DPPH radical scavenging assay

Radical scavenging activity of plant extracts against stable DPPH was determined spectrophotometrically. DPPH shows a strong absorption band at 517 nm. The solution of DPPH in Acetonitrile (6×10^{-5} M) was prepared daily, before UV-Vis measurements. 3 ml of this solution were mixed with 1 µl extract solution (extract: ethanol, 1:10 v/v).

For pair interactions, 1 µl extract solution consists of 0.5 µl of each extract.

The experiments were repeated for three times. The percentage of DPPH radical scavenging by the samples was calculated according to formula, % scavenging = $[\{A_i - A_f\}/A_i] \times 100$, where A_i control is the absorbance of DPPH radical, A_f sample is the absorbance of DPPH radical with extract after 30min.

3. Results and discussion

Comparing results of free radical scavenging percentage in the presence of ethanolic extracts of Sage, Red Cabbage, Walnut Leaf, Yellow Sweet Clover and Hawthorn one by one and mixtures of each pair of plants with same concentration at temperatures ranging from 25°C to 40°C, on the basis of data were measured by UV-Vis spectroscopy, are summarized in Table 1. The results provided in Table 1 show that the highest free radical scavenging percentage was the ethanolic extract of Sage at 25°C and with increased temperature decreased free radical scavenging percentage, while the lowest free radical scavenging percentage of Sage extract related to 40°C. Walnut leaf extract was more effective than 3 other single extracts against free radical and different temperatures have no significant effects on them. However, Red cabbage extract has weak free radical scavenging at all temperatures except for 25°C.

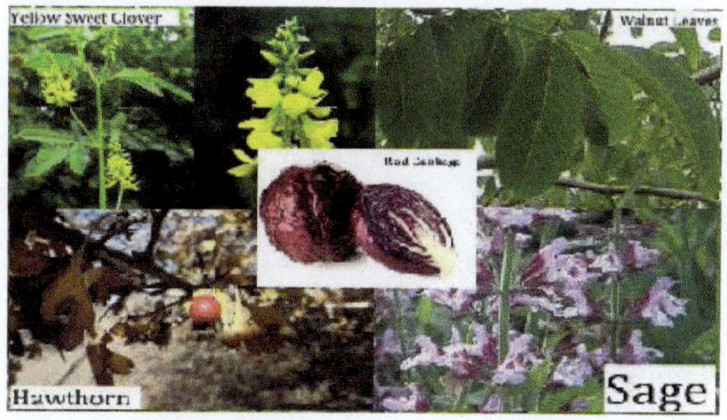

Fig.1. Medicinal plants

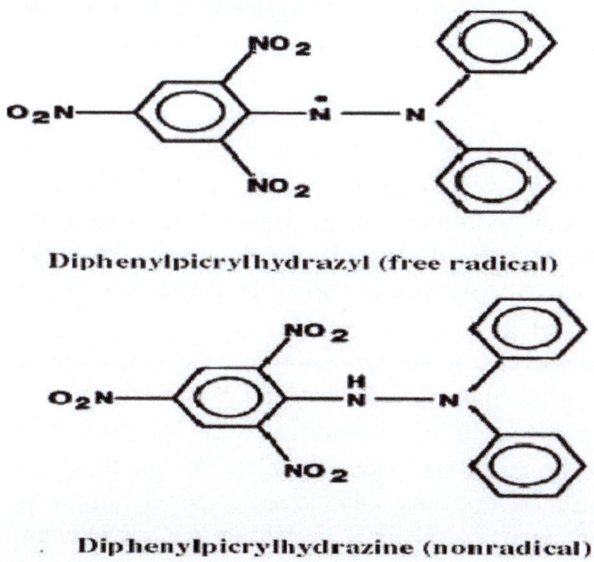

Fig.2. The structure of free radical and nonradical.

Table 1. Effect of temperature on the free radical scavenging.

Plant \ Temperature	25	28	31	34	37	40
Sage	96	78	56	26	25	23
Red Cabbage	66	27	18	30	18	26
Walnut Leaf	43	30	34	35	55	42
Yellow Sweet Clover	22	40	45.5	42	44	43
Hawthorn	27	31	35	37	40	55
Hawthorn & Yellow Sweet Clover	11	12	23.5	17	17	8
Sage & Yellow Sweet Clover	12	10	9.5	3.5	3	1
Sage & Hawthorn	19	17.5	21	21	12	21
Red Cabbage & Yellow Sweet Clover	22	16	14	16	17	18
Hawthorn & Red Cabbage	17	32.5	27	23.5	29	35
Walnut Leaf & Yellow Sweet Clover	22	18	14	21	31	35
Walnut Leaf & Red Cabbage	32	33	31	36	34	34
Walnut Leaf & Sage	13	25	17	27	29	31
Red Cabbage & Sage	23.5	29	19.5	25	23.5	22
Walnut Leaf & Hawthorn	17	9	8	1.6	16	18

The most scavenging percentage in mixture form is related to extract of Walnut Leaf and Red Cabbage at all temperatures. Overall, Free radical scavenging for mixtures of extracts reduced at all temperatures.

4. Conclusion

The determination of free radical scavenging percentage in ethanolic extracts of medicinal plants at different temperatures was done. Results show increasing or decreasing temperature doesn't have same effect on the free radical scavenging percentage at the presence of medicinal plants. So that, free radical scavenging in the presence of Saga increased with increasing temperature, while in the presence of Hawthorn decreased with increasing temperature but at the presence of Walnut Leaf, Red Cabbage, Yellow Sweet Clover, temperature doesn't have beneficial effects. The most free radical scavenging percentage are related to sage at 25°C, 28°C and 31°C, yellow sweet clover at 34°C, walnut leaf at 37°C and hawthorn at 40°C.Also this paper suggests that for preventing herb-herb interactions, medicinal plants as tea, food and fruit are used alone.

5. References

Ali, B.H., Blunden, G., Tanira, M.O. and Nemmar, A. 2008. Some phytochemical, pharmacological and toxicological properties of ginger (Zingiber officinale Roscoe): A review of recent research. *Food and Chemical Toxicology,* 46: 409-420.

Amarowicza, R., Pegg, R.B., Rahimi-Moghaddam, P., Barld, B. and Weil, J.A. 2004. Free-radical scavenging capacity and antioxidant activity of selected plant species from the Canadian prairies. *Food Chemistry,* 84: 551–562.

Anissi, J., Hassouni, M.E., Ouardaoui, A. and Sendide, K. 2014. A comparative study of the antioxidant scavenging activity of green tea, black tea and coffee extracts: A kinetic approach. *Food Chemistry,* 150: 438–447.

Atanassova, M., Georgieva, S. and Ivancheva, K. 2011. Total phenolic and total flavonoid contents, antioxidant capacity and biological contaminants in medicinal herbs. *The Journal of Chemical Technology and Metallurgy,* 46: 81-88.

Beal, M.F. 1995. Aging, energy and oxidative stress in neurodegenerative diseases. *Annals of Neurology,* 38: 357–366.

Boo, H.O., Heo, B.G. and Gorinstein, S. 2012. Analytical methods for enzyme and DPPH radical scavenging activities of natural pigments from some plants. *Food Analytical Methods,* 5: 1354–1361.

Chan, Y.C., Ali, A.S.M., Khairuddean, M., Khaw, K.Y., Murugaiyah, V. and Basiri, A. 2013. Synthesis and molecular modeling study of Cu (II) complexes derived from 2-(diphenylmethylene) hydrazinecarbothioamide derivatives with cholinesterase inhibitory activities. *Chinese Chemical Letters,* 24: 609–612.

Cheng, C.W., Fan, W., Ko, S.G., Song, L. and Bian, Z.X. 2010. Evidence-Based Management of Herb-Drug Interaction in Cancer Chemotherapy. *Explore New York,* 6: 324–329.

Daffodil, E.D., Lincy, P. and Mohan, V.R. 2014. Study of whole plant of vernonia cinerea less for in vitro antioxidant activity. *International Journal of Pharmaceutics,* 4: 172-178.

Dejica, C. Antioxidanti si terapie antioxidanta, (Ed.), *Editura Casa Cărţii de Ştiinţă Cluj-Napoca,* 2000; pp. 71-120.

Esmaeili, M.A. and Sonboli, A. 2010. Antioxidant, free radical scavenging activities of Salvia brachyantha and its protective effect against oxidative cardiac cell injury. *Food and Chemical Toxicology,* 48: 846–853.

Evans, W.E. and McLeod, H.L. 2003. Pharmacogenomics - Drug Disposition, Drug Targets, and Side Effects. *New England Journal of Medicine,* 6: 538-549.

Fasinu, P.S., Bouic, P.J. and Rosenkranz, B. 2012. An overview of the evidence and mechanisms of herb–drug interactions. *Frontiers in Pharmacology*, 3: 69.

Feher, J., Csomos, G. and Verechei, A. 1988. *Free radical Reactions in medicine*, Springer Verlag, Berlin-Heidelberg-New-York, pp. 11-46, 48-137.

Fu, W., Lei, Y.F., Cai, Y.L., Zhou, D.N. and Ruan, J.L. 2010. A new alkylene dihydrofuran glycoside with antioxidation activity from the root bark of *Morus Alba* L. *Chinese Chemical Letters,* 21: 821–823.

Ghasemi, K., Ghasemi, Y., Ehteshamnia, A., Nabavi, S.M., Nabavi, S.F., Ebrahimzadeh, M.A. and Pourmorad, F. 2011. Influence of environmental factors on antioxidantactivity, phenol and flavonoids contents of walnut (Juglans regia L.) green husks. *Journal of Medicinal Plants Research,* 5: 1128-1133.

Hajdu, S.I., Thun, M.J., Hannan, L.M. and Jemal, A. 2011. A note from history: landmarks in history of cancer, part1. *Cancer,* 117: 1097–102.

Halliwell, B. and Gutteridge, J.M.C. 1999. *Free radicals in biology and medicine*, third ed., Oxford University Press, Oxford, UK.

Hamdy Roby, M.H., Sarhana, M.A., Selima, K.A.H. and Khalel, K.I. 2013. Evaluation of antioxidant activity, total phenols and phenolic compounds in thyme (Thymus vulgaris L.), sage (Salvia officinalis L.), and marjoram (Origanum majorana L.) extracts. *Industrial Crops and Products,* 43: 827–831.

Harman, D. 1956. Aging: A theory based on free radical and radiation chemistry. *Journals of Gerontology Series A: Biological Sciences and Medical Sciences,* 11: 298–300.

Harman, D. 1992. Free radical theory of aging. *Mutation Research,* 275: 257–266.

Heo, B.G., Park, Y.J., Park, Y.S., Bae, J.H., Cho, J.Y., Park, K., Jastrzebskif, Z. and Gorinsteing, S. 2014. Anticancer and antioxidant effects of extracts from different parts ofindigo plant. *Industrial Crops and Products,* 56: 9–16.

Huang, K.X., Feng, Y.B., Yao, W., Yang, L.X., Wang, F., Li, H.B., Zeng, S., Gong, J.X., Hu, M.H., Zhao, Y., Wu, X.M., Li, X.K. and Qu, J. 2009. Evaluation of lipid peroxidation inhibition and free radical scavenging abilities of 5, 6, 7-trimethoxy dihydroflavonols. *Chinese Chemical Letters,* 20: 1187–1190.

Huang, X.Z., Yin, Y., Dai, J.H., Liang, H., Dai, Y. and Bai, L. 2010. Two new ceramides from the stems of Piper betle L. *Chinese Chemical Letters,* 21: 433–436.

Izzo,A.A. and Ernst,E. 2001. Interactions between herbal medicines and prescribed drugs A Systematic Review. *Journal of Alternative and Complementary Medicine,* 61 (15): 2163-2175.

Jaiswal, A.K., Gupta, S. and Abu-Ghannam, N. 2012. Kinetic evaluation of colour, texture, polyphenols and antioxidant capacity of Irish York cabbage after blanching treatment. *Food Chemistry,* 131: 63–72.

Jeong, S.Y., Kim, D.R., Kim, K.C., Nam, D.U. and Ahn Lee, S.C. 2004. Effect of seed roasting conditions on the antioxidant activity of defatted sesame meal extracts. *Food and Chemical Toxicology,* 69: 377–381.

Kähkönen, M.P., Hopia, A., Vuorela, H.J., Rauha, J.P., Pihlaja, K., Kujala, T.S. and Heinonen, M. 1999. Antioxidant activity of plant extracts containing phenolic compounds. *Journal of Agricultural and Food Chemistry,* 47: 3954-3962.

Kedare, S.B. and Singh, R.P. 2011. Genesis and development of DPPH method of antioxidant assay. *Journal of Food Science and Technology,* 48: 412–422.

Krishnaiah, D., Sarbatly, R. and Nithyanandam, R. 2011. A review of the antioxidant potential of medicinal plant Species. *Food and Bioproducts Processing,* 89: 217–233.

Lee, K.W., Hur, H.J., Lee, H.J. and Lee, Y.C. 2005. Antiproliferative effects of dietary phenolic substances and hydrogen peroxide. *Journal of Agricultural and Food Chemistry,* 53: 1990–1995.

Lugasi, A., Dworschák, E. and Kéry, A. 1998. Antioxidant and free radical scavenging properties of squeezed juice from black radish (Raphanus sativa L. var. niger) root. *Phytotherapy Research,* 12: 502-506.

Manek,R.A., Sheth, N.R.,Vaghasiya, J.D., Malaviya, S.V.,Jivani, N.V. and Chavda J. R. 2011. Study on Herb-herb Interaction Potential of *Glycyrrhiza glabra* with *Solanum xanthocarpum* and *Adhatoda vasica* on Mast Cell Stabilizing Activity. *International Journal of Pharmaceutics,* 7: 589-598.

Markert, C.L. 1968. Neoplasia: A Disease of Cell Differentiation. *Cancer Research,* 28: 1908-1914.

Mensor, L.L., Menezes, F.S., Leitão, G.G., Reis, A.S., Dos Santos, T.C., Coube, C.S. and Leitão, S.G. 2001. Screening of Brazilian plant extracts for antioxidant activity by the use of DPPH free radical method. *Phytotherapy Research,* 15: 127-130.

Miliauskas, G., Venskutonis, P.R. and Van Beek, T.A. 2004. Screening of radical scavenging activity of some medicinal and aromatic plant extracts. *Food Chemistry,* 85: 231–237.

Munari, C.C., Oliveira, P.F., Campos, J.C.L., Martins, S.P.L., Costa, J.C., Bastos, J.K. and Tavares, D.C. 2014. Antiproliferative activity of Solanum lycocarpum alkaloidic extract and their constituents, solamargine and solasonine, in tumor cell lines. *Journal of Natural Medicines,* 68: 236-241.

Packer, L., Rimbach, G. and Virgili, F. 1999. Antioxidant activity and biologic properties of a procyanidin-rich extract from pine (pinus maritima) bark, pycnogenol. *Free Radical Biology and Medicine,* 27: 704-724.

Parejo, I., Viladomat, F., Bastida, J., Rosas-Romero, A., Flerlage, N., Burillo, J.S. and Codina, C. 2002. Comparison between the Radical Scavenging Activity and Antioxidant Activity of Six Distilled and Nondistilled Mediterranean Herbs and Aromatic Plants. *Journal of Agricultural and Food Chemistry,* 50: 6882-6890.

Popescu, M., Ivopol, G., Dune, A., Ivopol, M. and Manea, S. 2011. Azeotropic distillation starting from fresh vegetable materials, an interesting alternative to simple extraction from vegetable dried sources. *Revista de Chimie –Bucharest,* 62: 1131-1135.

Rizea, G.D., Popescu, M., Ionescu, D., Mihele, D. and Manea, S. 2012. Comparative determinations of antioxidant free radical scavenging polyphenols in certain natural products by HPLC methods and UV-Vis spectrophotometry. *Revista de Chimie – Bucharest,* 63: 1085-1088.

Rock, C.L., Doyle, C., Demark-Wahnefried, W., Meyerhardt, J., Courneya, K.S., Schwartz, A.L., Bandera, E.V., Hamilton, K.K., Grant, B., McCullough, M., Byers, T. and Gansler, T. 2012. Nutrition and physical activity guidelines for cancer survivors. *CA: A Cancer Journal for Clinicians,* 62: 242-274.

Singh, B.K., Sharma, S.R. and Singh, B. 2009. Heterosis for mineral elements in single cross-hybrids of cabbage (Brassica oleracea var. capitata L.). *Scientia Horticulturae –Amsterdam,* 122: 32–36.

Singh, R.P., Murthy, K.N.C. and Jayaprakasha, G.K. 2002. Studies on the antioxidant activity of promegranate (Punica granatum) peel and seed extracts using in vitro models. *Journal of Agricultural and Food Chemistry,* 50: 81-86.

Sorensen. J.M. 2002. Herb – Drug, Food – Drug, Nutrient – Drug, and Drug – Drug Interactions: Mechanisms Involved and Their Medical Implications. *Journal of Alternative and Complementary Medicine,* 8: 293-308.

Tarirai, C., Viljoen, A.M. and Hamman, J. H. 2010. Reviews: Herb–drug pharmacokinetic interactions reviewed. *Expert Opinion on Drug Metabolism and Toxicology,* 6: 1515-1538.

Taveira, M., Pereira, D.M., Sousa, C., Ferreres, F., Andrade, P.B., and Martins, A. 2009. In vitro cultures of Brassica oleracea L. var. costata DC: Potential plant bioreactor for Antioxidant Phenolic Compounds. *Journal of Agricultural and Food Chemistry,* 57: 1247–1252.

Teresa San Miguel, M. Alfredo Martínez, J. and Vargas , E. 2005. Food–drug interactions in the summary of product characteristics of proprietary medicinal products. *European Journal of Clinical Pharmacology,* 61: 77-83.

Turkmen, N., Sari, F. and Velioglu, Y.S. 2006. Effects of extraction solvents on concentration and antioxidant activity of black and black mate tea polyphenols determined by ferrous tartrate and

Folin–Ciocalteu methods. *Food Chemistry*, 99: 835–841.

Van Wyk, B.E. and Wink, M. 2004. *Medicinal Plants of the World*, Timber Press, Portland, OR, Cambridge.

Velioglu, Y.S., Mazza, G., Gao, L. and Oomah, B.D. 1998. Antioxidant activity and total phenolics in selected fruits, vegetables, and grain products. *Journal of Agricultural and Food Chemistry,* 46: 4113–4117.

Williamson, E.M. 2005. Review, Interactions between herbal and conventional medicines. *Expert Opinion on Drug Safety,* 4: 355-378.

Williamson, E.M. 2003. Drug interactions between herbal and prescription medicines. *Drug Safety,* 26: 1075-1092.

Wink, M. and Abbas, S. 2013. *Epigallocatechin gallate (EGCG) from green tea (Camellia sinensis) and other natural products mediate stress resistance and slows down aging processes in Caenorhabditis elegans. In: Tea in health and disease prevention*. Elsevier, London, pp. 1105–1116.

Wink, M. and Van Wyk, B.E. 2008. *Mind-altering and poisonous plants of the world*, Timber Press, Portland, OR, London.

Yazdanparast, R. and Ardestani, A. 2007. In vitro antioxidant and free radical scavenging activity of Cyperus rotundus. *Journal of Medicinal Food,* 10: 667–674.

Yoo, M.K., Lee, H.C., Lee, H., Moon, B. and Lee, Y.C. 2008. Relative antioxidant andcytoprotective activities of common herbs. *Food Chemistry*, 106: 929–936.

Zeping, H., Xiaoxia, Y., Paul Chi Lui, H., Sui Yung, C., Paul Wan Sia, H., Eli, C., Wei,D., Hwee Ling,K. and Shufeng, Z. 2005. Herb-drug interactions: a literature review. *Drugs*, 65: 1239-1282.

Zhang, X.J., Liu, L.J., Song, T.T., Wang, Y.Q. and Yang, X.h. 2014. An approach based on antioxidant fingerprint–efficacy relationship and TLC bioautography assay to quality evaluation of Rubia cordifolia from various sources. *Journal of Natural Medicines,* 68: 448–454.

Zhou, X., Poon, J., Kwan, P., Zhang, R., Wang, Y., Poon, S., Liu, B. and Sze, D. 2010. *Novel Two-Stage Analytic Approach in Extraction of Strong Herb-Herb Interactions in TCM Clinical Treatment of Insomnia*. Vol. 6165. Lecture Notes in Computer Science. Springer Berlin Heidelberg. pp. 258-267.

Antimalarial activities of *Breynia Nivosa*

Jude E. Okokon*[1], koofreh Davis[2], Azare B. A[3]

[1]*Department of Pharmacology and Toxicology, Faculty of Pharmacy, University of Uyo,Uyo, Nigeria;*
*Email: *judeefiom@yahoo.com*

[2]*Department of Physiology, Faculty of Basic Medical Sciences, University of Uyo, Uyo, Nigeria;*

[3]*Department of Biological Sciences, University of Abuja, Nigeria;*

ARTICLE INFO

Topic: *Medicinal Plants*

Key words:

- ✓ Breynia nivosa
- ✓ *Antiplasmodial*
- ✓ *Antimalarial*
- ✓ *herbal remedy*

ABSTRACT

Background & Aim: Antiplasmodial activity of leaf extract of *Breynia nivosa* was evaluated to ascertain the folkloric claim of its antimalarial activity.
Experimental: The crude leaf extract (75 – 225 mg/kg), of *Breynia nivosa* was investigated for antiplasmodial activity against chloroquine sensitive *Plasmodium berghei* infections in mice. The antiplasmodial activity during early and established infections as well as prophylactic were investigated. Artesunate 5 mg/kg and pyrimethamine 1.2 mg/kg were used as positive controls. Thin films made from tail blood of each mouse were used to assess the level of parasitaemia of the mice.
Results & Discussion: The extract dose-dependently reduced parasitaemia induced by chloroquine sensitive *Plasmodium berghei* infection in prophylactic, suppressive and curative models in mice. These reductions were statistically significant ($p<0.001$). They also improved the mean survival time (MST) from 11 to 27 days relative to control ($p<0.01$ – 0.001). The activities of extract was comparable to that of the standard drugs used (pyrimethamine). The antiplasmodial and antipyretic effects may in part be mediated through the chemical constituents of the plant.
Industrial and practical recommendations: The plant, *Breynia nivosa,* possesses antimalarial property which can be exploited in the treatment of malaria.

1. Introduction

Breynia nivosa (W. Bull) Small syn. *Phyllanthus nivosus* W. G. Sm., *Breynia disticha* J.R.Forst. & G.Forst. (Euphorbiaceae), is a rounded shrub, about 2 m high, that is primarily used for its attractive foliage and found in villages and towns. It has mall, mottled, multi-colored variegated leaves with white, green and red coloration leaves (Smith, 1981). In southern Nigeria, it is used as chewing stick (Amadi *et al.*, 2007). Ethnomedically, *Breynia nivosa* is used in treating headaches, toothaches and tooth infections (Onyegbule *et al.*, 2014) and in the treatment of fever and malaria by the Ibibios of Niger Delta region of Nigeria. The leaf extract of the plant has been reported to contained flavonoids, tannins, alkaloids, glycosides and starch, saponins and proteins (Onyegbule *et al.*, 2007). Reported biological activities of the leaf include; antimicrobial (Amadi *et al*, 2007; Onyebule *et al.*, 2014), analgesic, anti-inflammatory, and antioxidant activities (Onyegbule *et al.*, 2014). In this study we report the animalarial activity of the leaf extract of *B. nivosa* to ascertain the folkloric uses of the plant as malarial remedy.

2. Materials and Methods

2.1. Plants collection

The plant material *Breynia nivosa* (leaves) was collected in a compound in Uyo metropolis, Akwa Ibom State, Nigeria in September, 2014. The plant was identified and authenticated by Dr. Margaret Bassey of Department of Botany and Ecological Studies, University of Uyo, Uyo, Nigeria. Hebarium specimen (FPUU) was deposited at Department of Pharmacognosy and Natural Medicine Herbarium.

2.2. Extraction

The plant parts were washed and shade-dried for two weeks. The dried plants' materials were reduced to powder using mortar and pistle. The powdered material was soaked in 50% ethanol. The liquid filtrates were concentrated and evaporated to dryness in vacuo 40°C using rotary evaporator. The extract (2g) was partitioned with a 50:50 mixture of distilled water and chloroform. The aqueous fraction was evaporated to dryness in a water bath at 60°C and the chloroform fraction air-dried. The ethanol extract, the aqueous and chloroform fractions were stored at - 4°C. until used in a refrigerator.

2.3. Animals

Albino Swiss mice (15 – 20g) of either sex were obtained from the University of Uyo animal house. They were maintained on standard animal pellets and water *ad libitum*. Permission and approval for animal studies were obtained from the College of Health Sciences Animal Ethics committee, University of Uyo.

2.4. Determination of median lethal dose (LD_{50})

The median lethal dose (LD_{50}) of the extract was estimated using albino mice by intraperitoneal (i.p) route using the method of Lorke (1983). This involved intraperitoneal administration of different doses of the extract (1000-5000 mg/kg) to groups of three mice each. The animals were observed for manifestation of physical signs of toxicity such as writhing, decreased motor activity, decreased body/limb tone, decreased respiration and death. The number of deaths in each group within 24 hours was recorded. The LD_{50} was calculated as geometrical means of the maximum dose producing 0% (a) and the minimum dose producing 100% mortality (b).

$$LD_{50} = \sqrt{ab}$$

2.5. Parasite inoculation

Each mouse used in the experiment was inoculated intraperitoneally with 0.2ml of infected blood containing about 1 x 10^{7} *P. berghei berghei* parasitized erythrocytes. The inoculum consisted of 5 x 10^{7} *P. berghei berghei* erythrocytes per ml. This was prepared by determining both the percentage parasitaemia and the erythrocytes count of the donor mouse and diluting the blood with isotonic saline in proportions indicated by both determinations (Odetola and Basir, 1980).

2.6. Drug administration

The drugs (artesunate and pyrimethamine), extract and fractions used in the antiplasmodial study were orally administered with the aid of a stainless metallic feeding cannula.

2.7. Evaluation of antiplasmodial activity of the extract

2.7.1. Evaluation of suppressive activity of the extract (4-day test).

This test was used to evaluate the schizontocidal activity of the extract, fractions and artesunate against early *P. berghei berghei* infection in mice. This was done as described by Knight and Peters (1980). Forty-two mice were randomly divided into five groups of six mice each. On the first day (D_O), the thirty mice were infected with the parasite and randomly divided into various groups. These were administered with the extract, fractions and artesunate. The mice group 1 were administered with the 112 mg/kg, the group 2, 224 mg/kg and group 3, 448 mg/kg of crude extract, groups 5 and 6 were administered with the 224 mg/kg of the aqueous and chloroform fractions respectively, while group 6 was administered with 5 mg/kg of artesunte (positive control), and 10 ml/kg of distilled water to group 7 (negative control) for four consecutive days (D_0 – D_3) between 8am and 9am. On the fifth day (D_4), thin blood film was made from tail blood. The film was then stained with leishman stain to reveal parasitized erythocytes out of 500 in a random field of the microscope. The average percentage suppression of parasitaemia was calculated in comparison with the controls as follows:

$$\frac{\text{Average \% parasitaemia in negative control} - \text{Average \% parasitaemia in Positive groups}}{\text{Average \% parasitaemia in negative control}}$$

2.7.2 Evaluation of prophylactic or repository activities of extract

The repository activity of the extract and pyrimethamine (daraprim) was assessed by using the method described by Peters (1965). The mice were randomly divided into five groups of six mice each Groups 1 - 3 were administered with 112, 224 and 448 mg/kg/day of the extract respectively, while group 4 – 7 were respectively given 224 mg/kg/day of the aqueous and chloroform fractions, 1.2 mg/kg/day of pyrimethamine (positive control) and 10 ml/kg of distilled water (negative control). Administration of the extract/drug continued for three consecutive days (D_0 – D_2). On the fourth day (D_3) the mice were inoculated with *P. berghei berghei.* The parasitaemia level was assessed by blood smears seventy-two hours later.

2.7.3 Evaluation of curative activities of extract (Rane's test)

This was used to evaluate the schizontocidal activity of the extract, fractions and artesunate in established infection. This was done as described by Ryley and Peters (1970). *P. berghei berghei* was injected intraperitoneally into another 30 mice on the first day (D_O). Seventy–two hours later (D_3), the mice was divided randomly into seven groups of six mice each. Various doses of the extract; 112 mg/kg, 224 mg/kg and 448 mg/kg were orally administered respectively to mice in groups 1-3, 224 mg/kg of the aqueous and chloroform fractions were administered to groups 4 and 5 respectively, 5 mg/kg/day of artesuante to the group 6 (positive control) and group 7 was given 10 ml/kg of distilled water (negative control). The extract and drugs were administered once daily for 5 days. Leishman's stained thin smears were prepared from tail blood samples collected on each day of treatment to monitor parasitaemia level. The mean survival time (MST) of the mice in each treatment group was determined over a period of 29 days (D_0 – D_{28}).

$$\frac{\text{No of days survived}}{\text{Total No. of days (29)}} \times 100 = \text{MST}$$

2.8 Statistical analysis and data evaluation

Data obtained from this work were analyzed statistically using Students' t-test and ANOVA (One- or Two- way) followed by a post test (Tukey-Kramer multiple comparison test). Differences between means will be considered significant at 1% and 5% level of significance i.e $P \leq 0.01$and 0.05.

3. Results and discussion

The median lethal dose (LD_{50}) was calculated to be 2242.07 mg/kg. The physical signs of toxicity included excitation, paw licking, increased respiratory rate, decreased motor activity, gasping and coma which was followed by death.

On the suppressive test, the extract and its fractions showed a dose-dependent chemosuppressive effect on the parasitaemia. These effects were statistically significant relative to the control ($p<0.001$). The chloroform fraction showed a high chemoinhibitory percentage of 69.86 % which was incomparable to that of the standard, artesunate, 5 mg/kg. (Table 1).

On the prophylactic/ repository activity test, the ethanol crude extract showed a dose-dependent reduction of parasitaemia in the extract-treated groups. These reductions were statistically significant relative to the control ($p<0.01$ - 0.001). The chloroform fraction demonstrated a high antiplasmodial activity which was significant ($p<0.001$) when compared to control but was incomparable to that exhibited by the standard drug, pyrimethamine, 1.2mg/kg. (Table 2).

On established infection, there was a progressive dose-dependent reduction of parasitaemia in all the extract/fraction-treated group relative to control. These reductions were statistically significant relative to the control ($p<0.001$) (Figure 1). Though the aqueous fraction and the highest dose of the crude extract (448 mg/kg) exhibited a high chemosuppression these were uncomparable to that of the standard, artesunate.

The crude extract and fractions demonstrated a significant ($p<0.001$) protective potentials on the animals as was seen in the mean survival time of the animals. The groups treated with chloroform and highest dose of the crude extract had a longer mean survival time, 24.92 ± 0.68 and 20.86 ± 0.78 days respectively,though less than that of the standard drug,artesunate (29.83 ± 0.12 days) (Table 3).

The major folkloric uses of *Breynia nivosa* have been in the treatment of headaches, toothaches and tooth infections (Onyegbule *et al.,* 2014) and in the treatment of fever and malaria. These prompted the need to evaluate the in vivo antiplasmodial potential of the crude leaf extract of *Breynia nivosa* to confirm its ethnobotanical uses.

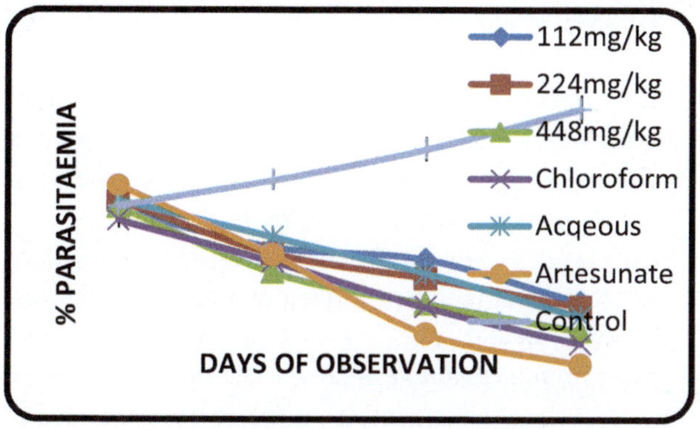

Figure 1: Curative effect of ethanolic leaves extract and fractions of *Breynia nivosa* on *Plasmodium berghei* established infection in mice.

Table 1. Suppressive activity of ethanolic leaves extract and fractions of *Breynia nivosa* on *Plasmodium berghei* infection in mice (4-day test)

Treatments	Dose (mg/kg)	Parasitaemia	% Chemosuppression
Normal saline	10ml/kg	23.00 ± 0.84	-
B. nivosa crude extract	112	12.3 ± 0.89[a]	46.52
	224	11.0 ± 0.58[a]	52.17
	448	9.3 ± 0.19[a]	59.56
Acqeous fraction	224	10.25 ± 1.02[a]	55.43
Chloroform fraction	224	6.93 ± 0.10[a]	69.86
Artesunate	5.0	3.98 ± 1.19[a]	82.69

Values are expressed as mean ± SEM. Significance relative to control [a]$p<0.001$, n = 6.

In this work, median lethal dose (LD_{50}) was determined to be 2242.07 mg/kg, and the extract was relatively safe (Homburger, 1989).

The antiplasmodial properties of the extract and its fractions were investigated using standard models. It was found that both the extract and its fractions significantly reduced the parasitaemia in suppressive, prophylactic and curative models in a dose - dependent fashion.

Table 2. Repository/Prophylactic activity of ethanolic leaves extract and fractions of *Breynia nivosa* on *Plasmodium berghei* infection in mice

Treatments	Dose (mg/kg)	Parasitaemia	% Chemosuppression
Control	10ml/kg	33.0 ± 1.57	-
B. nivosa leaf extract	112	25.37 ± 0.68[a]	23.12
	224	15.66 ± 0.40[a]	52.54
	448	13.33 ± 0.45[a]	59.60
Aqueous fraction	224	13.72 ± 1.04[a]	58.42
Chloroform fraction	224	9.34 ±0.26[a]	71.69
Pyrimethamine	1.2	3.16 ±0.93[a]	90.42

Values are expressed as mean ± SEM. Significance relative to control [a]$p<0.001$, n= 6.

Table 3. Mean survival time of mice receiving the various doses of ethanol leaves extract and fractions of *Breynia nivosa* during established *P.berghei* infections in mice.

Treatments	Dose (mg/kg)	MEAN SURVIVAL TIME(days)
Normal saline	10ml/kg	9.0±0.65
B. nivosa crude extract	112	13.43 ±0.53[ns]
	224	15.44± 0.82[a]
	448	20.86 ±0.78[a]
Chloroform fraction	224	24.92 ± 0.68[a]
Aqueous fraction	224	16.78 ± 0.44[a]
Artesunate	5.0	29.83± 0.12[a]

Values are essxpressed as mean ± SEM. Significance relative to control. [a]$p<0.001$, n = 6.

These results further confirm the ethnobotanical use of this plant. Some secondary metabolites of plants are said to have antiplasmodial activity. The leaf extract of the plant has been reported to contained flavonoids, tannins, alkaloids and saponins (Onyegbule *et al.,* 2007). Phytochemical compounds such as alkaloids and terpenes and their derivatives such as monoterpenes have been implicated in antiplasmodial activity of many plants (Philipson and Wright, 1991; Christensen and Kharazmi, 2001). Among these metabolites are flavonoids and triterpenoids such as quassinoids (Philipson and Wright, 1991; Christensen and Kharazmi, 2001; Kirby *et al.,* 1989). Flavonoids are reported to chelate with nucleic acid base pairing of the parasite (Lui *et al.,* 1992) and triterpenes like quassinoids are potent protein inhibitors (Liao *et al.,* 1976). These compounds (flavonoids and alkaloids) present in this plant extract may in part have contributed to the plasmocidal activity of this extract and therefore explained the mechanism of antiplasmodial effect of the extract and its fractions.

4. Conclusion

The results of this study demonstrated that *Breynia nivosa* possesses considerable antiplasmodial activity. These confirm its use to treat malaria and fever in folkloric medicine. Therefore, it would be interesting if the the active principle is isolated, identified and characterised.

5. Acknowledgement

The authors are grateful to Mr Nsikan Malachy of Pharmacology and Toxicology Department for his technical assistance.

6. References

Amadi, E.S., Oveka, C.A., Onveagba, R.A., Ugbogu, O.C., Okoli, I. 2007. Antimicrobial screening of *Breynia nivosus* and *Ageratum conzynoides* against dental caries organisms. *Journal of Biological Sciences.,* 7(2): 354 -358.

Christensen, S. B., Kharazmi, A. 2001. *Antimalarial natural products. Isolation, characterization and biological properties.* In. Bioactive compounds from natural sources: Isolation, characterization and biological properties. Ed. Tringali, C. London, Taylor & Francis. Pp.379- 432.

Homburger, F. 1989. *In vivo testing in the study of toxicity and safety evaluation.* In: A guide to general toxicology. Marquis J. K . (Ed). 2nd Edn Karger, New York

Kirby, G. C.,O'Neill, M. J., Phillipson, J. D., Warhurst, D. C. 1989. In vitro studies on the mode of action of quassinoids with against chloroquine resistant *Plasmodium falciparum. Biochemical Pharmacology.,* 38: 4367- 4374.

Knight, D. J., Peters, W. 1980. The antimalarial action of N- Benzyloxydihydrotriazines and the studies on its mode of action. *Annals of Tropical Medicine and Parasitology.,* 74,393 -404.

Liao, Y.F., Kupchan, S. M., Horwitz, S. B. 1976. Mode of action of antitumour compound bruceantin, an inhibitor of protein synthesis. *Molecular Pharmacology.,* 12: 167 – 176.

Lorke, D. 1983. A New Approach to Practical Acute Toxicity Testing. *Archieves of Toxicology.,* 54: 275-286.

Lui, K. C., Yang, S. C., Roberts, M. F. 1992. Antimalarial activity of *Artemisia annua* flavonoids from whole plants and cell cultures. *Plants Cell II., 637 - 640.*

Odetola, A., Basir, O. 1980. *Evaluation of Antimalarial properties of some Nigerian Medicinal Plants.* In: Sofowora A, Editor. Proceeding of African Bioscience Network, Federal Ministry of Science and Technology, Nigerian Society of Pharmacology and Drug Research and Production unit, University of Ife organized Workshop, Ife. pp. 275 – 283.

Onyegbule, F.A., Ilouno, I.O., Ikeh, C., Umeokoli, B.O., Eze, P.M. 2014. Evaluation of phytochemical constituents, analgesic, anti-inflammatory, antimicrobial and antioxidant activities of extracts of *Breynia nivosa* leaves. *Planta Med.,* 80 - LP18. DOI: 10. 1055/s-0034-1395078

Peters, W. 1965. Drug Resistance in *Plasmodium berghei. Experimental Parasitology.,* 17, 80-89.

Philipson, J. D., Wright C. W. 1991. Antiprotozoal compounds from plants sources. *Planta Medica.,* 57: 553-559.

Retnam K. R., DeBritto A. J. 1988. Preliminary phytochemical screening of three medicinal plants of tirunelveli hills. *Journal of Economy Texas Botany.,* 22: 42.

Ryley, J.F., Peters, W. 1970. The antimalarial activity of some quinolone esters. Annals of Tropical *Medicine and Parasitology*.,84: 209-222.

Smith A C. 1981. Flora Vitiensis nova: a new flora of Fiji. *National Tropical Botanical Garden, Lawai, Kauai, Hawaii*., 2: 466-467.

Evaluation of the essential oil composition and antioxidant activity of *Achillea eriophora* as a medicinal plant

Malek taher Maghsoodlou[1*], Jafar Valizadeh[2], Javad Mottaghipisheh[1], Nahid Rahneshan[1]

[1]*Department of Chemistry, University of Sistan and Baluchestan, Zahedan, Iran;*

[2]*Department of Biology, University of Sistan and Baluchestan, Zahedan, Iran;*

***Email:** *mt_maghsoodlou@chem.usb.ac.ir*

ARTICLE INFO

Topic: *Medicinal Plants*

Key words:
- ✓ Achillea eriophora
- ✓ *Essential oil*
- ✓ *Camphor*
- ✓ *Antioxidant activity*
- ✓ *Sistan*
- ✓ *Baluchestan*

ABSTRACT

Background & Aim: *Achillea* (Fam. Asteraceae) is a medicinal plant and different species of it have several uses in the folk medicine all around the world. *Achillea* species are used for feverish conditions, common cold, digestive complaints, slow healing wounds and skin inflammations. This study aims to investigate the essential oil composition and antioxidant activities from the aerial parts of *Achillea eriophora* collected from Khash city in Sistan and Baluchestan province.

Experimental: Chemical composition of the essential oils was obtained by hydro-distillation method using a Clevenger type apparatus and analyzed by GC/MS.

Results and Discussion: In the essential oil of *Achillea eriophora* 33 compounds representing 100%, were identified in which Camphor (21.55 %), Artemesia ketone (13.84%), Alpha-Thujone (11.85%), Borneole (8.94%), Yomogi alcohol (7.74%), 1,8-cineole (5.19%), Terpinene-4-ol (4.23%) and Myrtenol (3.10%) were the major constituents. In addition, the antioxidant activity of ethyl acetate and ethanolic extracts of *Achillea eriophora* was analyzed using the 1, 1-diphenyl-2- picrylhydrazyl (DPPH) free radical scavenging. According to antioxidant activity outcomes, the amount of IC50 of ethyl acetate and ethanolic extracts of the aerial parts of *Achillea eriophora* and also butylated hydroxyl toluene (BHT) as a standard was 245.20 ppm, 89.25 ppm and 45.58 ppm, respectively. Ultimately, it was highlighted that the antioxidant activity of ethyl acetate extract was weaker than ethanolic extract. The antioxidant activity of both of them were also weaker than BHT as a synthetic antioxidant. Some compounds like 1, 8-cineole and terpinen-4-ol can be responsible for antioxidant and antimicrobial activity, while Camphor and borneol have not been proven to be strong antioxidant agents as emphasized elsewhere.

Recommended applications/ industries: The results of the present study showed that *Achillea eriophora* from Sistan and Baluchestan may be considered as source of natural antioxidant to be used in medicinal and food products to promote human health and prevent diseases.

1. Introduction

In recent decades, the phytochemical constituents of plants have received much attention due to their potential use in nutraceuticals and drug industries. Spices and herbs are a part of daily food intake in many regions of the world. They have been used as natural sources of flavorings and preservatives (Bua-In and Paisooksantivatana, 2009; Jaimand and Rezaee, 2001; McKay and Blumberg, 2006). *Achillea* (Fam. Asteraceae) comprises more than 100 species, which are mainly distributed in Europe, Asia, Australia and North America (Rechinger, 1963). Nineteen species of this genus are found in different geographical and ecological regions of Iran (Asgarirad *et al.,* 2010; Gharibi *et al.*, 2011; Rustaiyan *et al.*, 1998). *Achillea* species have been used as anti-inflammatory, antispasmodic, diaphoretic, diuretic, emmenagogue agents and for treatment of hemorrhage, pneumonia, rheumatic pain, and wounds since ancient times (Ghasemi *et al.*, 2008). *Achillea* is rich in flavonoids, sesquiterpene lactones, and monoterpenoids which have antioxidant activities (Jaimand and Rezaee, 2001; Saeidinia *et al.*, 2005). The largest single component of volatile oil extracted from *Achillea millefoium* is chamazulene which has been shown to have anti-inflammatory and antiallergic effects (Nemeth and Bernath, 2008). Immunosuppressive effects on humoral immune responses have been reported with an aqueous extract of *Achillea talagonica* (Rezaeipoor *et al.*, 1999). To date *Achillea eriophora* has been analyzed from different parts of Iran such as Fars (Jaimand and Rezaee, 2007) and Shoushtar (Farhoudi and Mehrnia, 2013) for both the composition of essential oil and different pharmacological properties. But there are no reports of such an analysis on *Achillea eriophora* from Khash area in Sistan and Baluchestan, which is a geographical zone for medicinal plants. For this reason, the importance of this plant as an herbal medicine, the purpose of this study was to determine the comparative chemical compositions and antioxidant activities of the essential oils extracted the aerial parts of *Achillea eriophora.*

2. Materials and Methods

2.1. Plant Materials

Achillea eriophora was collected from Khash in Sistan and Baluchestan province during the flowering stage. Identification of the plant was done by the Medicinal and Ornamental plant Research Institute, University of Sistan and Baluchestan, Zahedan, Iran. Collected plant materials were dried in the shade and the aerial parts were separated from the roots.

2.2. Isolation of the Essential Oil

The aerial parts of *Achillea eriophora* were dried and milled into a fine powder. The extraction procedure used was hydrodistillation using a Clevenger type apparatus. For the extraction, 500 g of the cleaned, air-dried and powdered of the aerial parts of *Achillea* eriophora were hydrodistilled in a Clevenger type apparatus for 4h. The essential oil was dried over anhydrous Na_2SO_4 (Merk), stored in a dark glass bottle and kept at 4 °C until analysis.

2.3. GC/MS Analysis

The essential oils were analyzed on an Agilent 6890 gas chromatograph interfaced to an Agilent 5973 N mass selective detector (Agilent Technologies, Palo Alto, USA). The GC column was HP-5MS fused silica capillary with a (5% phenyl) – polymethylsiloxane stationary phase, film thickness of 0.25μm, a length of 30 m and an internal diameter of 0. 25 mm. The data were acquired under the following conditions: initial temperature was 60°C; velocity programming 3°C/min; injector temperature 280 °C and detector temperature 280 °C. The carrier gas was helium at a flow rate of 1 ml/min and the split ratio was 1:15. For GC–MS detection, an electron ionization system with ionization energy of 70 eV was used. The retention indices were calculated for all volatile constituents by using retention time of n-alkanes which were injected after the essential oil under the same condition. The components were identified by comparing retention indices with those of standards. The results were also confirmed by comparing their mass spectra with the published mass spectra or Wiley library.

2.4. Preparation of ethyl acetate and ethanolic extracts

A portion of dried plant material (10 g) was extracted with ethanol and ethyl acetate at room temperature for 24 hours and, then filtered using Whatman No.42 filter paper to remove debris. After filtration and solvent evaporation, extracts were stored in sealed vials at 4 °C until biological testing.

Table 1. Chemical composition of the *Achillea eriophora* essential oil from Khash.

compound	%[1]	RI[2]	compound	%	RI
Artemesia triene	0.328	923	Terpinen-4-ol	4.236	1174
Comphene	0.354	946	Alpha-Terpineol	0.649	1186
Dehydrocineole	0.527	993	Myrtenol	3.105	1194
Yomogi alcohol	7.745	999	Cis-p-Mentha-1(7), 8-dien-2-ol	0.351	1227
Alpha- Terpinene	1.314	1014	2 (5H)-Furanone,5-(2-methyl-3-methylen-4-buthyl)-	1.034	1268
P-Cymene	0.585	1020	Bornyl acetate	0.645	1287
1,8-cineole	5.190	1028	Lavandulyl aetate	0.435	1288
Gamma-Terpinene	1.562	1054	Terpinen-4-ol-acetate	0.362	1229
Artemesia ketone	13.849	1080	Eugenol	0.328	1356
Artemesia alcohol	3.646	1080	Methyl eugenol	2.111	1403
Terpinolen	0.451	1086	Lungi pinocarvone	0.415	1569
Alpha-Thujone	11.854	1103	Caryophyllene oxide	0.366	1582
Beta-Thujone	3.126	1116	3-phenyl propenoic acid, 3-methyl buthyl ester	0.601	1593
Cis-p-Menth-2-en-1-ol	0.431	1118	Benzen propanoic acid, 2-penthyl ester	0.692	1594
Comphor	21.559	1141	Caryophylla 4(12), 8(13)-dien-5-beta-ol	0.319	1639
Pinocarvone	1.863	1160	Exacyclotetradecan-2-1,14-methyl	1.018	1650
Borneol	8.948	1165	-	-	-

1. compound percentage
2. Retention indices

2.5. Antioxidant evaluation

2.5.1. DPPH radical-scavenging activity

The DPPH radical scavenging activity of the extracts from the aerial parts of *Achillea eriophora* were measured according to the procedure described by Brand-Williams (Brand-Williams et al., 1995). Briefly, 1 ml samples of various concentrations of the extracts in ethanol and ethyl acetate were separately added to a 1 ml solution of DPPH radical in ethanol (final concentration of DPPH was 0.1 mM). The mixture was shaken vigorously and allowed to stand in the dark at room temperature for 30 minutes. Then, the absorbance of the resulting solution was measured at 517 nm using a UV-Vis, Specords 100 spectrophotometer. Inhibition of free radical DPPH was calculated as percentage [IP (%)] as follows: IP (%) = 100 × (A blank - A sample) / A blank

Where: Ablank: absorption of blank sample; A sample: absorption of testing extract solution.

The antioxidant activity of the extracts was expressed as the IC50. IC50 values (ppm) denote the concentration of sample, which is required to scavenge 50% of DPPH free radicals. This was obtained by interpolation and using linear regression analysis. For the calculation of these values, Microsoft Excel software was used. Percent inhibition after 30 minutes was plotted against concentration, and the equation for the line was used to obtain the IC50 value. A lower IC50 value indicates greater antioxidant activity. The synthetic antioxidant Butylated Hydroxy Toluene (BHT) was also used as positive control.

3. Results and discussion

3.1. Chemical composition of the essential oil

The oils were isolated by hydro-distillation and analyzed by capillary gas chromatography, using flame ionization and mass spectrometric detection. Determination of individual components was based on comparing their relative retention times with those of authentic samples on HP-5MS capillary column, and their mass spectra of peaks to be matched with those obtained from authentic samples and/ or the Wiley NIST 7 library spectra and existing data (Adams, 2007). The obtained results of the identified compounds in the essential oil from the aerial parts of *Achillea eriophora* with their percentage and coefficient of quarts (RI) were shown in Table 1. The yield of volatile oil of *Achillea* eriophora was 2.1 % (v/w). The chromatographic analysis of the extracted volatile oil of *Achillea eriophora* revealed the presence oxygenated monoterpens (86.88%), hydrocarbon monoterpens (5.121 %), other oxygenated compounds (3.553 %), oxygenated sesquiterpenes (0.781 %) and as other compounds (3.664 %). The high content of oxygenated compounds might explain the characteristic and fragrant odor of the oil. The results showed in the essential oil of *Achillea eriophora* 33 compounds representing 100 %, were identified in which Camphor (21.55 %), Artemesia ketone (13.84%), Alpha-Thujone (11.85 %), Borneole (8.94 %), Yomogi alcohol (7.74%), 1,8-cineole (5.19%), Terpinene-4-ol (4.23 %) and Myrtenol (3.10 %) were the major constituents.

Chemical composition of the essential oil of *Achillea* species growing in different geographical locations has been extensively studied. Farhoudi and Mehrnia (2013) reported sabinene (21.1 %), 1, 8-Cineole (18.3 %), ά – bisabolol (10.6%), terpinene-4-ol (8.6 %), α-pinene (6.7 %), β-pinene (4.0 %), p-Cymene (3.21 %) and chamazulene (2.1 %) as the major compounds in *Achillea eriophora* essential oil from Shoushtar (Farhoudi and Mehrnia, 2013). The comparision of chemical compositions of *Achillea eriophora* from Shoushtar and Khash was presented in Table 2. Saberi-ameli *et al.* (2007) identified 32 components in the oil of *Achillea eriophora* from Kerman. The major components were Camphor (46.43 %), 1, 8-Cineole (9.85 %), Alpha-Thujone (8.16 %), Comphen (4.88 %) and Beta-Thujone (4.66%) (Saberi-ameli *et al.*, 2007). In another studies Nadim *et al.* (2001) and Rustaiyan *et al.* (1998) found sabinene, α-pinene, 1, 8-cineole, chamazulene, borneol, β-pinene and terpinine-4-ol as the major chemical compounds in *Achillea* species essential oil (Nadim *et al.*, 2001; Rustaiyan *et al.*, 1998). The comparison of results showed 1, 8-cineole was a main compound in species of *Achillea* but with different percentages. In addition, Camphor (46.43 %) and 1, 8-Cineole (9.85 %) which appeared as major constituents in the oil of *Achillea eriophora* from Kerman were present in low concentration (Camphor 21.59 % and 1, 8-cineole 5.19 %) in *Achillea eriophora* from Sistan and Baluchestan. Whereas the amount of Camphor and 1, 8-Cineole components in the plant which collected from Shoushtar was 0.86 % and 18.3 %, respectively. Although α-pinene, β-pinene and sabinene have been reported as main compounds in many species of *Achillea*, but there were not identified in *Achillea eriophora* from Sistan and Baluchestan. In total, great quantitative and qualitative variations in volatile composition of *Achillea eriophora* were seen between this and other studies. These variations may be due to the influence of geographical differences, environmental conditions, physiological differences, different extraction, analytical procedures and genetic factors (Kokkini *et al.*, 2004; Hassanpouraghdam *et al.*, 2010).

3.2. Antioxidant Activity

Medicinal plants that traditionally used in folk medicine are particularly interesting for investigation of their antioxidant effects. A number of methods and modifications have been proposed for antioxidant activity assessment. In this study, the antioxidant activity of ethyl acetate and ethanolic extracts of Achillea eriophora was analyzed using the 1, 1-diphenyl-2- picrylhydrazyl (DPPH) free radical scavenging. The reduction ability of DPPH radical formations was determined by the decrease in its absorbance at 517 nm induced by antioxidants. Antioxidant effects on DPPH radical scavenging are seemed to be related to their hydrogen donating ability. DPPH is a stable free radical and accepts an electron or hydrogen radical to become a stable diamagnetic molecule (Soares *et al.*, 1997). The results indicated, the amount of IC50 of ethyl acetate and ethanolic extracts of the aerial parts of Achillea eriophora and also butylated hydroxyl toluene (BHT) as a standard was 245.20 ppm, 89.25 ppm and 45.58 ppm respectively, which showed the antioxidant activity of the of ethanolic extract was higher than ethyl acetate extract. The antioxidant activity of both of them was also weaker than butylated hydroxyl toluene as a synthetic antioxidant. Ho (2010) reported some chemical compounds like 1, 8-cineole and terpinen-4-ol can be responsible for antioxidant and antimicrobial activity (Ho, 2010). Although, Camphor and borneol have been reported as main compounds in *Achillea eriophora* from Sistan and Baluchestan but none of them have been proven to be strong antioxidant agents as emphasized elsewhere.

Table 2. The comparision of chemical composition of the *Achillea eriophora* essential oil from Khash and Shoush

Compound	% Khash	% Shoushtar	Compound	% Khash	% Shoushtar
Artemesia triene	0.328	-	Terpinen-4-ol	4.236	8.6
Comphene	0.354	-	Alpha-Terpineol	0.649	0.64
Dehydrocineole	0.527	-	Myrtenol	3.105	-
Yomogi alcohol	7.745	-	Cis-p-Mentha-1(7), 8-dien-2-ol	0.351	-
Alpha- Terpinene	1.314	-	2 (5H)-Furanone,5-(2-methyl-3-methylen-4-buthyl)-	1.034	-
P-Cymene	0.585	3.21	Bornyl acetate	0.645	-
1,8-cineole	5.190	18.3	Lavandulyl aetate	0.435	-
Gamma-Terpinene	1.562		Terpinen-4-ol-acetate	0.362	-
Artemesia ketone	13.849		Eugenol	0.328	0.44
Artemesia alcohol	3.646		Methyl eugenol	2.111	-
Terpinolen	0.451		Lungi pinocarvone	0.415	-
Alpha-Thujone	11.854	0.71	Caryophyllene oxide	0.366	-
Beta-Thujone	3.126		3-phenyl propenoic acid, 3-methyl buthyl ester	0.601	-
Cis-p-Menth-2-en-1-ol	0.431	0.34	Benzen propanoic acid, 2-penthyl ester	0.692	-
Camphor	21.559	0.86	Caryophylla 4(12), 8(13)-dien-5-beta-ol	0.319	-
Pinocarvone	1.863	-	Exacyclotetradecan-2-1,14-methyl	1.018	-
Borneol	8.948	1.73	-	-	-

Moreover, Antioxidant activity is usually due to phenolic compounds which are presented in stem and leaves more than flowers due to their synthesis and metabolism process in these parts of the plant. However, the phenolic compounds which are responsible for antioxidant activity, need to be investigated in other studies.

4. Conclusion

This study indicated that *Achillea eriophora* from Sistan and Baluchestan may be used as a valuable source for pharmaceutical and cosmetic purposes and perfume industries. It also can considered as a source of natural antioxidant to be used in medicinal and food products to promote human health and prevent diseases. However, further studies are needed to be performed to investigate the antioxidant activity of *Achillea* eriophora from Khash in Sistan and Baluchestan province by different in vitro tests.

5. Acknowledgments

We are thanksful to the university of Sistan and Baluchestan Research council for the partial support of this research.

6. Conflict of interest

There is not any conflict of interest in this study.

7. References

Adams, R.P. 2007. *Identification of essential oils components by gas chromatography/mass spectrometry*, 4th ed. Allured Business Media: Carol Stream, IL, USA, pp. 1–804.

Asgarirad, H., Pourmorad, F., Hosseinimehr, S.J., Saeidnia, S., Ebrahimzadeh, M.A. and Lotfi, F. 2010.

In vitro antioxidant analysis of *Achillea tenuifolia. African Journal Biotechnology,* 9: 3536-354.

Brand-Williams, W., Cuvelier, M.E. and Berset, C. 1995. Use of a free radical method to evaluate antioxidant activity. *Food Science and Technology,* 28: 25-30.

Bua-In, S. and Paisooksantivatana, Y. 2009. Essential oil and antioxidant activity of Cassumunar Ginger (Zingiberaceae: *Zingibermontanum*) collected from various parts of Thailand. *Kasetsart Journal,* 43: 467-475.

Farhoudi, R. and Mehrnia, M.A. 2013. The essential oil composition and antioxidant activity of *Achillea* spp. growing in the Southwest of Iran. *Journal of Medicinal Plants and By-products,* 2: 123-130.

Gharibi, S., Rahimmalek, M., Mirlohi, A., Majidi, M.M. and Tabatabaei, B.E. 2011. Assessment of genetic diversity in *Achillea millefolium* subsp. millefolium and *Achillea millefolium* subsp. elbursensis using morphological and ISSR markers. *Journal of Medicinal Plant Research,* 5: 2413-2423.

Ghasemi, Y., Khalaj, A., Mohagheghzadeh, A. and Khosaravi, A. 2008. Composition and in vitro antimicrobial activity of the essential oil of *Achillea eriophora. Chemistry of Natural Compounds,* 44: 663-665.

Hassanpouraghdam, M.B., Akhgari, A.B., Aazami, M.A. and Emarat-Pardaz, J. 2010. New menthone type of *Mentha pulegium* L. volatile oil from Northwest Iran. *Czech Journal of Food Science,* 29: 285-290

Ho, J.C. 2010. Chemical composition and bioactivity of essential oil of seed and leaf from *Alpiniaspeciosa* grown in Taiwan. *Journal of the Chinese Chemical Society,* 57:758-757.

Jaimand, K. and Rezaee, M.B. 2001. Comparative study of the essential oils of three *Achillea* species from Iran. *Journal of Essential Oil Research,* 13: 354-356.

Jaimand, K., Rezaee, M.B. 2007. Investigation on chemical constituents of essential oils from *Achillea* eriophora DC by Distillation methods. Iranian Journal of Medicinal and Aromatic Plants Research, 20: 90-98.

Kokkini, S., Hanlidou, E., Karousou, R. and Lanaras, T. 2004. Clinal variation of *Mentha pulegium* essential oils along the climatic gradient of Greece. *Journal of Essential Oil Research,* 16: 588-593.

McKay, D.L. and Blumberg, J.B. 2006. A review of the bioactivity and potential health benefits of chamomile tea (*Matricaria recutita* L.). *Phytotherapy Research,* 20: 519-530.

Rechinger, K.H. 1963. *Flora Iranica,* No. 158. Akademische Druke Verlags antalt, Wien, Austria, pp. 49-71.

Nadim, M.M., Malik, A.A., Ahmad, J. and Bakshi, S.K. 2001. The essential oil composition of *Achillea millefolium* L. cultivated under tropical condition in India. *World Journal of Agricultural Science,* 7: 561-565.

Nemeth, E. and Bernath, J. 2008. Biological activities of yarrow species (*Achillea* spp.). *Current Pharmacutical Design,* 14: 3151-67.

Rezaeipoor, R., Saeidnia, S. and Kamalinejad, M. 1999. Immunosuppressive activity of *Achillea talagonica* on humoral immune responses in experimental animals. *Journal of Ethnopharmacology,* 65: 273-6.

Rustaiyan, A., Komeilizadeh, H. and Shariatpanahi, M.S. 1998. Comparative study of the essential oils of three *Achillea* Species from Iran. *Journal Essential Oil Research,* 10: 207-209.

Saberi-ameli, S., Sadipour, A., Ghelichnia, H., Amanzadeh, Y. and Kazemi-gourti, M. 2007. Phytochemical analysis of *Achillea eriophora* DC from Khebr, national park of Kerman by GC/MS. *3rd Conference on Medicinal Plants,* Shahed University, Tehran, pp. 557 - 8.

Saeidinia, S., Gohari, A.R., Yassa, N. and Shafiee, A. 2005. Composition of the volatile oil of *Achillea conferta* DC. From Iran. *Daru,* 13: 34-36.

Soares, J.R., Dinis, T.C., Cunha, A.P. and Almeida, L.M. 1997. Antioxidant activities of some extracts of *Thymus* zygis. *Free Radical Research,* 26: 469-78.

Rosa foetida Herrm. flowers as a future natural antibacterial agent against the main cause of skin burn wound infections, *Pseudomonas aeroginosa*.

Maedeh Rezghi[1], Seyyed Reza Hoseinidoust[2], Jinous Asgarpanah[1]*

[1]*Department of Pharmacognosy, Faculty of Pharmacy, Pharmaceutical Sciences Branch, Islamic Azad University, Tehran – Iran (IAUPS);*

[2]*Department of Microbiology, Faculty of Pharmacy, Pharmaceutical Sciences Branch, Islamic Azad University, Tehran – Iran (IAUPS);*

***Email:** *taxolfa@yahoo.com*

ARTICLE INFO

Topic: *Medicinal Plants*

Key words:
- ✓ *Antibacterial*
- ✓ Pseudomonas aeruginosa
- ✓ *Rosa foetida*
- ✓ *Skin burn wounds*

ABSTRACT

Background & Aim: Belongs to Rosaecea family, *Rosa foetida* is one the Persian native plants which has not been investigated biologically. As it is traditionally used topically as poultice to treat infectious skin burns, the present paper focused on the assessment of the antibacterial activities of different extracts of *R. foetida* flowers against the main cause of skin burn wounds infections, *Pseudomonas aeruginosa*.
Experimental: The antibacterial activity and MIC value determination were investigated by cup plate method and micro plate dilution method respectively.
Results: All *R. foetid* extracts had inhibition activity on the growth of *P. aeruginosa* of which the aqueous and methanol extracts exhibited the strongest activities. Inhibition zone diameter and MIC values of the concentration of 125 mg/ml of both extracts were found to be somehow the same as those of the standard drug, Imipenem/Cilastatin (8/8 μg/ml).
Recommended applications/industries: Results demonstrated that the plant is effective against the standard and pathogenic strains of *P. aeruginosa* and could be a potential source of effective natural antibacterial compounds to be applied in further phytochemical and invivo biological studies.

1. Introduction

Burn wound infections are a serious complication of thermal injury and there are about 12000 deaths per year due to thermal injury. Although presently more patients with burns die of pneumonia than of burn wound infection, burn wound sepsis remains an important infectious complication in this population (Weinstein and Mayhall, 2003). Since the most common causes of burn wound infections were bacteria, burn wounds were treated by the exposure method, with application of topical antimicrobials and antibiotics to the burn wound surface. *Pseudomonas aeruginosa* plays a prominent role as an etiological agent involved in serious infections in burned patients (Sutter and Hurst, 1966; Kominos and Charles, 1972).

It is well-recognized as a pathogen which exhibits inherent drug resistance and represents a leading cause of morbidity due to burn wound infection (Eckert *et al.*, 2006). Reports of *P. aeruginosa* infection analyses in Burn Centers and Hospitals of Tehran to estimate their frequency and antibiotic susceptibility showed that the frequency of *P. aeruginosa* resistance to most of antibiotics including gentamicin, ceftizoxime, carbenicillin, cephaothin and ceftazidime was over 90% (Rastegar Lari *et al.*, 1998). Reports from another study in a major burn center in Tehran showed that all *P. aeruginosa* strains were multi drug resistant. The percentage of resistance to tested antibiotics was: imipenem 97.5%, amikacin 90%, piperacillin 87.5%, ceftizoxime 72.7%, gentamicin 67.5%, ciprofloxacin 65%, ceftriaxone 60%, and ceftazidime 57.5% (Ranjbar *et al.*, 2011). According to the previous reports, there is a pressing need for alternative therapeutics against this pathogen and additional studies are required to find antibacterial prophylaxis and new substitutes for current bacterial-resistant antibiotics.

Iran is one of the countries having endemic *Rosa* species and *Rosa foetida* Herrm. is one of the species widely spread throughout the country from Western to central and southern parts (Amin, 2005). *Rosa* species are well known for their medicinal and cosmetic properties. *Rosa* species are reported to have antibacterial, anti-inflammatory and diuretic properties (Mahmood *et al.,* 1996; Brinkworth *et al.*, 1992; Frederick *et al.*, 2002). The commercial significance of *R. damascena* lies particularly in rose oil which has a high international demand, and Iran is one of the major producers of this oil and the related aromatic water called "Golab" in Persian (Loghmani-Khouzani *et al.,* 2007). Rose hips which are rich in Vitamin C (300-4000 mg/100 g) (Ercisli, 2007) and antioxidants also have market demand for their role in enhancing the body immune system against infections and particularly the common cold.

A native plant to Iran, *Rosa foetida* Herrm. (Rosaceae family) has yellow flowers without scent which some find objectionable. Since there were no yellow rose native to Europe, its introduction from Persia was an important addition to the cultivation of roses, and it is now an important contributor to the stock of cultivated roses (Forsyth, 2007). Its common name is Persian yellow rose and is wildly distributed in Kurdistan Mountains, west of Iran. The decoction of the petals is used in Iranian traditional medicine as anti-diarrhea and for treatment of stomach disorders. It is topically used as a poultice to treat burns especially the burn wound infections. It is also used traditionally in some foods as a yellow color agent. Reports on *Rose foetida* flowers volatile oil composition have been published and hydrocarbons including n-nonadecane, 1-heptadecene and n-dodecanoic acid were the main group of constituents in the oil (Asgarpanah *et al.*, 2014). Since there have been no attempts to study the antibacterial activity of *R. foetida* flowers against the main cause of burn wound infections, *P. aeruginosae* up to now, we prompted to evaluate the antimicrobial properties of methanol, chloroform and aqueous extracts of *R. foetida* flowers against *P. aeruginosa* standard strain and five pathogen clinical strains isolated from patients suffering burn wound infection. This investigation is done to confirm the biological basis for the folkloric use of these flowers as natural antibacterial agent for treatment of burn wound infections.

2. Materials and Methods

2.1. Plant material

Fresh flowers of *R. foetida* were collected in June 2012 from Divandarreh, in Kurdistan Province, Iran: (N35°54′, E 32°46′, 1850 m). Specimen was identified by Dr. G.H. Amin and voucher was deposited in the Herbarium of Pharmaceutical Sciences Branch, Islamic Azad University (IAU), Tehran under code number 7042 AUPF.

2.2. Extraction Procedure

2 kg of chopped fresh petals were separately extracted by percolator apparatus using methanol, chloroform and water. Each extraction repeated for 3 times. The methanol and chloroform extracts were concentrated by rotary evaporator apparatus and the solvent removed to produce a dark brown gummy solid. The aqueous extract concentrated and dried by leaving it in room temperature. All extracts were kept in sterile vials in a dark and cool place for further tests.

Table1. The inhibition zone diameter of *Rosa foetida* flowers extracts[a].

	Diameter of zone of inhibition (mm)															
	MTE (mg/ml)					**ATE (mg/ml)**					**CTE (mg/ml)**					**Imi./Cil. (8/8 μg/ml)**
	1000	500	250	125	62.5	1000	500	250	125	62.5	1000	500	250	125	62.5	
P. aeruginosa[b]	20.6	18.6	16.0	13.8	10.3	20.3	19.5	17.6	14.3	10.1	13.3	12.5	8.5	-	-	15.6
Sample 1[c]	20.0	18.1	15.5	13.0	10.1	20.8	19.3	17.3	13.5	9.5	13.0	12.3	10.0	-	-	17.3
Sample 2	21.3	19.5	17.0	15.8	12.0	20.8	19.0	16.8	14.0	11.1	12.3	8.6	-	-	-	17.0
Sample 3	27.6	25.5	24.0	22.1	20.3	26.1	23.6	20.8	18.0	14.0	11.1	10.5	8.5	-	-	13.2
Sample 4	17.6	16.3	14.6	12.8	10.8	19.5	17.1	15.8	13.0	11.6	10.5	9.6	8.1	-	-	14.3
Sample 5	21.6	19.3	16.1	13.8	10.0	21.5	19.3	16.3	13.6	10.0	10.0	8.3	-	-	-	17.4

[a]Zone of inhibition, including the diameter of the well (6mm); mean value of three independent experiments.
MTE=Methanol total extract; ATE=Aqueous total extract; CTE=Chloroform total extract
Imi./Cil.=Imipenem/Cilastatin
[b]Standard *P. aeruginosa* strains
[c]Samples 1-5 are 5 different clinical isolates of *P. aeruginosa*

2.3. *Test Organisms*

One Gram-negative bacterium *Pseudomonas aeruginosa* (PTCC25823) obtained from Persian type culture collection (PTCC) of Iranian Research Organization for Science and Technology accompany with five clinical pathogen *P. aeruginosa* strains isolated from the patients suffering burn wound infections taken for this study.

2.4. *Antibacterial activity*

Antibacterial activities of *R. foetida* flowers extracts of were investigated against 6 bacterial strains by the cup plate method (Fazly-Bazzaz *et al.*, 2005). An overnight bacterial culture equal to 0.5 McFarland standard (1.5 x 108 CFU/ml) was used to culture on Muller-Hinton agar plates. The wells were made on agar plates with 5mm diameter. 1000, 500, 250, 125 and 62.5 mg of the each extract were separately dissolved in 1 ml water (for aqueous extract) and DMSO 10% (for methanol and chloroform extracts) and then filtered and 80 μl of each solution was added to each well. Imipenem/Cilastatin (8/8 mg/ml) was used as positive control for tested microorganisms. 80 μl of DMSO 10% served as negative control. The plates incubated at37°C for 24h. The diameter of zone of inhibitions was detected in each plate. The experiments carried out 3 times and the results were presented as mean±SD.

2.5. *Minimum Inhibitory Concentration (MIC)*

After confirmation the antibacterial activity in the extracts MIC of each was determine by testing 10 concentrations of the extracts against sensitive tested bacteria by the micro plate dilution method. The reconstituted extracts were separately diluted to give concentrations of 500 mg/ml, 250 mg/ml, 125 mg/ml, 62.5 mg/ml, 31.25 mg/ml, 15.62 mg/ml, 7.81 mg/ml, 3.90 mg/ml, 1.95 mg/ml and 0.97 mg/ml. The lowest concentration of the extract that could inhibit the bacterial growth was considered as MIC (Mehregan *et al.*, 2008). As the same, Imipenem/Cilastatin and DMSO 10% were used as positive and negative controls, respectively.

3. Results and discussion

According to Table 1, all *R. foetida* extracts had inhibition effect on the growth of *P. aeroginosa* among which the aqueous and methanol extracts exhibited significant activities. Observed antibacterial activity by 125 mg/ml concentrations of methanol and aqueous extracts were somehow equal to the antibacterial activity of the standard drug Imipenem/Cilastatin (8/8 mg/ml). MIC values of the extracts determined and as the *Tab. 2* the lowest MIC values observed by methanol and aqueous extracts.

Occurrence of bacterial infections especially infections caused by *P. aeruginosa* in skin burns is a serious problem. Regarding to development of antibacterial drug resistance of pathogen *P. aeruginosa* and side effects exhibited by the drugs used for skin burn infections, there is a great demand alternative and effective chemotherapeutic agents. Use of medicinal herbs in the treatment of *P. aeruginosa* infections is an old practice in many parts of the world. Plants contain a spectrum of secondary metabolites that their importance as antimicrobial agents against this bacterial strain has been emphasized by several works.

As the flowers of the native species *R. foetida* is used traditionally as a disinfectant and antibacterial agent in dermatitis, skin disorders and especially in skin burn wounds, we prompted to evaluate the antibacterial activities of methanol, aqueous and chloroform extracts of the flowers against the standard *P. aeruginosa* strain and five pathogenic strains isolated from different patients suffered skin burn wounds. All the extracts had inhibition activity on the growth of all six studied strains among which the methanol and aqueous ones with dose of 125 mg/ml had the most significant effects by the same inhibition zone diameters to those of the standard drug. The MIC values were also determined as the same.

As the results, it is concluded that the flowers possess polar constituent which were extracted in aqueous and methanol solvents. It is confirmed by weak antibacterial activity observed by chloroform extract against all studied *P. aeruginosa* strains. This extract contained non/semi polar compounds which had low antimicrobial activity in this study.

Phytobiological evaluations of *Rosa* species have found that the most possess moderate to strong antibacterial activities against human pathogenic bacterial strains including *P. aeruginosa* (Tambekar and Mankar, 2006) and colorful petals including red, yellow and orange ones possess natural resistance to microbial attack. (Zhang *et al.*, 2011). Literature survey revealed that these properties were maybe due to complex mixtures of polar organic compounds especially the flavonoids (Velioglu and Mazza, 1991) and lack of violet, yellow or red flowers in some *Rosa* species was due to the absence of these compounds (Katsumoto *et al.*, 2007).

Table 2. Minimum inhibitory concentration (MIC) of *Rosa foetida* flowers extracts[a].

	MIC (mg/ml)		
	MTE	ATE	CTE
P. aeruginosa[b]	62.5	62.5	500
Sample 1[c]	62.5	125	250
Sample 2	31.25	31.25	500
Sample 3	31.25	31.25	500
Sample 4	62.5	31.25	500
Sample 5	62.5	62.5	1000

[a]All determinations were done in triplicate.
MTE=Methanol total extract; ATE=Aqueous total extract;
CTE=Chloroform total extract
Imi./Cil.=Imipenem/Cilastatin
[b]Standard *P. aeruginosa* strains
[c]Samples 1-5 are 5 different clinical isolates of *P. aeruginosa*

4. Conclusion

Results show that *R. foetida* possess reliable antibacterial activities against the main cause of skin burn wounds infections, *P. aeruginosa* (the standard and pathogenic strains). This plant could be a good choice for further invivo biological investigations especially on the infectious skin burns and future phytochemical studies, identification and structure elucidation of the responsible compounds is suggested.

5. Acknowledgments

Supports from Pharmaceutical Sciences Branch, Islamic Azad University (IAU) is gratefully acknowledged.

6. References

Weinstein, R.A., Mayhall, C.G. 2003. The Epidemiology of Burn Wound Infections: Then and Now. *Clin Infect Dis.*, 37 (4): 543-550.

Sutter, V.L., Hurst, V. 1966. Sources of *Pseudomonas aeruginosa* Infection in burns: Study of wound and rectal cultures with phage typing. *Annal Surg.*, 163(4): 597-602.

Kominos, S.D., Charles, E. 1972. Mode of transmission of *Pseudomonas aeruginosa* in a burn unit and an intensive care unit in a general hospital. *Appl Environ Microbiol*., 23(2): 309-312.

Eckert, R., Brady, K.M., Greenberg, E.P., Qi, F., Yarbrough, D.K., He, J., McHardy, I., Anderson, M.H., Shi, W. 2006. Enhancement of antimicrobial activity against *Pseudomonas aeruginosa* by coadministration of G10KHc and Tobramycin. *Antimicrob Agents Chemother*., 50(11): 3833-3838.

Rastegar Lari, A., Bahrami Honar, H., Alaghehbandan, R. 1998. *Pseudomonas* infections in Tohid Burn Center, Iran. *Burns*., 24(7): 637-641.

Ranjbar, R., Owlia, P., Saderi, H., Mansouri, S., Jonaidi-Jafari, N., Izadi, M., Farshad, S., Arjomandzadegan, M. 2011. Characterization of *Pseudomonas aeruginosa* strains isolated from burned patients hospitalized in a major burn center in Tehran, Iran. *Acta Med Iran*., 49(10): 675-679.

Amin, G. 2005. *Popular Medicinal Plants of Iran*. Tehran University of Medical Sciences Publishing. Tehran, Iran, pp 232.

Mahmood, N., Piacente, S., Pizza, C., Burke, A., Khan, A.I., Hay, A.J. 1996. The anti-HIV activity and mechanisms of action of pure compounds isolated from *Rosa damascena*. Biochem. Biophys. *Res. Comm*., 229: 73-79.

Brinkworth, R.I., Stoermer, M.J., Fairlie, D.P. 1992. Flavones are inhibitors of HIV-1 protease. *Biochem. Biophys. Res. Comm*., 188: 631-637.

Frederick, C., Wagner, A., Morvillo, N. 2002. Randomly amplified polymorphic and DNA (RAPD) analysis of the musk roses (*Rosa moschata*). *Prac. Fla. State Hort. Soc*., 115: 117-119.

Loghmani-Khouzani, H., SabziFini, O., Safari, J. 2007. Essential oil composition of *Rosa damascena* Mill cultivated in central Iran. *ScientiaIranica*., 14(4): 316-319.

Ercisli, S. 2007. Chemical composition of fruits in some *Rose* (*Rosa* spp.) species. *Food Chem*., 104: 379-384.

Forsyth, H.K. 2007. *The Constant Gardener: A Botanical Bible*. The Miegunyah Press. Carlton, Australia, pp 150.

Asgarpanah, J., Ziarati, P., Safialdinardebily, M. 2014. The volatile oil composition of *Rosa foetida* Herrm. flowers growing wild in Kurdistan province (Iran). *J. Essent Oil Bear Plants*., 17 (1): 169 – 172.

Fazly-Bazzaz, B.S., Khajehkaramadin, M., Shokooheizadeh, H.R. 2005. Antibacterial activity of *Rheum ribes* extract obtained from various plant parts against clinical isolates of Gram-negative pathogens. *Iran J Pharm Res*., 2: 87-91.

Mehregan, H., Mojab, F., Pakdaman, S.H., Poursaeed, M. 2008. Antibacterial activity of *Thymus pubescence* methanolic extract. *Iran J Pharm Res*., 7(4): 291-295.

Tambekar, D.H., Mankar, S.S. 2006. Studies on antimicrobial spectrum of *Rose* petals against bacterial pathogens. *Asian J Microbiol Biotechnol Environ Sci*., 8(2): 367-372.

Zhang, W., Abdel-Rahman, F.H., Saleh, M.A. 2011. Natural resistance of rose petals to microbial attack. *J Environ Sci Health B*., 46(5): 381-393.

Velioglu, Y.S., Mazza, G. 1991. Characterization of flavonoids in petals of *Rosa damascena* by HPLC and spectral analysis. *J Agric Food Chem*., 39 (3): 463–467.

Katsumoto, Y., Fukuchi-Mizutani, M., Fukui, Y., Brugliera, F., Holton, T.A., Karan, M., Nakamura, N., Yonekura-Sakakibara, K., Togami, J., Pigeaire, A., Tao, G.Q., Nehra, N.S., Lu, C.Y., Dyson, B.K., Tsuda, S., Ashikari, T., Kusumi, T., Mason, J.G., Tanaka, Y. 2007. Engineering of the *Rose* Flavonoid Biosynthetic Pathway Successfully Generated Blue-Hued Flowers Accumulating Delphinidin. *Plant Cell Physiol*., 48(11): 1589-1600.

Chemical composition of the volatile oils of three Lamiaceae species growing wild in North of Iran

Salar Hafez Ghoran[1]*, Boshra Azadi[2], Hidayat Hussain[3]

[1]*Department of Chemistry, Faculty of Sciences, Golestan University, Gorgan 4913815739, Iran;*
*Email: ***S.Hafezghoran@gu.ac.ir and S_Hafezghoran@yahoo.com**

[2]*Phytochemistry Department, Faculty of Medicinal Chemistry, Pharmaceutical Sciences Branch, Islamic Azad University, Tehran, Iran;*

[3]*UoN Chair of Oman's Medicinal plants and Marine Natural products, University of Nizwa, Nizwa, Sultanate of Oman;*

ARTICLE INFO

Topic: *Medicinal Plants*

Key words:

- ✓ Satureja macrantha
- ✓ Ziziphora persica
- ✓ Lavandula stoechas
- ✓ *Essence*
- ✓ *Lamiaceae*

ABSTRACT

Background & Aim: The Lamiaceae or Labiatae (commonly referred to as the mint or deadnettle family) are an exceedingly large and widespread of flowering plants (Angiospermae). Most member of Lamiaceae plants are used in Iranian folk medicine as stimulant, antiseptic, aphrodisiac, stomachic, expectorant, carminative, anti-diarrheic and anti-bacterial. The aim of the present work was to obtain a better insight into the nature of essential oil.

Experimental: The essences of three Lamiaceae species viz., *Satureja macrantha* C.A. Mey., *Ziziphora persica* Bunge, and *Lavandula stoechas* L. obtained by hydro-distillation method of flowers growing wild in the north of Iran. The study led to the identification of 67 components by a combination HP-5 GC-FID and GC-MS analytical techniques and the oil yields were 1.3 %, 1.64 %, and 1.16 % on fresh flowers, respectively.

Results & Discussion: The chemical components of *S. macrantha* were found to contain mainly: Carvacrol (43.3 %), γ-Terpinene (24.1 %) and *p*-Cymene (21.6 %). On the other hand the major oil components for *Z. persica* were Isopulegone (46.6 %), followed by *p*-mentha-1(7),8-diene (16.4 %), 1,8-Cineole (7.0 %), Isomenthol (5.5 %) and Isoledene (3.3 %), accounting for 98.0 % of the total components. Camphor (61.5 %), 1,8-Cineole (10.1 %), Fenchone (4.2 %) and Linalool (3.8 %) were found to be the major constituents of the oil of *L. stoechas*. The essential oils of *S. macrantha*, *Z. persica*, and *L. stoechas* were identified by much larger amount of monoterpenes (96.52 %, 89.31 %, and 93.49 %, respectively) and sesquiterpenes (1.87 %, 8.10 %, and 5.04 %, respectively).

Industrial and practical recommendations: Based on the results of this study, the chemical variations of three volatile oils might be correlated with geographical regions and environmental conditions (temperature, humidity, interaction with other species and etc.) play a significant role in biosynthesis of the components of the oil

1. Introduction

Volatile oils, essential oils or ethereal oils are usually obtained from the appropriate plant material by steam distillation. If certain components are unstable at these temperatures, however, then other, less harsh techniques, such as expression or solvent extraction, may be employed. These oils, which typically contain a complex mixture of low boiling-point components, are widely used in flavoring, perfumery, and aromatherapy (Isman, 2000). *Satureja macrantha* C. A. Mey., *Ziziphora persica* Bunge, and *Lavandula stoechas* L. are three species of aromatic herbs of the family Lamiaceae (=Labiatae) and are widely distributed in the northern part of Iran.

Satureja species grow in different geographical areas of Iran. There are 12 annual and perennial species (eight species are endemic of Iran), which have been used as a foodstuff and traditional medicine. *S. macrantha* C. A. Mey.; is a small shrub divided in western, northwestern and northern parts of Iran (Mozaffarian, 2013).

There are four species of *Ziziphora* genus which grow in Iran and other countries such as Afghanistan, Armenia, Pakistan, Turkey, and Turkmenistan (Mozaffarian, 2013). Moreover *Ziziphora* species are present in high altitude areas in Iran, especially northern and eastern parts. *Z. persica* Bunge: is an edible medicinal plant, which the aerial parts used in foods to offer flavor and aroma (Ozturk *et al.*, 1995). Furthermore the volatile oils of *Z. persica* have antibacterial activity, which can be used as conservative in foods, to protect them from pathogens (Ozturk & Ercisli, 2006).

Lavandula species are important members of family Lamiaceae, which are mainly cultivated for their essential oils. There are three species of *Lavandula* genus, which are wildly distributed in north of Iran (Golestan province) (Mozaffarian, 2013). The dried flowers of *L. stoechas* have been used in perfumery, cosmetics, food processing and traditional medicine because of their various biological activities such as antifungal (Angioni *et al.*, 2006), antibacterial (Goren *et al.*, 2002; Bouzouita *et al.*, 2005). Moreover the volatile oils of *L. stoechas* were shown effective cytotoxic activity on COL-2 (human colon cancer) (Goren *et al.*, 2002).

Interestingly the extracts of three investigated plants are used in folk medicine as stimulant, antiseptic, aphrodisiac, stomachic, expectorant, and carminative, anti-diarrheic, anti-bacterial and also have anti-inflammatory activity (Ozturk *et al.*, 1995; Goren *et al.*, 2002; Ozturk & Ercisli, 2006; Beikmohammadi, 2011). The aim of the present work was to obtain a better insight into the nature of essential oil of three Lamiaceae herbs from north of Iran (Golestan province) by using GC-FID and GC/MS.

2. Materials and Methods

2.1. Plant material

The aerial parts of *S. macrantha*, *Z. persica*, and *L. stoechas* were collected in full flowering stages in August 2013 from Golestan province, Iran. Voucher specimens (No. 6240, No. 6241, and No. 6238, respectively) have been deposited in the Herbarium of the faculty of biology (Golestan University, Gorgan, Iran). Plant specimens were identified by Dr. Mohammad Fatemi from that institute. The dried flowering aerial parts for three herbs were individually extracted by hydro-distillation method using Clevenger-type apparatus for 4-5 hours to give the following yield (w/w): 1.3%, 1.04%, and 1.16%, respectively. Anhydrous sodium sulfate was used to remove water after extraction and the volatile oils stored in refrigerator at 4°C.

2.1. Isolation procedure of S. macrantha, Z. persica, and L. stoechas essential oil

The determination of retention data and the area percentage of the identified oil components are mentioned in Table 1. The experiments were analyzed by an Agilent 7890A gas chromatograph (manufactured by America) equipped with a 30 m × 0.32 *i.d.*, 0.25 μm film thicknesses with silica HP-5 column (capillary). In addition, GC-MS was measured in Hewlett Packard 5975C GC-MS system with a HP-5 fused silica column using the aforementioned chromatographic conditions (Table 1).

2.3. Identification and characterization of the volatile oil constituents

The retention indices (RI) for three herbs oil were individually determined by conjunction of the sample with containing the homologous series of C_8 to C_{26} *n*-alkanes (Van del Dool & Kratz, 1963). The constituents of *S. macrantha*, *Z. persica*, and *L. stoechas* oils were identified by their retention indices compared with data published in the literature (Adams, 2001), computer library (NIST/NIH libraries) and Wiley library (Massada, 1976). Finally, the percentage of each oil component was carried out by peak area normalization measurement.

3. Results and discussion

The essential oil compounds of *S. macrantha, Z. persica*, and *L. stoechas* were analyzed by using GC-MS analysis. The yield oils (yellow liquids) were 1.3 %, 1.04 %, and 1.16 % (w/w), based on dry weights, respectively. Finally, 67 components were identified in three Lamiaceae species (see Tables 2).

Twenty-eight compounds were identified form the essential oils of *S. macrantha*. The major components of the essential oils of *S. macrantha* were carvacrol (43.02%), γ-terpinene (24.1%) and *p*-cymene (21.6%). The high percentages of carvacrol and p-cymene proved that this essential oil clearly belongs to the aromatic chemo-type (see Table 2). According to the previous studies, Sefidkon and Jamzad studied the oil of *S. macrantha*, which collected in northeast of Iran (Khorasan), consists of p-cymene (25.8%), limonene (32.3%) and thymol (8.1%) (Sefidkon & Jamzad, 2005). The relative quantities of γ-terpinene and p-cymene are noticeably smaller in the *S. macrantha* from Turkey but carvacrol (64.4%) was higher (Azaz *at al*., 2005). Golestanian *S. macrantha* oil has carvacrol as the most abundant component, while volatile oil of *S. macrantha* obtained from the northwest of Iran (Urmia); contains spathulenol (14.0%), vanillin (13.4%) and *p*-cymene (12.3%), as the main constituents (Gohari *et al*., 2006).

Moreover, 32 components, representing 98.09 % of the oil content of Golestanian *Z. persica* were characterized, which are mentioned in Table 2. It is interesting to note that the most abundant compounds were isopulegone (46.6%), followed by *p*-mentha-1(7),8-diene (16.4%), 1,8-Cineole (7.0%), isomenthol (5.5%) and isoledene (3.3%).

The *Z. persica* oil consisted of 31.6% monoterpene hydrocarbons, 7.3% monoterpene alcohols, 0.7% monoterpene esters, 7.0% monoterpene ethers, 49.3% monoterpene ketones and 8.1% sesquiterpenes. It has been reported by Dembitskii *et al* that major component of the essential oils of *Z. persica* was pulegone and that species was collected from Kazakh and Azerbaijanian (Dembitskii *et al*., 1994). Moreover, the major components of the essential oils of Turkey origin *Z. persica* were (+)-pulegone (79.3%), limonene (6.8%) and piperitenone (4.2%). On the other hand, Golestanian *Z. persica* oils were identified by high percentage of monoterpene ketone, such as isopulegone. These data indicated that monoterpene ketones (isopulegone and pulegone) are mainly chemo-type for *Z. persica* in Iran, Turkey, Kazakhstan and Azerbaijan (Dembitskii *et al*., 1994; Ozturk & Ercisli, 2006), while *Z. persica* from the eastern parts of Iran is mostly monoterpene alcohol chemo-type, with high contents of neomenthol (22.5%) and *p*-menth-3-en-8-ol (18.1%) (Rustaiyan *et al*., 2006).

Essential oil compounds of *Z. persica* from Golestan constitute the first report on savory oil of the isopulegone chemo-type.

Table 2 reports the chemical constituents of *L. stoechas*. Thirty-seven components were identified, which accounted for 98.55% of the total volatile fraction in the *L. stoechas* aerial parts. In a research on *Lavandula* essential oils, Angioni *et al* (2006) noted the enormous variability in the chemical compositions of *L. stoechas*. In spite of the variability, there are some apparent chemical constituents. Not only are there fenchone-rich, camphor-rich, myrtenyl acetate-rich, α-pinene-rich and camphene-rich chemotypes as previously noted by Angioni *et al*, but also in Golestanian *L. stoechas*, Camphor was the main compound, accounting 61.32%, followed by 1,8-Cineole, fenchone, linalool and borneol (10.08%, 4.21%, 3.77% and 3.19%, respectively).

β-Selinene, β-eudesmol, camphene and α-pinene were the most representative components. The Grecian *L. stoechas* essential oil obtained from aerial parts were identified by fenchone (30.9%), camphor (9.6%) and 1,8-cineole (8.1%), and it was rich in pinocarvyl acetate (10.2%) (Kokkalou, 1988). The Tunisian essential oil from aerial parts of *L. stoechas* was characterized by the low amount of 1, 8-cineole (4.9%), but it was rich in fenchone (68.2%) (Bouzouita *et al*., 2005).

Table 1. Temperature programming for determination of retention data and the area percentage of *Satureja macrantha* C. A. Mey; *Ziziphora persica* Bunge and *Lavandula stoechas* L.

Treatment	Rate (°C/min)	Column temperature (°C)	Holding time (min)	Injector temperature (°C)	Detector temperature (°C)	Flow rate (mL/min)	Carrier gas
		50	3	250	260	1	Helium
S. macrantha	4	250	0				
	5	280	3				
		50	10	250	260	1	Nitrogen
Z. persica	4	200	0				
	10	270	5				
		60	4	250	260	1	Nitrogen
L. stoechas	3	100	2				
	4	260	0				

Table 2. Chemical components of the essential oils of *Satureja macrantha*, *Ziziphora persica*, and *Lavandula stoechas* from north of Iran (Golestan province).

Volatile Compounds [a]	LRI [b]	*S. macrantha*	*Z. persica*	*L. stoechas*	Method of identification [c]
Tricyclene [d]	923	0.43	-	-	MS, RI
α-Thujene [d]	930	1.19	0.14	-	MS, RI
α-Pinene	939	0.58	0.85	1.07	MS, RI, Std
Camphene [d]	951	0.24	0.33	1.21	MS, RI
Verbenene [d]	967	-	1.76	0.38	MS, RI
β-pinene	979	0.21	2.35	0.96	MS, RI, Std
Myrcene [d]	991	-	0.25	-	MS, RI
p-Mentha-1(7),8-diene [d]	1002	-	16.4	-	MS, RI
α-Phellandrene [d]	1005	0.23	-	-	MS, RI
δ-3-Carene [d]	1011	0.09	0.79	-	MS, RI
α-Terpinene [d]	1017	2.94	-	0.34	MS, RI
o-Cymene [d]	1022	-	-	0.32	MS, RI
p-Cymene [d]	1025	21.6	0.82	0.21	MS, RI
β-Phellandrene [d]	1026	0.17	0.17	0.25	MS, RI
Limonene [d]	1029	0.28	0.84	-	MS, RI
1,8-Cineole	1031	0.11	6.96	10.08	MS, RI, Std
β-Trans-ocimene [d]	1054	-	-	0.32	MS, RI
γ-Terpinene	1062	24.09	-	-	MS, RI, Std
Trans-4-thujanol [d]	1064	0.11	-	-	MS, RI
β-Terpinene [d]	1071	-	0.81	-	MS, RI
trans-Linalool oxide [d]	1084	-	-	0.75	MS, RI
Fenchone	1087	-	-	4.21	MS, RI, Std
α-Terpinolene [d]	1088	0.07	0.21	-	MS, RI
Linalool	1098	-	-	3.77	MS, RI, Std
α-Thujone [d]	1105	-	0.47	0.49	MS, RI
Chrysanthenone [d]	1123	-	0.53	-	MS, RI
α-Campholene aldehyde [d]	1132	-	-	0.15	MS, RI
Camphor	1143	-	-	61.32	MS, RI, Std
p-Menthone [d]	1147	-	1.54	-	MS, RI
Isopulegone	1153	-	46.58	-	MS, RI, Std
Pinocarvone [d]	1160	-	-	0.24	MS, RI
Borneol	1165	0.3	0.53	3.19	MS, RI, Std
Terpinen-4-ol [d]	1177	0.29	0.74	0.33	MS, RI
Isomenthol [d]	1182	-	5.54	-	MS, RI
Myrtenol [d]	1194	-	-	0.16	MS, RI

Myrtenal [d]	1195	-	-	0.37	MS, RI
Eucarvone (Verbenone) [d]	1204	-	-	0.18	MS, RI
cis-Carveol [d]	1226	-	-	0.34	MS, RI
Carvone [d]	1239	-	-	0.39	MS, RI
Cuminaldehyde [e]	1242	-	-	056	MS, RI
Geraniol	1249	-	-	0.57	MS, RI, Std
2′,4′-Dimethylacetophenone [d]	1255	-	0.21	-	MS, RI
Phellandral [d]	1273	-	-	0.4	MS, RI
Anethole [d]	1282	-	-	0.19	MS, RI
Thymol [d]	1290	0.09	-	-	MS, RI
p-cymen-7-ol [d]	1295	-	-	0.37	MS, RI
Carvacrol	1298	43.02	0.49	-	MS, RI, Std
Terpinen-4-ol acetate [d]	1340	0.25	-	-	MS, RI
α-Cubebene [d]	1348	-	0.31	-	MS, RI
Isoledene [d]	1373	-	3.33	-	MS, RI
β-Bourbonene [d]	1384	-	0.7	-	MS, RI
β-Cubebene [d]	1388	0.1	-	-	MS, RI
α-Cedrene [d]	1411	1.04	0.97	-	MS, RI
β-Caryophyllene [d]	1419	0.11	-	-	MS, RI
Iridomyrmecin [d]	1436	-	0.68	-	MS, RI
β-Farnesene [d]	1440	-	-	0.3	MS, RI
α-Humulene	1455	0.15	-	-	MS, RI, Std
Selina-4,11-diene [d]	1475	-	0.24	-	MS, RI
γ-Gurjunene [d]	1477	0.19	2.16	-	MS, RI
β-Selinene [d]	1489	-	-	1.25	MS, RI
β-Bisabolene	1505	-	-	0.45	MS, RI, Std
δ-Cadinene [d]	1523	0.15	-	0.16	MS, RI
α-Cadinene [d]	1538	-	0.23	-	MS, RI
Germacrene B	1561	0.2	0.16	-	MS, RI, Std
Caryophyllene oxide [d]	1582	-	-	1.05	MS, RI
β-Eudesmol [d]	1649	-	-	1.3	MS, RI
α-Bisabolol [d]	1685	0.36	-	0.36	MS, RI
Farnesol	1732	-	-	0.17	MS, RI, Std
Monoterpene hydrocarbons		52.12	25.72	5.06	
Oxygenated Monoterpenes		44.17	63.59	88.45	
Sesquiterpene hydrocarbons		2.94	8.10	2.16	
Oxygenated Sesquiterpene		0.27	-	2.88	
Other		-	0.68	-	
Total identified		98.5 %	98.09 %	98.55 %	

[a] Compounds are listed in order of their elution from a HP-5MS column using homologous series of C_8 to C_{26} *n*-alkanes. [b] LRI, literature retention indices on HP-5MS column. [c] Method of identification: MS, by comparison of the mass spectrum with those of the computer mass libraries; RI, by comparison of RI with those from the literature; Std, by injection of an authentic sample. [d] Tentatively identified according to the mass spectrum (MS) and by comparison of RI with the literature (LRI).

However, the essential oil obtained from *L. stoechas*, harvested in a different Turkish region, appeared to be of a peculiar chemotype characterized by the presence of pulegone (40.4%), menthol (18.1%), menthone (12.6%) and 1,8-cineole (3.9%) (Goren *et al*., 2002). Overall, the Golestanian *L. stoechas* essential oil analyzed in this study showed a lower content of fenchone and the presence of borneol in quite high with respect to literature data.

4. Conclusions

The incompatibility between the results mentioned in different literature on *S. macrantha*, *Z. persica* and *L. stoechas* could still be logical due to the influence of several factors mentioned such as experimental conditions, the climate conditions, harvest conditions, and geographical source (Kokkalou, 1988; Goren *et al.*, 2002; Bouzouita *et al.*, 2005; Sefidkon & Jamzad, 2005; Angioni *et al.*, 2006; Gohari *et al.*, 2006; Rustaiyan *et al.*, 2006). Interestingly α-pinene, camphene, β-pinene, p-cymene, β-phellandrene, 1,8-cineole, borneol and terpinen-4-ol were present in three investigated species viz., *S. macrantha, Z. persica*, and *L. stoechas*.

According to many studies, the chemical variations of *S. macrantha*, *Z. persica*, and *L. stoechas* volatile oils - given the same species with similar part of plant and method of distillation - might be correlated with geographical regions and environmental conditions (temperature, humidity, interaction with other species and etc.) play a significant role in biosynthesis of the components of the oil. It should also be noted that the chemical composition of an essential oil prepared from the same organ of one species varies to same degree according to the ecological conditions under which the herb has grown.

5. Acknowledgement

The authors are grateful to Golestan University (GU) for partial support of this work.

6. References

Adams, R.P. 2001. Identification of essential oil components by gas chromatography/quadruple mass spectroscopy. Allured Publishing Co. Carol Stream, Illinois.

Angioni, A., Barra, A., Coroneo, V., Dessi, S. and Cabras, P. 2006. Chemical composition, seasonal variability, and antifungal activity of *Lavandula Stoechas* L. ssp. *Stoechas* essential oils from stem/leaves and flowers. *Journal of Agricultural and Food Chemistry*, 54: 4364-4370.

Azaz, A.D., Kurkucoglu, M., Satil, F., Baser, K.H.C. and Tumen, G. 2005. *In vitro* antimicrobial activity and chemical composition of some *Satureja* essential oils. *Flavour and Fragrance Journal*, 20: 587-591.

Beikmohammadi, M. 2011. The evaluation of medicinal properties of *Ziziphora clinopodioides*. *World Applied Science Journal*, 12: 1635-1638.

Bouzouita, N., Kachouri, F., Hamdi, M., Chaabouni, M.M., Ben Aissa, R., Zgoulli, S., Thonart, P., Carlier, A., Marlier, M. and Lognay, G.C. 2005. Volatile constituents and antimicrobial activity of *Lavandula stoechas* L. oil from Tunisia. *Journal of Essential Oil Research*, 17: 584-586.

Dembitskii, A.D., Bergalive, E.Sh. and Kyazimov, I.M. 1994. Chemical composition of the essential oils of *Ziziphora* growing under various ecological conditions. *Chemistry of Natural Compounds*. 30: 673-675.

Gohari, A.R., Hadjiakhoondi, A., Sadat-Ebrahimi, E., Saeidnia, S. and Shafiee, A. 2006. Composition of the volatile oils of *Satureja spicigera* C. Koch Boiss. and *S. macrantha* C. A. Mey from Iran. *Flavour and Fragrance Journal*, 21: 510-512.

Goren, A. C., Topcu, G., Bilsel, G. and Bilsel, M. 2002. The chemical constituents and biological activity of essential oil of *Lavandula Stoechas* ssp. *Stoechas*. *Zeitschrift fur Naturforschung C*, 57: 797-800.

Isman, M.B. 2000. Plant essential oil for pest and disease management. *Crop Protection*, 19: 603-608.

Kokkalou, E. 1988. The constituents of the essential oil from *Lavandula stoechas* growing wild in Greece. *Planta Medica*. 54: 58-59.

Mozaffarian, V. 2013. Identification of medicinal and aromatic plants of Iran. Farhang Moaser. Tehran.

Ozturk, Y., Aydin, S., Tecik, B. and Baser, K.H.C. 1995. Effects of essential oils from certain *Ziziphora* species on swimming performance in mice. *Phytotherapy Research*, 9: 225-227.

Ozturk, S. and Ercisli, S. 2006. The chemical composition of essential oil and *in vitro* antibacterial activities of essential oil and methanol extract of *Ziziphora persica* Bunge. *Journal of Ethnopharmacology*, 106: 372-376.

Massada, Y. 1976. Analysis of essential oil by gas chromatography and mass spectrometry. John Wiley and Sons Inc.: New York.

Rustaiyan, A. H., Jazmad, M., Masoudi, S. and Ameri, N. 2006. Volatile constituents of *Nepeta heliotropifolia* Lam., *Mentha mozzaffarianii* Jamzad and *Ziziphora persica* Bunge. three *Labiatae* herbs growing wild in Iran. *Journal of Essential Oil Research*, 18: 348-351.

Sefidkon, F. and Jamzad, Z. 2005. Chemical composition of the essential oil of three Iranian *Satureja* Species (*S. mutica*, *S. macrantha* and *S. intermedia*). *Food Chemistry*, 91: 1-4.

Van del Dool, H. and Kratz, P.D. 1963. A generalization of the retention index system including linear temperature programmed gas-liquid partition chromatography. *Journal of Chromatography A*, 11: 463-471.

Effect of *Thymus vulgaris* extract on systemic antibody responses against Influenza and Newcastle disease vaccine in broiler chickens

Forough Talazadeh[1*], Mansoor Mayahi[1], Hossein Najafzade Varzi[2], Hadis Norouzizade[2]

[1]*Department of Clinical Sciences, Faculty of Veterinary Medicine Shahid Chamran University of Ahvaz- Iran;*
[*]**Email:** *ftalazade@gmail.com*

[2]*Department of Basic Sciences, Faculty of Veterinary Medicine Shahid Chamran University of Ahvaz- Iran;*

ARTICLE INFO

Topic: *Veterinary*

Key words:

- ✓ *Avian Influenza Virus (AIV)*
- ✓ *Thyme extract*
- ✓ *Immune response*
- ✓ *Newcastle disease virus*
- ✓ *Broiler chickens*

ABSTRACT

Background & Aim: The recent study was conducted to investigate the effects of Thyme extract in drinking water on immune response of broiler chickens.

Experimental: A total of 245 day-old broiler chicks were purchased and 20 chicks were bled for determination maternal antibody and remaining chicks divided into 5 equal groups. Chickens of group A, B and C received 0.1%, 0.15% and 0.2% of Thyme extract in drinking water for all of the period of experiment, respectively. Chickens of group D did not receive Thyme extract but vaccinated against Newcastle and Influenza diseases. Chickens of group E were kept as control group and did not receive Thyme extract and Newcastle and Influenza diseases vaccines. Chickens of group A, B, C and D were vaccinated with live Newcastle vaccine (B1 strain) intraocularly and AI-ND killed vaccine (subtype H9N2) subcutaneously of neck back. Blood samples were collected before vaccination as well as on days 14, 28 and 35 after vaccination. Ten chickens of each group were bled randomly and antibody titer against Newcastle and Influenza vaccine virus was determined by HI test.

Results & Discussion: Results indicted that the extract had no effect on antibody response against Newcastle vaccine virus, but 14 days after vaccination, receiving of 0.2% of extract, significantly increased the specific antibody response against Influenza vaccine compared to all groups.

Industrial and practical recommendations: Herbs that are rich in flavonoids such as thyme (*Thymus vulgaris*) extend the activity of vitamin C, act as antioxidants and may therefore enhance the immune function.

1. Introduction

Nowadays, using antibiotics at sub-therapeutic levels has caused concerns about antibiotic residues in the animal productions which lead to the development of drug-resistant bacteria in animals and human. Thus, medical and public concerns focused on the complete removal of the antibiotics from animal feed in the European Union at the beginning of 2006 (Nollet, 2005; Wakeman, 2005; Cervantes, 2006). Therefore, poultry industry has been looking for the substances that could replace antibiotic growth promoters (AGP) in the feed (Bach Knudsen, 2001). Application of feed additives has two objectives: controlling pathogenic microorganisms and enhancing beneficial microorganisms in the digestive content of the gut (Vahdatpour *et al.*, 2011). Recently some alternative components such as probiotics, prebiotics, organic acids and phytogenics fed additive have been introduced instead of antibiotics (Patterson and Burkhoder, 2003; Ricke, 2003). Recent bans and restrictions on the use of animal antibiotic growth promoters stimulated interest in bioactive secondary metabolites of plant source as alternative performance enhancers (Greathead, 2003). Medicinal plants and their essential oils have been used extensively in food products, perfumery, dental and oral products due to their different medicinal properties (Suppakul *et al.*, 2003). Also in poultry production, it's very important to improve immunity so as to prevent infectious diseases. A variety of such factors as vaccination failure, infection by immune suppressive diseases, and abuse of antibiotics can induce immunodeficiency. Utilization of immunostimulants is a solution to improve the immunity of animals and to decrease their susceptibility to infectious disease (Liu, 1999). Herbs that are rich in flavonoids such as thyme (*Thymus vulgaris*) extend the activity of vitamin C, act as antioxidants and may therefore enhance the immune function (Manach *et al.*, 1996; Cook and Samman, 1996). *Thymus vulgaris* is a medicinal herb in the *Lamiaceae* family, cultivated worldwide for culinary, cosmetic perennial and medical purposes. This species has special functions such as antispasmodic, expectorant, antiseptic, antimicrobial and antioxidant (Hertrampf, 2001; Abu-Darwish *et al.*, 2009). Thymol (5-methyl-1-2-isopropyl phenol) and carvacrol (5-isopropyl-2-methyl phenol) are the main phenolic components in Thymus vulgaris (Masada, 1976). Thyme (extract, oil, and the major components) have shown antibacterial activity against the *Clostridium botulinum, Clostridium perfringens*, *Bacillus subtilis*, *Salmonella sonnei, Escherichia coli*, *Helicobacter pylori*, *Salmonella typhimurium*, *Bacillus cereus*, *Listeria monocytogenes, Campylobacter jejuni* and *Salmonella enteric* reported in previous literatures (Nevas *et al.*, 2004; Fan and Chen, 2001; Tabak *et al.*, 1996; Juven *et al.*, 1994; Ultee *et al.*, 2000; Friedman *et al.*, 2002; Thakare, 2004). Performance promoting effects of essential oil, extract, powder or principal components of thyme have been demonstrated in poultry (Al-Kassie, 2009; cross *et al.*, 2007, Al-Mashhadani *et al.*, 2011; Lee *et al.*, 2003; Bolukbasi and Erhan., 2007; El-Ghousein and El-Beitawi., 2009). For example, supplementation of 200 ml Thyme extract per 1000 liter drinking waters in broiler chickens led to improvement of body weight gain and feed conversion ratio (Feisi and Bijanzad., 2010). Moreover, Rahimi *et al.* (2011) reported that dietary Thyme extract solution (0.1%) in water increased the performance and *lactic acid* counts whereas reduced the *Escherichia coli* numbers ($p < 0.05$). A variety of factors such as vaccination failure, infection by immune suppressive diseases, and abuse of antibiotics can induce immunodeficiency. Utilization of immunostimulants is one solution to improve the immunity of animals and to decrease their susceptibility to infectious disease (Liu, 1999). Herbs that are rich in flavonoids such as thyme (*Thymus vulgaris*) extend the activity of vitamin C, act as antioxidants and may therefore enhance the immune function (Manach *et al.*, 1996; Cook and Samman, 1996). The current study was conducted to evaluate the potential of applying different levels of Thyme extract (*Thymus vulgaris*) on systemic antibody responses against Influenza and Newcastle disease vaccine in broiler chickens.

2. Materials and Methods

2.1. Chickens

A total of 245 day-old broiler chicks (Ross 308) were procured. All chickens were divided into 5 groups and raised under standard conditions. Chickens of group A, B, C and D were submitted to vaccinations against AIV and NDV.

2.2. Vaccinia

Hitchner B1 vaccine Cevac®, AI- ND killed vaccine (subtype H9N2).

2.3. Thyme extract

Thymus vulgaris aqueous extract was purchased commercially as solution (Dineh Iran - The Group of Pharmaceutical, Hygienic & Food industries (P.J.S)). The product contained 5 mg thymol per 5 ml of the solution.

2.4. Experimental design

Chickens of group A, B and C received 0.1%, 0.15% and 0.2% of Thyme extract respectively in drinking water for all of the period of experiment. Chickens of group D did not receive Thyme extract but vaccinated against Newcastle and Influenza diseases. Chickens of group E were kept as control group and did not receive Thyme extract and Newcastle and Influenza diseases vaccines. Chickens of group A, B, C and D were vaccinated with live Newcastle vaccine (B1 strain) intraocularly and AI-ND killed vaccine (subtype H9N2) subcutaneously of neck back.

2.5. Blood collection and serological tests

Blood samples were collected before vaccination as well as on days 14, 28 and 35 post vaccination. Ten chickens of each group were bled randomly and antibody titer against Newcastle and Influenza vaccine virus was determined by HI test. Blood samples were drained from the brachial vein and sera were separated, identified and frozen at -20° C until the serological tests were performed. Serum samples were analyzed by Hemagglutination inhibition test (HI) to detect antibodies against AIV and NDV (Alexander *et al.*, 1983).

2.6. Microplate heamagglutination inhibition (HI) assay

Beta procedure of micro-plate HI test was performed in U-bottomed 96-well microtiter plates with 1% chicken erythrocytes to determine the antibody level of the sera samples collected from the chicks of different groups. The test was conducted using constant 4HA unit AIV and ND virus and diluted.

2.7. Statistical analysis

The titers obtained by HI were submitted to analysis of variance using the Statistical Package for social Sciences (SPSS) version 18.0 program. One Way ANOVA LSD Test were performed to determine the significant differences in HI titers of chickens of each group after vaccination. Means were compared at a significance level of 5%.

3. Results and discussion

Results of Table 1, indicated that before vaccination, there was no significant difference between all groups. On the other hand, 14, 28 and 35 days after vaccination, there was no significant difference between groups A, B, C as compared to the group D ,but groups A, B, C and D had significant difference as compared to the group E ($P < 0.05$). The results of present study showed that Thyme extract had no effect on antibody response against Newcastle vaccine virus.

The results of Table 2, indicated that before vaccination, there was not any significant difference between all groups, whereas 14 days after vaccination, there was significant difference between group C and all groups. Antibody titers in groups A, B, and C were higher than group D and E on the 28 and 35 days after vaccination, but there was not any significant difference between groups A, B, C as compared to group D. 14, 28 and 35 days after vaccination, group C has the highest antibody levels. The results of present study showed that14 days after vaccination, receiving of 0.2% of Thyme extract, significantly increased the specific antibody response to avian Influenza vaccine compared to all groups. In poultry industry, it's very important to improve immunity so as to prevent infectious diseases. A variety of such factors as vaccination failure, infection by immune suppressive diseases, and abuse of antibiotics can induce immunodeficiency. Utilization of immunostimulants is one solution to improve the immunity of animals and to decrease their susceptibility to infectious disease (Liu, 1999). Herbs that are rich in flavonoids such as thyme (*Thymus vulgaris*) extend the activity of vitamin C, act as antioxidants and may therefore enhance the immune function (Manach *et al.*, 1996; Cook and Samman, 1996). In agreement with our results, Teymouri Zadeh *et al.* (2009) reported no significant difference in antibody responses to red blood cell and Newcastle disease viruses no between 0.1% *thymus vulgaris* extract received birds and control group (Teymouri Zadeh *et al.*, 2009). None of the immune related parameters such as antibody titer against Newcastle, Influenza viruses and sheep red blood cell, heterophil to lymphocyte ratio and albumin to globulin ratio were differed significantly in broilers treated with 5 and 10 g/kg thyme powder while compared with control birds (Toghyani *et al.*, 2010). Furthermore, Rahimi *et al.* (2011) reported that dietary thyme extract (0.1%) soluble in water increased performance and *lactic acid* counts and reduced *E.coli* numbers but did not affect immune system compared with control group ($P<0.05$) (Rahimi *et al.*,2011).

Table 1. The effect of Thyme extract on HI antibody titer against Newcastle disease virus in broiler chicks.

groups	Days after vaccination			
	0	14	28	35
A (0.1%)	6.7±0.29	2.37±0.9 ^{C*}	4±0.8^{E}	3.04±0.2^{E}
B (0.15%)	6.7±0.29	2.19±0.35 ^{C}	4.1±0.9^{E}	3.25±0.53^{E}
C (0.2%)	6.7±0.29	3.25±0.9 ^{ABDE}	4.3±0.9^{E}	3.47±0.4^{E}
D (vaccinated)	6.7±0.29	2.05±0.7 ^{C}	3. 5±0.3^{E}	2.9±0.37^{E}
E (unvaccinated)	6.7±0.29	1.85±0.35 ^{C}	-	-

Different superscripts in the same column represent significant difference ($p < 0.05$).
*Mean ± standard deviation

Table 2. Effect of probiotic on HI antibody titer against avian Influenza disease virus.

groups	Days after vaccination			
	0	14	28	35
A (0.1%)	6.05±0.8	4.1±0.87^{e*}	5.54±0.82 ^{e}	4.72±0.9 ^{e}
B (0.15%)	6± 0.15	4.6±0.96 ^{e}	5.09±0.75 ^{e}	4.5±0.89^{e}
C (0.2%)	6.13±0.57	4.6±0.84 ^{e}	5.02±0.9^{e}	4.5±0.42 ^{e}
D (vaccinated)	5.9±0.33	4± 0.85 ^{e}	5.1±0.56 ^{e}	4.63±0.48 ^{e}
E (unvaccinated)	6.1±0.19	1.7±0.82^{abcd}	- ^{abcd}	- ^{abcd}

Different superscripts in the same column represent significant difference ($p < 0.05$).
*Mean ± standard deviation

The beneficial effects of thyme plant on bacterial and fungal activities and also potent antioxidant properties of major components of thyme essential oil such as thymol and carvacrol has been reported (Vincent 2002; Basilico and Basilico 1999). Considering the thyme characteristics, we anticipated that an increase in immune response of chicks would be observed. The lower results of thyme extract on immune system is probably related to the dose of additives, type of thyme, possess and preparation period and also vaccination program times and stimulator material that used in our study. Regarding this fact that a few reports are available on the impact of thyme or thyme component on bird immune response, more studies will be needed to investigate thyme extract immonomodulatory properties and principal components (Thymol and carvacol) on broiler health.

4. Conclusions

In conclusion, the results of the present study showed that supplementation of 0.1, 0.15 and 0.2% thyme extract in drinking water did not improve the systemic antibody responses against Newcastle disease vaccine in broiler chickens in the whole experimental period but 14 days after vaccination, receiving of 0.2% of Thyme extract significantly increased the specific antibody response against Influenza vaccine virus compared to all groups.

5. References

Abu-Darwish, M.S., Abu-Dieyeh, Z.H., Batarseh, M., Al-Tawaha, A.R.M and Al-Dalian, S.Y.A. 2009. Trace element contents and essential oil yields from wild thyme plant (*Thymus serpyllum.* L) growth at different natural variable environments, Jordan. *Journal of Food Agriculture and Environment*, 7: 920-924.

Al-Kassie, G.A.M. 2009. Influence of two plant extracts derived from thyme and cinnamon on broiler performance. *Pakistan Veterinary Journal*, 29:169-173.

Al-Mashhadani, E., Farah, H., Al-Jaff, K., Farhan, Y. M. and AL-Mashhadani, H.E. Effect of anise, thyme essential oils and their mixture (EOM) on broiler performance and some physiological traits. 2011. *Egyptian Poultry Science*, 31(2): 481-489.

Bach Knudsen, K.E. 2001. Development of antibiotic resistance and options to replace antimicrobials in animal diets. *Proceedings of the Nutrition Society*, 60:291-299.

Basilico, M.Z. and Basilico, J.C. 1999. Inhibitory effects of some spice essential oils on Aspergillus ochraceus NRRL 3174 growth and ochratoxin A production. *Letter Applied Microbiology*, 29: 238-24

Bolukbasi, S., Erhan, M. 2007. Effect of dietary Thyme (*Thymus vulgaris*) on laying hens performance and *Escherichia coli* (*E. coli*) concentration in feces. *International journal of natural and engineering science*, 1(2): 55-58.

Cervantes H. 2006. Banning antibiotic growth promoters: Learning from the European experience. *Poultry International*, 45: 14-15.

Cook, N. C. and Samman, S. 1996. Flavonoids-chemistry, metabolism, cardio protective effects, and dietary sources. *Journal of Nutrition and Biochemistry,* 7: 66-76.

Cross, D.E., McDevitt, R.M., Hillman, K. 2007. Acamovic. The effect of herbs and their associated essential oils on performance, dietary digestibility and gut microflora in chickens from 7 to 28 days of age. *British Poultry Science*, 48: 496–506.

El-Ghousein, S.S and N.A. Al-Beitawi. 2009. The effect of feeding of crushed Thyme (*Thymus vulgaris*) on growth, blood constituents, and gastrointestinal tract and carcass characteristics of broiler chickens. *Journal of Poultry Science*, 46: 100-104

Fan, M and J. Chen. 2001. Studies on antimicrobial activity of extracts from thyme. *Wei Sheng Wu Xue Bao*, 41: 499-504.

Feizi, A., Bijanzad, P. 2010. Evaluating the Effects of *Thymus vulgaris* extract on Growth Performance Parameters in Broiler Chicken. *Journal of Veterinary Medicine*, 12: 39-45.

Friedman M., Henika, P. R. and Mandrell, R. E. 2002. Bactericidal activities of plant essential oils and some of their isolated constituents against *Campylobacter jejuni*, *Escherichia coli*, *Listeria monocytogenes*, and *Salmonella enterica*. *Journal of Food Protection*, 65:1545-1560.

Greathead, H. 2003. Plants and plant extracts for improving animal productivity. *Proceedings of the Nutrition Society*, 62:279-290.

Hertrampf, J.W. 2001. Alternative antibacterial, performance promoters. *Poultry International*, 40:50-52.

Juven, B. J., Kanner, J., Schved, F. and Weisslowicz, H. 1994. Factors that interact with the antibacterial action of thyme essential oil and its active constituents. *Journal of Applied Bacteriology*. 76:626-631.

Lee, K. W., Everts, H., Kappert, H. J., Frehner, M., Losa, R. and Beynen, A. C. 2003. Effects of dietary essential oil components on growth performance, digestive enzymes and lipid metabolism in female broiler chickens. *British Poultry Science*, 44: 450-457.

Liu, X. Y. 1999. Stress and Immunity. In: "*Poultry Immunology*", (Ed.): Yin, T. B.China Agriculture Press, Beijing, China, 230–252.

Manach, F., Regerat, F. and Texier, O. 1996. Bioavailability, Metabolism and Physiological Impact of 4-oxo-flavonoids. *Nutrition Research*, 16: 517-44.

Masada, Y. 1976. Analysis of oils by gas chromatography and mass spectrometry. Johan Wiley and Sons.

Nevas, M., Korhonen, A. R., Lindstrom, M., Turkki, P. and Korkeala, H. 2004. Antibacterial efficiency of finnish spice essential oils against pathogenic and spoilage bacteria. *Journal of Food Protection*, 67: 199-202.

Nollet, L. 2005. AGP alternatives-part I. EU close to a future without antibiotic growth promoters. *World Poultry*, 21: 14-15.

Patterson, J.A., Burkholder, K.M. 2003. Application of prebiotics and probiotics in poultry production. *Poultry Science*, 82: 627–631.

Rahimi, S., Teymouri Zadeh, Z., Karimi Torshizi, M. A., Omidbaigi, R. and Rokni, H. 2011. Effect of the Three Herbal Extracts on Growth Performance, Immune System, Blood Factors and Intestinal Selected Bacterial Population in Broiler Chickens. *Journal of Agricultural Science and Technology*, 13: 527-539

Ricke, S.C. 2003. Perspectives on the use of organic acids and short chain fatty acids as antimicrobials. *Poultry Science* , 82: 632–639.

Suppakul, P., Miltz, J., Sonneveld, K. and Bigger, S. W. 2003. Antimicrobial properties of basil and its possible application in food packaging. *Journal of Agricultural and Food Chemistry*, 51: 3197- 3207.

Tabak, M., Armon, R., Potasman, I. and Neeman, I. 1996. *In vitro* inhibition of Helicobacter pylori by extracts of thyme. *Journal of Applied Bac*teriology, 80: 667-672.

Teymouri Zadeh, Z., Rahimi, S.H., Karimi Torshizi, M.A., Omidbaigi, R. 2009. *Iranian Journal of Medicinal and Aromatic Plants*, Vol 25, No. 1.

Thakare, M. 2004. Pharmacological screening of some medicinal plants as antimicrobial and feed additive, M.S Thesis, Virginia Polytechnic Institute and State University, Blacksburg, Virginia USA.

Toghyani, M., Tohidi M,Gheisari, A., Tabeidian, S. 2010. Performance, immunity, serum biochemical and hematological parameters in broiler chicks fed dietary thyme as alternative for an antibiotic growth promoter. *African Journal of Biote*chnology, 9(40): 6819-6825.

Ultee, A., Slump. R. A., Steging, G. and Smid, E. J. 2000. Antimicrobial activity of carvacrol toward *Bacillus cereus* on rice. *Journal of Food Protection*, 63: 620-624.

Vahdatpour, T., Nikpiran, H., Babazadeh, D., Vahdatpourand, S. & Jafargholipour, M.A. 2011. Effects of Protexin ®, Fermacto ® and combination of them on blood enzymes and performance of Japanese quails (Coturnix Japonica). *Annals of Biological Researches*, 2: 283-291.

Wakeman, G.W. 2005. AGP alternatives- Part II. Dietary strategies to influence bacterial microflora. *World Poultry*, 21: 28-29.

Vincent, H.V. 2002. Carvacrol and thymol reduce swine waste odour and pathogens stability of oils. *Current Microbiology*, 44: 38-43.

11

Anti-diabetic and hypolipidaemic activities of *Solenostemon monostachyus*

Jude E. Okokon[1]*, Louis U. Amazu[2], Lucky L. Nwidu[3]

[1]*Department of Pharmacology and Toxicology, Faculty of Pharmacy, University of Uyo, Uyo – Nigeria;*

Email: *judeefiom@yahoo.com

[2]*Department of Pharmacology and Therapeutics, College of Medicine, Evans Enwerem University, Orlu Campus, Imo State;*

[3]*Department of Pharmacology and Toxicology, Faculty of Pharmacy, Niger Delta University, Wilberforce Island, Bayelsa State;*

ARTICLE INFO

Topic: *Pharmacology*

Key words:

- ✓ Solenostemon monostachyus
- ✓ *Anti-diabetic*
- ✓ *hypolipidemic*
- ✓ *diabetes*

ABSTRACT

Background & Aim: *Solenostemon monostachyus* has remain invincible in Ibibio ethnomedicine for the management of numerous ailment including diabetes mellitus. Many of these ethnomedicinal claims are yet to be pharmacologically verified. The purpose of this study therefore was to subject the extract/fractions of *Solenostemon monostachyus* used in folkloric management of diabetes to scientific assay.

Experimental: The crude extract and fractions of *S. monostachyus* (75 -225 mg/kg) were evaluated for antidiabetic activity in alloxan – induced diabetic rats. The antidiabetic activity during acute and prolong studies were investigated. Glibenclamide, 10 mg/kg, was used as positive control. The Blood Glucose Level (BGL) was measured by using a glucometer and the various lipids level were estimated using Randox diagnostic kits.

Results & Discussion: Treatment of alloxan diabetic rats with the extract/fractions caused a significant ($p<0.001$) reductions in BGL of the diabetic rats both in acute and prolong treatment (two weeks). The activities of extract and fractions were comparable to that of glibenclamide in prolonged study. *S. monostachyus* treatment showed considerable lowering of serum total cholesterol, triglycerides, LDL cholesterol, VLDL cholesterol and an increase in HDL cholesterol in the treated diabetic group.

Industrial and practical recommendations: These results suggest that the extract of *S. monostachyus* possesses anti-diabetic and hypolipidaemic effect on alloxan-induced diabetic rats which can be exploited in the management of diabetes.

1. Introduction

Solenostemon monostachyus P. Beauv (family Lamiaceae) is an important herb that is widespread in West and Central Africa. It occurs as an annual weed in anthropogenic habitats and rocky savannahs. It is slightly succulent, aromatic and grows up to 100 cm tall (Mba and Menut, 1994). The aerial parts of the plant are used in various decoctions traditionally by the Ibibios of the Niger Delta of Nigeria to treat stomach ulcer, fever/malaria (Ajibesin *et al.*, 2008; Adebayo and Krettli, 2011), hemorrhoid and other inflammatory diseases. The decoction of the plant is also used to treat hypertension as well as a diuretic (Koffi *et al.*, 2009). The infusion of the leaves is used to treat diabetes in part of Nigeria and Côte d'Ivoire (Olabanji *et al.*, 2008; Djama *et al.*, 2012), Phytochemical studies on *Solenostemon monostachyus* leaves have revealed the presence of water, proteins, lipids, glucids, calcium, phosphate (Buisson *et al.,* 1965), essential oil (Mve-Mba *et al.*, 1994) and phyto-constituents such as diterpenoids (Toshio *et al.* 1980), flavonoids, coumarin, polyphenol (Datte *et al.,* 2010; N'guessan *et al.,* 2011). The leaf essential oil of *S. monostachyus* has been reported to contain; β-pinene, oct-1-en-3-ol, β-caryophyllene, octan-3-ol and (*E, E*)-α-farnesene (Mvé-Mba *et al.,* 1994). The plant has been reported to possess antimicrobial (Ekundayo and Ezeogu, 2006), antioxidant (Datte *et al.*, 2010; N'guessan *et al.,* 2011; Okoko and Ere, 2012), antihypertensive (Fidele *et al.,* 2012) and antiulcer activities (Okokon *et al.*, 2015). We report the antidiabetic and hypolipidaemic activities of *Solenostemon monostachyus* in alloxan induced diabetic rats to provide scientific basis for it use in traditional medicine to treat diabetes and associated diseases.

2. Materials and Methods

2.1. Plants collection

The plant material *Solenostemon monostachyus* (aerial parts) was collected in a farmland in Uruan area, Akwa Ibom State, Nigeria in August, 2014. The plant was identified and authenticated by Dr. Margaret Bassey of Department of Botany and Ecological Studies, University of Uyo, Uyo, Nigeria. Herbarium specimen (FPUU 573) was deposited at Department of Pharmacognosy and Natural Medicine Herbarium.

2.2. Extraction

The plant aerial parts were washed and shade-dried for two weeks. The dried plants' materials were reduced to powder using mortar and pistle. The powdered material was soaked in 50% ethanol. The liquid filtrates were concentrated and evaporated to dryness in vacuo 40°C using rotary evaporator. The extract (2g) was partitioned with a 50:50 mixture of distilled water and chloroform. The aqueous fraction was evaporated to dryness in a water bath at 60°C and the chloroform fraction air-dried. The ethanol extract, the aqueous and chloroform fractions were stored at - 4°C. until used in a refrigerator.

2.3. Phytochemical Screening

Phytochemical screening of the crude extract was carried out employing standard procedures and tests (Trease and Evans, 1989, Sofowora, 1993), to reveal the presence of chemical constituents such as alkaloids, flavonoids, tannins, terpenes, saponins, anthraquinones, reducing sugars, cardiac glycosides among others.

2.4. Animals

Albino male rats (110 – 130 g) of either sex were obtained from the University of Uyo animal house. They were maintained on standard animal pellets and water *ad libitum*. Permission and approval for animal studies were obtained from the College of Health Sciences Animal Ethics committee, University of Uyo.

2.5. Determination of median lethal dose (LD_{50})

The median lethal dose (LD_{50}) of the extract was estimated using albino mice by intraperitoneal (*i.p*) route using the method of Lorke (1983). This involved intraperitoneal administration of different doses of the extract (100-1000 mg/kg) to groups of three mice each. The animals were observed for manifestation of physical signs of toxicity such as writhing, decreased motor activity, decreased body/limb tone, decreased respiration and death. The number of deaths in each group within 24 hours was recorded. The LD_{50} was calculated as geometrical means of the maximum dose producing 0% (a) and the minimum dose producing 100% mortality (b).

$$LD_{50} = \sqrt{ab}$$

2.6. Evaluation of anti-diabetic and hypolipidemic activity of the Extract and fractions

2.6.1. Induction of diabetes and animal treatment: Diabetes was induced in 24 h fasted animals (male rats) by a single intraperitoneal injection of a freshly prepared solution of alloxan monohydrate (150 mg/kg) in ice cold 0.9% saline (NaCl) solution. The animals were given 2 ml of 5% dextrose solution using orogastric tube immediately after induction to overcome the drug induced hypoglycemia. 72 hours later, rats with blood glucose level (BGL) above 200 mg/dl were considered diabetic and selected for the experiment.

The animals were randomly divided into seven groups of 6 rats each and treated as follows:
Group I: Diabetic rats administered *Solenostemon monostachyus* extract (75 mg/kg/day) orally for 14 days.
Group II: Diabetic rats given *Solenostemon monostachyus* extract (150 mg/kg/day) orally for 14 days.
Group III: Diabetic rats administered orally with *Solenostemon monostachyus* extract (225 mg/kg/day) for 14 days.
Group IV: Diabetic rats administered orally with chloroform fraction of *C. lutea* (150 mg/kg/day) for 14 days.
Group V: Diabetic rats administered orally with aqueous fraction of *Solenostemon monostachyus* (150 mg/kg/day) for 14 days.
Group VI: Diabetic rats given Glibenclamide (10 mg/kg/day) for 14 days orally.
Group VII: Diabetic control rats receiving normal saline (10 ml/kg) for 14 days.

The change in body weight and fasting BGL of all the rats were recorded at regular intervals during the experimental period. For acute study, the BGL was monitored after 1, 3, 5 and 7h of administration of a single dose of the extract and at the end of 1, 3, 5, 7 and 14 days for prolonged treatments. The BGL was monitored in the blood of the diabetic rats by tail tipping method. The blood was dropped on the dextrostix reagent pad. This was inserted into microprocessor digital blood glucometer and the readings were recorded (WHO, 1980).

2.7. Evaluation of hypolipidemic activity of the extract and fractions

After 14 days of treatments with the extract/fractions (24 h after the last dose), the rats were anaesthetized with ethyl ether vapor and the blood was collected through cardiac puncture into sample bottles devoid of anticoagulant. The samples were centrifuged at 1000 rpm for 15mins to obtain the sera. Serum cholesterol, triglyceride and High Density Lipoprotein (HDL) levels were measured by enzymatic colorimetric methods using Randox diagnostic kits. All samples were analyzed with a wine light Unicam spectrophotometer. The concentrations of low density lipoprotein (LDL) and very low density lipoprotein (VLDL) were calculated from the formula of Friedwald *et al.,* (1972). These analyses were done at Department of Chemical Pathology, University of Uyo Teaching Hospital, (UUTH), Uyo.

2.8. Statistical analysis

All the group data were statistically analyzed with one – way ANOVA, followed by Tukey – Krammer multiple comparison posttest. Values of $p<0.01$ were considered significant.

3. Results and discussion

Phytochemical screening of the crude extract of *Solenostemon monostachyus* revealed that the crude extract contained tannins, saponins, cardiac glycosides, anthraquinones, flavonoids, steroids and terpenes, alkaloids and phlobatannins.

The median lethal dose (LD_{50}) was calculated to be 748.331 mg/kg. The physical signs of toxicity included excitation, paw licking, increased respiratory rate, decreased motor activity, gasping and coma which was followed by death

There were observable changes in the body weight of treated and untreated alloxan-induced diabetic rats. Treatment of alloxan-induced diabetic rats with ethanol crude extract/fractions of *Solenostemon monostachyus* or glibenclamide considerably improved the weights of treated diabetic rats compared to untreated diabetic rats (Table 1).

The crude extract (75–225 mg/kg) produced dose-dependent reductions in blood glucose level (BGL) alloxan-induced diabetic rats relative to control during acute studies. These effects were statistically significant ($p < 0.05 – 0.001$) and progressed for 7 hours (Table 2). The effect of the highest dose of the extract (225 mg/kg) at the end of 7 hr as well as that of chloroform fraction were more significant than that of the standard drug, glibenclamide (Table 2).

On prolonged treatment (14 days), the extract produced sustained reductions of BGL in diabetic rats. These reductions were significant ($p < 0.05 - 0.001$) when compared to control (Table 3). The effect of the highest dose of the extract and that of the chloroform fraction was comparable to that of standard drug, glibenclamide, 10 mg/kg, on day 14.

Table 1. Effect of ethanolic extract/fractions of *Solenostemon monostachyus* on body weights of alloxan - induced diabetic rats.

Treatment	Dose (mg/kg)	Day 0	Day 15	Change in body weight
Control	0.2ml	126.8 ± 8.65	102.5±6.20	- 24.30
Extract	75	122.4 ±5.14	124.1±4.35	1.70
	150	126.2 ±8.11	130.5± 7.42	4.33
	225	125.8 ±6.55	130.5±9.52	4.70
Chloroform fraction	150	126.8±9.86	133.4±9.67	6.60
Aqueous fraction	150	124.8±6.65	131.5±8.54	6.70
Glibenclamide	10	128.6±7.16	138.3±5.21	9.70

Data are represented as mean ± SEM. (n=6) .

Table 2. Effect of ethanol extract and fractions of *Solenostemon monostachyus* aerial parts on blood glucose level of alloxan-induced diabetic rats during acute study.

Treatment	Dose	Blood glucose level (mg/dl) in hours				
	(mg/kg)	0hr	1hr	3hr	5hr	7hr
Control	0.2ml	240.4± 5.82	245.0± 4.33	250.0± 5.22	258.4 ± 6.65	254.2± 6.26
Crude extract	75	235.2 ± 3.19	231.2 ± 3.64	224.2 ± 3.90[a]	215.0 ± 7.28[a]	218.0 ± 6.89[b]
	150	240.4 ± 5.68	236.4 ± 6.30	220.2 ± 3.12[c]	194.0 ± 14.10[c]	187.4±.4.10[c]
	225	242.8± 6.77	234.7 ± 3.48	211.8 ± 2.84[c]	188.9 ± 2.43[c]	175.4±2.58 [c]
Chloroform fraction	150	237.2 ± 4.90	229.3 ± 4.37	197.0± 5.26 [c]	161.0 ± 3.69[c]	157.6± 2.70[c]
Aqueous fraction	150	243.4±7.60	223.6 ± 5.12	215.0 ± 9.22[c]	196.2± 10.00[c]	184.8±8.99[c]
Glibenclamide	10	242.4± 4.36	235.2 ± 3.24	216.4± 3.18[c]	197.8 ± 9.25[c]	180.0 ± 3.17[c]

Data are expressed as mean ± SEM. Significant at [a]p< 0.05, [b]p< 0.01, [c]p< 0.001. When compared to control. (n=6).

Table 3. Effect of ethanol extract and fractions of *Solenostemon monostachyus* aerial parts on blood glucose level of alloxan-induced diabetic rats during prolonged treatment

Treatment	Dose in	Blood glucose level (mg/dl) in days			
	(mg/kg)	Day 0	Day 1	Day 7	Day 14
Control	0.2ml	240.4± 5.82	254.0± 7.31	260.0 ± 9.34	267.2 ± 10.67
Crude extract	75	235.2 ± 3.19	222.2± 9.38	186.2 ± 10.78 [a]	139.4 ± 8.33[c]
	150	240.4 ± 5.68	186.5±6.64 [c]	140.4 ± 8.12 [a]	95.6± 4.15 [c]
	225	242.8± 6.77	185.6± 8.26 [c]	135.5± 8.10[a]	82.2 ± 2.26 [c]
Chloroform fraction	150	237.2 ± 4.90	202.3 ± 10.38 [b]	120.0± 10.14[a]	85.8± 5.98 [c]
Aqueous fraction	150	243.4±7.60	212.5 ± 9.63 [a]	146.8 ± 8.84 [a]	118.6 ± 5.96 [c]
Glibenclamide	10	242.4± 4.36	175.2 ± 8.20 [c]	106.0 ± 11.76 [a]	80.2 ± 6.44 [c]

Data are expressed as mean ± SEM. Significant at [a]p<0.05; bp< 0.01,cp<0.001 when compared to control (n = 6).

Table 4. Effect of ethanolic leaf extract and fractions of *Solenostemon monostachyus* on serum total cholesterol, triglycerides, HDL – cholesterol, LDL – cholesterol and VLDL – chol of alloxan- induced diabetic rats.

Drug	Dose mg/kg	Average Serum lipids profile (mMOL/L)				
		Total Cholesterol	Triglycerides	HDL Cholesterol	LDL Cholesterol	VLDL Chol
Control(Normal saline)	0.2ml	4.22±0.14	2.40±0.17	0.74±0.11	2.21±0.14	1.20±0.17
Crude Extract	75	3.92±0.37 [c]	2.10±0.12	1.02±0.14	1.52±0.20	0.92±0.04[c]
	150	3.71±0.12 [c]	1.49±0.28[a]	1.16±0.18[c]	1.12±0.16	0.74±0.06[c]
	225	3.24±0.15 [a]	1.25±0.31[c]	1.38±0.15[c]	1.05±0.06[c]	0.68±0.12[c]
Chloroform fraction	150	3.31±0.26 [c]	1.28±0.26[c]	1.58±0.12[c]	0.68±0.11	0.59±0.09[c]
Aqueous fraction	150	3.40±0.14 [c]	1.35±0.23[c]	1.50±0.15[b]	0.86±0.12[c]	0.45±0.05[c]
Glibenclamide	10	3.02±0.18[c]	1.05±0.48 [c]	1.60±0.14[c]	0.55±0.12[c]	0.42±0.08[c]

Data are expressed as mean ± SEM. Significant at [a]$p < 0.05$, [b]$p < 0.01$, [c]$p < 0.001$. When compared to control (n=6).

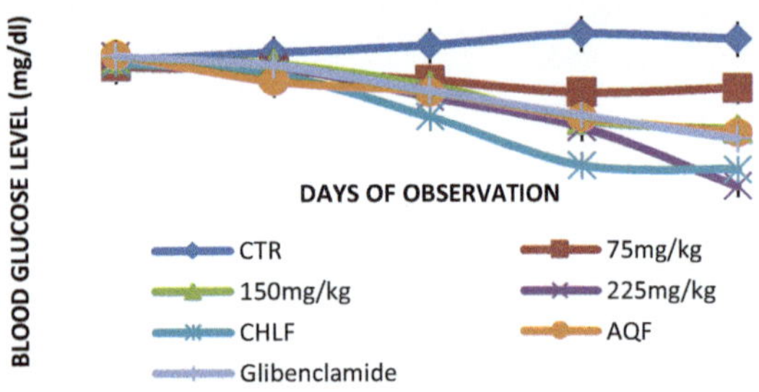

Fig. 1. Blood glucose level in days of observation.

Solenostemon monostachyus leaves are used in different decoctions to treat diabetes in parts of Nigeria and Côte d'Ivoire (Olabanji *et al.*, 2008; Djama *et al.*, 2012). In this study, evaluation of antidiabetic and hypolipidemic activities of *Solenostemon monostachyus* aerial parts extract/fractions (75-225 mg/kg) were carried out in alloxan-induced diabetic rats. The extract which showed moderate toxicity was observed to demonstrate significant antidiabetic and hypolipidemic activities in alloxan-induced diabetic rats following treatment with the extract for two weeks.

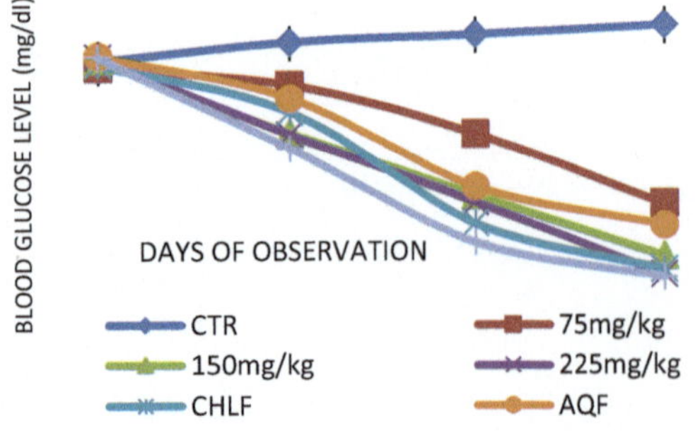

Fig. 2. Blood glucose level in days of observation.

Repeated administration of the extract and fractions of *Solenostemon monostachyus* aerial parts for a period of 2 weeks to diabetic rats caused significant decrease in BGL of treated diabetic rats compared to untreated diabetic rats. These results corroborate those of Amaechi *et al.,* (2015) who worked on streptozotocin-induced diabetic rats using a single dose and reported significant antidiabetic activity of the leaf extract of *S. monostachyus*. Thus confirming strongly the antidiabetic potentials of this plant as claimed in ethnomedicine. Secondary metabolites of plants such as polysaccharides (Tomoda *et al.,* 1985), terpenes and tannins (Reher *et al.,* 1991), steroids (Ivorra *et al.,* 1989), and alkaloids (Karawya and Wahab, 1984) have been reported to possess antidiabetic activity. Phytochemical studies of the *Solenostemon monostachyus* revealed the presence of terpenes, saponins, tannins and alkaloids as well as coumarins, polyphenols, monoterpenes, diterpenoids and sesquiterpenes (Toshio *et al.,* 1980; Mvé-Mba *et al*., 1994; Datte *et al*., 2010; N'guessan *et al.*, 2011). These constituents may in part be responsible for the observed significant activity of this extract either singly or in synergy with one another. Sulphonylureas cause hypoglycemia by stimulating insulin secretion from the pancreas and these compounds are potent in mild alloxan induced diabetes and inactive in intense alloxan induced diabetes whereby nearly all β –cells have been destroyed (Yallow *et al.,* 1960). The reduction in BGL of the diabetic rats by glibenclamide in this study portrays an insevere state of diabetes. The body weights of the treated diabetic rats were found to increase significantly contrary to those of untreated diabetic rats. Diabetes is associated with a severe loss in body weight due to loss or degradation of structural proteins (Rajkumar *et al.,* 1991). Treatment of the diabetic rats with extract/fractions of *Solenostemon monostachyus* remedied this condition. Several mechanisms of antidiabetic action of plants have been reported. Some plants' extracts are reported to exert hypoglycemic action by potentiating the insulin effect, either by increasing the pancreatic secretion of insulin from the cells of islets of langerhans or its release from bound insulin (Pari and Amarnath, 2004). While others act through extra pancreatic mechanisms by inhibition of hepatic glucose production (Edduoks *et al.*, 2003) or corrections of insulin resistance (Hu *et al.,* 2003). These extract and fractions may have acted through one of the above mechanisms.

Elevations of serum lipids levels are usually observed during severe diabetes and have been implicated in the development of artherosclerosis (Minorava *et al.,* 2000). In this study also, the serum lipids (total cholesterol, triglycerides, LDL and VLDL) levels of the extract treated diabetic rats were found to be significantly reduced, except that of HDL which was increased, following 2 weeks of treatment with the extract as against that in the untreated diabetic rats in this study. This result is in agreement with the report of Amaechi *et al*., (2015), who reported similar activity with the leaf extract of the plant though employing a single dose. Diabetes–induced hyperlipidemia is attributable to excess mobilization of fat from the adipose due to the under utilization of glucose (Krishnakumar *et al.,* 2000). The alleviation of the diabetic state due to the administration of the extract may have increased the utilization of glucose, thereby depressing the mobilization of fat. Also, the plant extract may have stimulated lipoprotein lipase activities resulting in decrease of plasma triglyceride and probably, increase the uptake of triglyceride from plasma by skeletal muscle and adipose tissues (El-Hazmi and Warsy, 2001).

Phytochemical compounds like phenols, tannins, alkaloids, steroids, cardiac glycosides, flavonoids and terpenes present in this extract have been reported to exert antilipidemic activity (Tandon, 2005). They may in part be responsible for the hypolipidemic activity of this extract.

4. Conclusions

The results of this study show that ethanol extract/fractions of *Solenostemon monostachyus* aerial part possessed antidiabetic and hypolipidemic properties. This confirmation justifies its use in ethnomedical medicine for the treatment of diabetes.

5. Acknowledgement

The authors are grateful to Ms. Sifon Akpan of Department of Pharmacology and Toxicology for her technical assistance.

6. References

Adebayo, J.O., Krettli, A.U. 2011. Potential antimalarials from Nigerian plants: A review. *J Ethnopharm.*, 133: 289 –302.

Ajibesin, K.K., Ekpo, B.A., Bala, D.N., Essien, E.E., Adesanya, S.A. 2008. Ethnobotanical survey of Akwa Ibom State of Nigeria. *J Ethnopharm* 115: 387 – 408.

Amaechi, D., Udosen, E.O., Edet, E.E., Asanga, E.E., Mbakwe, I.E. 2015. Lipid profile status of streptozotocin induced diabetic rats treated with ethanolic leaf extract of *Solenostemon monostachyus. J. Med Plts Res*., 9(8): 289 – 293.

Amazu, L.U., Antia, B.S., Okokon, J.E. 2015. Antiulcer activity of *Solenostemon monostachyus. The J. Phytopharmacol.,* 4(2): 97 – 101

Buisson, P. 1965. Plantes alimentaires de l'Ouest Africain: Etude botanique, biologique et chimique. Leconte, Marseille, France., 568 pp.

Datte, J.Y., Kpahe, F., Offoumou, A.M. 2010. Acute toxicity and antioxidant activity of hydroethanolic extract of *Solenostemon monostachyus* P. Beauv. Leaves. *J compl integr med.*, Vol 7 Art. 45.

Djama, A.A., Kouassi Goffri, M.C., Koua, A.A., Ofosu, F.G., Aboh, I.J .2012. Heavy Metal Analysis of Some Anti-diabetic Medicinal Plants in Côte d'Ivoire. *Current Research Journal of Biological Sciences*., 4(5): 633-637.

Desai, P.D., Ganguly, A.K., Govindahari, T.R., Joshi, B.S., Kamat, V.N., Mande, A.H., Mohammed, P.A., Nagle, S.K., Nayak, R.H., Saksena, A.K., Sathe, S.S., Vishwanathan, N. 1966. Chemical investigation of some Indian plants; Part II. *Ind J Chem*., 4: 457.

Ekundayo, E.O., Ezeogu, L.I. 2006. Evaluation of antimicrobial activities of extracts of five plants used in traditional medicine in Nigeria. *Intern. J. Trop. Med.*, 1: 93-96.

El-Hazmi, M.A., Warsy, A.S. 2001. Evaluation of serum cholesterol and triglyceride levels in 1-6-year-old Saudi children. Journal of Tropical Pediatrics., 47: 181-185.

Fidele, K.Z., Andre, K.B., Yao, D.J., Michel, O.A. 2012. Action of hydroethanolic leaves extract of *Solenostemon monostachyus* (lamiaceae) on cardiovascular system of mammalians: blood pressure lowering effects. *Intl J Pharm Biol Sci.,* 2(3): 310-320.

Edduoks, M., Jouad, H., Maghrani, M., Lemhadri, A., Burcelin, R., 2003. Inhibition of endogenous glucose production accounts for hypoglycemic effect of *Spergularaia purpurea* in streptozotocin mice. *Phytomedicine* 10:594 – 599.

Ghosal, S., Singh, A.K., Govindachari, T.R., Joshi, B.S., Kamat, V.N., Manmade, A.H., Mohammed, P.A., Nagle, S.K., Nayak, R.H., Saksena, A.K., Sathe, S.S., Vishwanathan, N. 1974. Chemical investigation of some Indian medicinal plants: Part II. *Ind J Chem.,* 4: 457.

Hu, X., Sato, J., Oshida, Y., Xu, M., Bajotto, G., Sato, Y. 2003. Effect of Goshajinki-Gan(Chinese herbal medicine:Niu-Che-Sen-Qi-Wan) on insulin resistance in streptozotocin induced diabetic rats.*Diabetes Res and Clin Pract.,* 59: 103 – 111.

Ivorra, M. D., Paya, M., Villar, A. 1989. A review of natural products and plants as potential antidiabetic agents. *J. Ethnopharmacol.,* 27: 243-275.

Karawya, M.S., Wahab, S.A. 1984. Diphenylamine, an antihyperglycaemic agent from onion and tea. *J. Nat. Prod.,* 47: 775-780.

Krishnakumar, K., Augustti, K.T., Vijayammal, P.L. 2000. Hypolipidaemic effect of *Salacia oblonga* Wall. root bark in streptozotocin diabetic rats. *Med. Science* 28: 65-67.

Kirtikar, K.R., Basu, B.D. 1999. Indian Medicinal Plants. 2nd edition. Bishen Sing Mahendra Pal Sing, Dehhradun, pp. 1655 – 1656.

Koffi, N., Marie –Solange, T., Emma, A.A., Noel, Z.G. 2009. Ethnobotanical study of plants used to reat arterial hypertension in traditional medicine, by abbey and Krobou population of Agboville (Cote d'ivoire).*Eur. J. Sci. Res.*, 35: 85-98.

Mba, C.E., Menut, C. 1994. Aromatic plants of tropical Central Africa. *Flav Frag J.*, 9: 315-317.

Mve-Mba, C.E., Menut, C., Lamaty, G., Zollo, P.H.A., Tchoumbougnang. 1994. Aromatic plants of tropical central Africa. Part XIX. Volatile components from leaves of two lamiaceae from Cameroon: *Leucas deflexa* Hook. and *Solenostemon monostachyus* (P.Beauv.) Briq. *Flav Frag J.,* 9(6): 315-317

N'Guessan, H.A., Dago, D.C.E., Mamyrbekova-Bekro, J.A., Békro, Y.A. 2011. CCM d'extraits selectifs de 10 plantes utilisées dans le traitement traditionnel de l'hypertension arterielle en Côte d'Ivoire. *Eur J Sci Res.*, 66 (4): 575-585.

Mironova, M.A., Klein, R.L., Virella, G.T., Lopes-Virella, M.F. 2000. Antimodified LDL antibodies, LDL – containing immune complexes and susceptibility of LDL to in vitro oxidation in patients with type-2 diabetes. *Diabetes.,* 49: 1033 – 1049.

Okoko, T., Ere, D. 2012. Antioxidant activities of *Solenostemon monostachyus* leaf extract using *in vitro* methods. *Sci Res Essays.,* 7(6): 621-626.

Olabanji, S.O., Omobuwajo, O.R., Ceccato, D. 2008. Accelerator-based analytical technique in the study of some antidiabetic medicinal plants of Nigeria. *Nucl. Instr. Meth. Phys. Res.,* 266: 2387-2390.

Pari, L., Amarnath, S. 2004. Antidiabetic activity of *Boerhavia diffusa* L.: effect on hepatic key enzymes in experimental diabetes. *J. Ethnopharmacol.,* 91: 109-113.

Rajkumar, L., Govindarajulu P. 1991. Increased degradation of dermal collagen in diabetic rats.*Ind J.Exp Biol,* 29: 1081 – 1083.

Reher, G., Slijepcevic, M., Krans, L. 1991. Hypoglycaemic activity of triterpenes and tannins from *Sarcopoterium spinosum* and two *Sanguisorba species*. *Planta. Med,* 57:A57-A58.

Sofowora, A. 1993. Medicinal Plants and Traditional Medicine in Africa. 2nd ed. Spectrum Books Limited, Ibadan, Nigeria.

Tandon, S. 2005. Phytochemicals and cardiovascular health.*Current R and D High.*, 28: 18 – 22.

Toshio, M., Peter, R., Conrad, H.E. 1980. Structures of six Coleons (Diterpenoids) from *Solenostemon monostachyus* (P. Beauv.) Briq. (Labiatae). *Helvetica Chimica Acta*- 63, Fasc.1-Nr.9

Tomoda, M., Shimada, K., Konno, C., Hikino, H. 1985. Structure of Panaxan B, A hypoglycaemic glycan of *Panax ginseng* roots. *Phytochem*, 24:2431-2433.

Effect of Sucrose Replacement by Stevia as a Non-Nutritive Sweetener and Bulking Compounds on Physiochemical Properties of Foodstuffs

Alaleh Nikooie[1], Amir Pouya Ghandehari Yazdi[1*], Mina Shamsaei[2], Leila Sedaghat Boroujeni[3]

[1]*Department of Food Science and Technology, Shahrekord Branch, Islamic Azad University, Sharekord, Iran;*
[*]**Email:** ***foodtechnology43@yahoo.com***

[2]*Department of Food Science and Technology, Khorasgan Branch, Islamic Azad University, Isfahan, Iran;*
[3]*Department of Food Science and Technology, Science and Research Branch of Tehran, Islamic Azad University, Tehran, Iran;*

ARTICLE INFO

Topic: *Medicinal Plants*

Key words:

- *Stevia*
- *Physiochemical properties*
- *Food products*
- *Sweetener*

ABSTRACT

Background & Aim: Changes in lifestyle, decrease in physical exercise along with incidence of obesity, hypertension and cardiovascular diseases indicate a need for low calorie formulations. The sweetness of Stevia, a natural sweetener, is estimated to be 300 times as much as that of sugar. Extraction of stevia leaves is considered a promoter of calorie balance and a beneficial part of a healthy diet. Stevia is also used to treat diabetes, obesity, tooth decay, hypertension, exhaustion and depression.

Experimental: Regarding the aforementioned applications and critical role of sucrose in the creation of texture, color and taste, the replacement of sucrose is an important issue. Most researches indicate the fact that sugar-free products are not pleasant and acceptable; thus, the presence of sugar is inevitable i.e. in case of complete substitution, concurrent consumption of both sugar and stevia (different combinations) seemingly gives it more flavors and makes it the most demanded product. This article reviews effective parameters in sucrose substitution with stevia and the results obtained from it.

Industrial and practical recommendations: Its bitter aftertaste can diminish its consumption in food formulation; however, other flavoring agents and fillers can modify this problem. With regard to its high sweetness (300 times as much as sucrose), its consumption is low and thus it is economically justifiable. Using this sweetener in daily industries, fruit juices and confectioneries as a sucrose substitute is possible with respect to the research findings.

1. Introduction

Nowadays, changes in lifestyle, reduction of physical education and exercise, and incidence of diseases such as obesity and cardiovascular problems are all factors in obligation of production low calorie foods and decrease of sucrose consumption due to incidence of diabetes and its undesirable effects on the body (Glicksman and Farkas, 1966). Since obesity is a complicated disorder with both environmental and genetic reasons, its incidence due to quick changes in lifestyle and increase of fatty foods consumption has increasingly grown in the Middle Eastern countries, and recently, it is considered a prevalent reason for mortality. In Iran, incidence of obesity in children and teenagers is 8.8% and 4.5%, respectively (Farokhzad and Bagheri, 2004). Overall, using nonnutritive sweeteners as a possible solution to the prohibition of obesity has widely been taken into consideration by researchers.

1.1. Stevia

Stevia, which refers to all products from *Stevia rebaudiana* (Carakostas *et al.*, 2008), is a natural sweetener practically used in pharmaceutical industries (Mogra and Dashora, 2009; Ahmed *et al.*, 2011). Stevioside was first extracted by Bertoni, and after that by a French chemist (Ahmed *et al.*, 2011; Jaroslov *et al.*, 2007). Stevia sweetness is estimated to be 300 times as much as that of sugar cane (Ghosh *et al.*, 2008; Koyama *et al.*, 2003; Laribi *et al.*, 2012). Stevia is native to Brazil and Paraguay (named Paraguay sweet plant). The most abundant varieties include *Stevia eupatoria, Stevia ovate, Stevia plummerae, Stevia rebaudiana, Stevia salicifolia,* and *Stevia serrata* (Curry and Roberts, 2008). Stevia is diploid with 11 paired chromosomes (Brandle *et al.*, 1998). Studies have shown that stevia can be a replacement for some/all sugar sources with acceptable physical and eventual properties but no remarkable side effects (Madan *et al.*, 2012). So far, 9 diterpenic glycoside compounds have been identified in *Stevia rebaudiana* structure with a common skillet (figure 1) (Reddy *et al.*, 2005). These compounds compose 5-10% of dried leaves and heat-sensitive; besides, they are 200-300 times as sweet as sugar beet (Ahmed *et al.*, 2011). This partial sweetness arises from diterpen glycosides, which seem to occur due to the difference in remained carbohydrates in carbons number 13 and 19, common in hardness of aglicon steviol. A new method of extraction and refinery of these compounds and their pharmacokinetical investigation has been reported by Chatsudthipon and Muanprasate (Thomas and Glade, 2010). Most processes are accompanied by using organic solvents and coagulators, in some cases, chromatography or chelating agents along with extracting solvents have also been used. However, all previously mentioned processes have complicated processes, which need modifications in order to lessen the use of chemicals, extra steam, color and flavor. Direct effect of stevioside (low concentration) in transferring Glucose in skeletal organs was investigated and the results revealed that insulin activities improve (Ahmed *et al.*, 2011) and thus it can be concluded that stevia extract is considered a beneficial part of healthy lifestyles in diet (Thomas *et al.*, 2010). Stevia is used to cure diabetes, obesity, tooth decay, hypertension, exhaustion and depression (Mogra and Dashora, 2009; Ghosh *et al.*, 2008; Goyal and Goyal, 2010). Stevioside and Rebadioside A, polyphenolic compounds of stevia extract, are non-decay e.g. sucrose solution causes tooth decay in rat's infants while no decay has been observed in stevioside consumption. Stevioside also has inhibited S. Mutans, the main organism of tooth decay, along with low acid secretion condition (Thomas and Glade, 2010); besides, it has been recommended as an inhibitor of microorganisms' growth in the mouth (Fatemi, 2007). Table 1 depicts researches on sucrose replaced with Stevia as a non-nutritive sweetener in various products.

1.2. Investigation of sucrose replacement with stevia on color and microstructural properties of food products

Regarding the key role of sucrose in creation of color in browning processes, three color indexes including L* ‹a*, and b* were used to investigate products' color where L* is brightness ranges from 0(darkness)-100(light reflection). Positive amounts of a* refer to red and its negative amounts to green; moreover, positive amounts of b* are related to yellow and negative amounts to blue (Ghandehari Yazdi *et al.*, 2013). Substitution of sucrose with Stevioside in biscuits significantly brightens treatments in two levels of %50 and %100 replacement (Vatankhah *et al.*, 2014). Besides, results obtained from the presence of stevioside-maltodextrin in 4 levels of substitution including %25, %50, %75 and %100 showed that samples became brighter so that the least amount of browning index was related to treatment including %100 stevioside-maltodextrin (Omidvar *et al.*, 2014). Brightness arose from substitution also have found in apple jam where Stevioside-Arabic Gum caused an increase in L* and a decrease in a* (Ghandehari yazdi *et al.*, 2014a), while in mango jam, the presence of stevioside led to an increase in L*, b*, and C* with no change in a* (Basu *et al.*, 2013); moreover, in another study on mango jam containing %50 sucrose, %0.27stevioside during 20 days of storing, the amount of L* and b* has been constant while a* has significantly decreased (Yoosefi Asl *et al.*, 2012). Reduction of color by stevioside-sorbitol in cake and stevioside-xylitol in combined gel of rice flour and chitosan has been reported as well (Manisha *et al.*, 2012; Torres *et al.*, 2013). Brightening surface due to sucrose replacing by stevioside and thus increase of L* and b* and decrease of b* have been reported in Naneghandi (an Iranian bread) (Vatankhah *et al.*, 2013). Unlike reviewed results from literature, increase in malt beverage color due to steviosde-CMC as a sucrose replacer has been observed (Nasiri *et al.*, 2013). Reduction of L* ،a* and b* has been reported in sucrose substitution with a mixture of stevioside-bulky agents in chocolate (Shah *et al.*, 2010). Sucrose replacement with stevioside-tragacanth on Ghotab caused an increase in color intensity (Ghandehari Yazdi *et al.*, 2014b). Observed differences in the obtained results arose from using different bulky agents such as alcoholic sugars, digestible compounds like poly dextrose and indigestible compounds like cellulose (Bullock *et al.*, 1992) in the presence of maltodextrin due to its high molecular weight with outer reducing groups, Millard, Caramelization and browning reaction occur less._Therefore, its consumption with dietary sweetener reduces color (Ghandehari Yazdi *et al.*, 2013). Color intensity increased by using tragacanth associated with stevioside because of galactronic acid as its main chain and presence of some pentose like fructose, pyranose, Galactose, Xylose, L Arabinose. Former sugars participate in caramelization and Millard and increase the browning index. On the other hand, increase in tragacanth amount accelerates water binding; thus, during frying time, more water is lost, water activity is reduced; and consequently, dry solid increases leading to an increase in caramelization (Ghandehari Yazdi *et al.*, 2014b). Microstructure of sucrose-replaced products has been investigated in some studies; e.g. study on microstructure of Ghotab showed an increase in roundness amount and number of holes (Ghandehari Yazdi *et al.*, 2014c); however, in the same study on sucrose replaced by stevioside-tragacanth, the obtained results were the opposite. This is thought to be because of the type of filler. Microstructure study on mango jam showed that produced pectin gel from sucrose was well distributed and had a homogenous structure while substitution creates a non-homogenous with thick matrix. In fact, sucrose molecule can place among the matrix gaps i.e. sucrose itself has no role in gel production but its chemical structure affects the size of produced matrix while bigger sizes of stevioside molecules lead to a non-homogenous structure (Basu *et al.*, 2013).

1.3. Investigation of sucrose replacement with stevia on physiochemical and rheological properties of food products

Due to its high amount of proteins and thus high water-holding capacity, Stevia can make soups, pastes, and bakery products swell. Oil absorption capacity is related to entrapment of oil into the matrix, and stevia leaves powder shows appropriate oil absorption (Lemus-Monadca *et al.*, 2012). Stevia extracts have the capability of heat resistance more than 200°C, and high resistance in 100°C for 1 hour as well (Kroyer *et al.*, 2010). Unlike alcoholic sugar, stevia's sugars are heat resistance with the capability of keeping their sweetening property; thus, stevia can be a suitable replacer for sugar in formulations (Jaroslov *et al.*, 2007; Carino *et al.*, 2006), and it is stable in pH=3-9 (Brandle *et al.*, 1998). In substitution of sucrose with stevia-inulin in milk chocolate, viscosity decreased while increase in inulin caused an increase in viscosity so that in treatment containing %6 inulin and % 100 substitutions, no significant differences were observed in comparison to control (Rad *et al*, 2012). In another study on chocolate sucrose replaced with a mixture of stevia, maltodextrin and polydextrose, physical factors including hardness, melting point and rheological properties in prepared treatment with different inulin polymerization degree including HP (DPav ≥23, long chain inulin), HPX (DPav ≥ 23, longchain inulin with low solubility) and GR (DPav ≥10) were investigated. Obtained results revealed that hardness of HPX remarkably decreased, no significant difference was found in melting point of HP, and the amount of viscosity in HP treatment was more than others. The best model in describing data was Herschel Bulkey model (Shah *et al.*, 2010). Shorideh *et al.* (2013) produced a low calorie dark chocolate with functional properties from a mixture of stevia-inulin-tagatose. In sucrose replaced with stevia milk shake (mixture of kiwi, banana and apple), there was no effect on the amount of acidity, vitamin C and pH, while it affected the amount of total soluble solid (Alizadeh *et al.*, 2014a). Stevia also has no effect on the amount of ash, fat, protein, density, apparent viscosity, while it increases water activity because sucrose replacement reduces hydrogen bonds, and thus free water increases thickness, pH and moisture amount along with spread ability and diameter (Vatankhah *et al*, 2013a). Results obtained from Texture analyzer indicate an increase in flexibility and a decrease in hardness.

Table 1. Replacing of saccharose by Stevia as non-nutritive sweetener in food products.

Product	Percent replacement	Additional compound	Reference
Halva masghati lari (an Iranian confectionary)	50%	Maltodextin	(Omidvar *et al.*, 2014)
Saffron beverage	25%	-	(Hashemi *et al.*, 2014)
Mango jam	25%	Sucrlose	(Basu *et al.*, 2013)
Ice Cream	4.65 gr Stevia, 13.95 gr Sucrose in the formulations	-	(Alizadeh *et al.*, 2014b)
Apple jam	100%	Arabic gum	(Ghandehari Yazdi *et al.*, 2014)
NanGhandi (an Iranian bread)	50%	-	(Vatankhah *et al.*, 2013a)
Fruit based Milk shake	100%	-	(Alizadeh *et al.*, 2014a)
Quince jam	50%(0.27% in the Formulations)	Pectin	(Yousefi Asl *et al.*, 2012a)
Malt beverages	25-50%	CMC gum	(Nasiri *et al.*, 2013)
Choclate	-	inulin or polydextrose	(Shah *et al.*, 2010)
Ghotab(an Iranian confectionary)	100%	Tragacanth Gum	(Ghandehari Yazdi *et al.*, 2014b)
Biscuit	50%	-	(Vatankhah et al., 2014)
Products powder	0.05% in the Formulations	Sucralose	(Shokouhi, 2013)
Orange beverage	75%	-	(Ajeli *et al.*, 2014)
Cream	-	Flavors(Vanilla, Cocoa, Saffron)	(Bagheri *et al.*, 2013)
Cake	0/4% weight of flour	Isomalt	(Hematian Soraki and Rahimi Ahmadabad, 2013)

Omidvar *et al.* (2014) found that in sucrose replacement with stevioside in Halva Masghati, hardness and stickiness increased while cohesiveness, gumminess and brittleness decreased. Additionally, substitution of sucrose in cream revealed that texture integrity and acidity increase but synersis decreased (Bagheri *et al.*, 2013). In the case of sucrose replacing by stevia-CMC in malt beverage, it has no effect on the amount of pH despite increase in ash, BX, total solid and density and increase in viscosity (Nasiri *et al.*, 2013). Replacing of sucrose with steviosided-sucralose in mango jam indicates that the amount of consistency coefficient and yield stress has decreased but flow index has increased (Basu *et al.*, 2103). Consistency coefficient and decrease in yield stress was also found in sugar replaced with stevioside-Arabic Gum in apple jam; however, the amount increased when the Gum increased. Additionally, it is thought that replacement due to reduction of sugar amount and lack of free water inhibition, and obtaining a softened pectin structure led to a decrease in hardness (Ghandehari Yazdi *et al.*, 2014a). Sucrose substitution in ice cream caused an increase in volume, a decrease in viscosity and BX (Alizadeh *et al.*, 2014b). Reduction of hardness was also observed in replacing sucrose with stevioside-tragacanth treatment in Dietary Ghotab (Ghandehari Yazdi *et al*, 2014b). Stevioside affects chemical properties of food e.g. stevia extraction due to the presence of compounds called Rebadiana and steviolbioside (Wheeler *et al.*, 2008), and flavonoids, Alcaloids, xantophyls, hydroxyl cinamic acid as well (De Oliveira *et al.*, 2008; Delshadian *et al.*, 2012) have antioxidant activity.

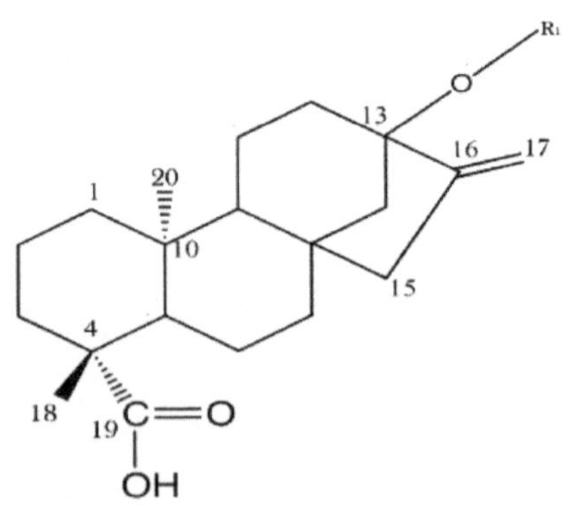

Fig. 1. Stevia structure (Reddy *et al.*, 2005)

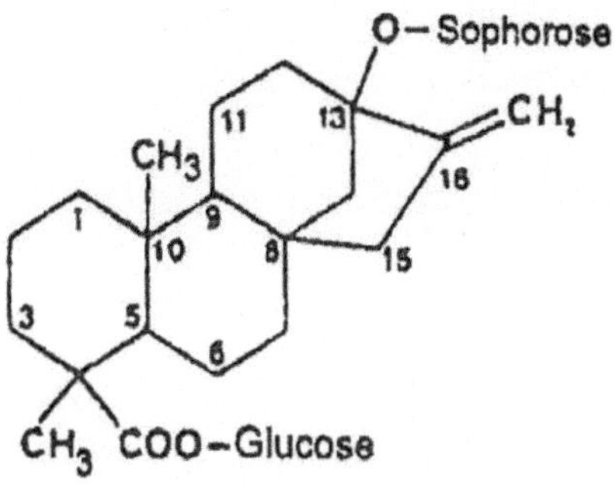

Fig. 2. Stevioside structure (Keramat, 2008)

Investigation of peroxide index in biscuit revealed an inverse relationship between peroxide index and stevia concentration (Hamzeloei *et al.*, 2008). These results are in agreement with those obtained in peroxide value in stevia replaced treatments of cocoa milk (Delshadian *et al.*, 2012).

1.4. Investigation of sensorial properties of food products

Due to its association with some essential oils like tanans and flavenoides, and recently considering the presence of stevioside or rebadioside A (with less effect than stevioside) (Mogra & Dashora, 2009), Stevia extract creates a bitter aftertaste (Keramat, 2008). Since flavor is a paramount issue in consumer acceptability, researches focus on investigation of substitution effects on the occurrence of possible aftertastes e.g. observation of significantly bitter taste in Halva Masghati samples containing %50 replacement (Omidvar *et al.*, 2014). In addition, results obtained from substitution in Gel powers (Shokouhi Torghi, 2013), dietary cream (Bagheri *et al,* 2013), apple jam (Ghandehari Yazdi *et al*, 2013a), and cake (Hematian Soraki *et al*, 2013) were in agreement with the latter. Using flavoring agents or powdery fillers is a way of detracting or removing aftertaste (Hematian soraki *et al*, 2013; Bagheri *et al*, 2013).

1.5. Investigation of stevioside on the calorie of food products

While sucrose and other conventional sweeteners are easily absorbed, participate in metabolism, and thus increase body weight, researches have shown that stevia extract with 2.7 kcal/g, barely contributes to body metabolism, and plays a role in the reduction of intake energy (Lemus-Mondaca *et al.*, 2012). In fact, this calorie reduction arises from sugar substitution with stevia e.g. calorie amount in Halva Masghati (an Iranian confectionery) sample containing %100 stevioside-maltodextrin has decreased from 4500 cal/g to 3500 cal/g (Omidvar *et al.*, 2014). This calorie reduction is also found in saccharoe replaced with stevia in fruit juice in both control and free sugar treatment, which were 338.9 and 194 kcal/100g, respectively (Alizadeh *et al.*, 2014a). In addition, the presence of stevia instead of sugar diminished calorie amount from 143.03 to 105.25 in ice cream (Alizadeh *et al.*, 2014b).

4. Conclusion

Antioxidant properties and being secure and low calorie make stevia a nonnutritive sweetener in food products. However, its bitter aftertaste can diminish its consumption in food formulations, but other flavoring agents and fillers can modify this problem. Most researches indicate the fact that products free of sugar do not have enough desirability and acceptability; hence, the presence of sugar is inevitable i.e. in case of complete substitution, concurrent consumption of both sugar and stevia (different combinations) seemingly makes it more favorable and a must-be-purchased product.

5. References

Ahmed, B., Hossain, M., Islam, R., Kumar Saha, A. and Mandal, A. 2011. A Reivew on natural sweetener plant stevia having medicinal and commercial importance. *Agronomski glasnik*, 73(1-2):75-91.

Ajeli, A., Arian Far, a, and Safari, O. 2014. Application of Stevia natural sweetener to replace sucrose in Oranges beverage and Evaluation physicochemical and sensory characteristics. *Third national Conference on Food Science and Technology, Quchan,* Islamic Azad University of Quchan, Iran. *http://www.civilica.com/Paper GHOCHANFOOD03 GHOCHANFOOD03_043.html.*

Alizadeh, M., Azizi-lalabadi, M., Hojat-ansari, H. and Kheirouri, S. 2014a. Effect of Stevia as a Substitute for Sugar on Physicochemical and Sensory

Properties of Fruit Based Milk Shake. *Journal of scientific research and reports*, 3(11):1421-1429.

Alizadeh, M., Azizi-Lalabadi, M. and Kheirouri, S. 2014b. Impact of using stevia on physicochemical, sensory, rheology and glycemic index of soft ice cream. *Food and Nutrition Sciences*., 5(4).

Bagheri, F., Radi, M and Amiri, S. 2013. Cream diet produced by using a sweetener. *Twenty-first National Congress of Food Science and Technology*, Shiraz, Shiraz University, Iran. *http://www.civilica.com/Paper-NCFOODI21-NCFOODI21_627.html.*

Balsini, S., Najafi, a. and Hadad khodaparast. (2008). Membrane separation method for the sweetener from the leaves of Stevia. *The second of National Conference functional food. Tehran, Tarbiat Modares University, Iran.* pp 532-534. *http://www.civilica.com/Paper-FUNCFOOD02-FUNCFOOD02_071.html.*

Basu, S., Shivhare, U. S. and Singh, T. V. 2013. Effect of substitution of stevioside and sucralose on rheological, spectral, color and microstructural characteristics of mango jam. *Journal of Food Engineering*, 114: 465-476.

Brandle, J. E., Starratt, A. N. and Gijzen, M. 1998. Stevia rebaudiana: its agricultural, biological, and chemical properties. *Canadian Journal of Plant Science*, 78(4):527-533.

Bullock, L. M., Handel, A. P., Segall, S. and Wasserman, P. A. 1992. Replacement of simple sugars in cookie dough. *Food technology*, 46: 82-86.

Carakostas, M. C., Curry L. L., Boileau, A. C. and Brusick, D. J. 2008. Overview: the history, technical function and safety of rebaudioside A, a naturally occurring steviol glycoside, for use in food and beverages. *Food and Chemical Toxicology*, 46(7):1-10.

Carino, R,. Hernandez, C., Torres, V., Gonzaleaz, A., Arriaga, A. and Madrigal, B. 2006. Antimutagenicity of Stevia Pilosa and Stevia Eupatoria evaluated with the ames test. *Journal of Toxicology in vitro*, 691-697.

Curry, L. L. and Roberts, A. 2008. Subchronic toxicity of rebaudioside A. *Food and Chemical Toxicology*, 46: S11-S20.

Delshadian, Z., Mohammadi, R., Rouhi, M., Homayouni Rad, A. and Mortazavian, A. M. 2013. Effect of using stevia sweetener on peroxide value of chocolate milk. *Iranian Journal of Nutrition Sciences & Food Technology*, 7(5):107-113.

De Oliveira, B. S. H., Stiirmer, J. L. C. S., De Souza Filho, J. D. and Ayub, R. A. 2008. Plant growth regulation activity of steviol and derivatives. *Phytochemistry*, 69:1528-1533.

Farokhzad, H. and Bagheri, A. 2001. Obesity and hazard factors of Cardiovascular in Iranian children. *Iranian journal of Diabetes and lipid*, 2: 175-183

Fatemi, H. 2007. *Food Chemistry*. Sahami enteshar co Publication. pp 449-450.

Ghandehari Yazdi, A. P., Hojjatoleslami, M., Keramat, J. and Jahadi, M. 2013. A Study On The Influences Of Replacing sucrose with Sucralose-Maltodextrin Mixture On the Rheological Properties and the amount of Calories in Ghotab- A Traditional Confectionary. *Journal of Food Science and new technologies*, 1(2):42-58.

Ghandehari yazdi, A. P., Hojjatoleslami, M., Keramat, J. and Shariati, M. A. 2014a. Replacing Sucrose by Stevoioside and Adding Arabic Gum: investigation of Rheological Properties of Apple Jam. *Journal of Applied Science and Agriculture*, 9(2):508-513.

Ghandehari Yazdi, A. P., Hojjatoleslami, M., Keramat, J. and Jahadi, M. 2014b. Effect of Sucrose Replacement with dietary sweetener Stevioside and adding Tragacanth Gum on Rheological and Micro-structural Properties of Ghotab-Traditional Confectionary. *Journal of innovation of in food Science and technology*, 6(3):97-106.

Ghandehari Yazdi, A. P., Hojjatoleslami, M., Sedaghat, L. and Shariati, M. A. 2014c. Study on the Effect of Saccharose Replacement by Mixture of Maltodextrin-Stevioside on Microstructre Properties of Ghotab. *International Journal of Farming and Allied Sciences*, 6:679-682.

Ghosh, S., Subudhi, E. and Nayak, S. 2008. Antimicrobial assay of Stevia rebaudiana Bertoni leaf extracts against 10 pathogens. *International Journal of Integrative Biology,* 2(1):27.

Glicksman, M. and Farkas, E. 1966. Gums in artificially sweetened foods. *Food Technology*, 20: 58-60.

Goyal, S.K.and Goyal, R.K. 2010. Stevia (Stevia rebaudiana) a bio-sweetener: a review. *journal of food sciences and nutrition*, 61(1):1-10.

Hamzeluie, M., Mirzayi, H. and Ghorbani, M. 2001. Evaluation effects of evaluation of sugar replace by glycosidic sweeteners of stevia on the peroxide index in biscuit. *Agriculture and natural resources*, 16(1).

Hashemi, N., Rabiei, H., Tavakolipour, H. and Gazrani, S. 2014. Evaluation of Physico-chemical and rheological characteristics of Saffron beverage based on sweetener Stevia. *Twenty-second National Congress of Food Science and Technology. Gorgan, Gorgan University of Agricultural Sciences and Natural Resources, Iran. http://www.civilica.com/Paper-NCFOODI22-NCFOODI22_354.html.*

Hematian Soraki, A. and Rahimi Ahmadabad, F. 2013. The effect of sucralose, Stevia and isomalt sweeteners in diabetic cakes. *Twenty-first National Congress of Food Science and Technology*, Shiraz, Shiraz University, Iran. *http://www.civilica.com/Paper-NCFOODI21-NCFOODI21_1609.html.*

Jaroslov, P., Brabora, H. and Tuulia, H. 2007. Characterisation Of Steviol Rebaudiana By Choprehensive Tow Dimensional Liquid Chromatography Time Of Flight Mass Spectrometry. *Journal of Chromatography A*, 1150: 85-92.

Keramat, J. 2007. *An introduction to food chemistry*. Isfahan University of Technology, Isfahan province of Iran. pp 189-390.

Koyama, E., Kitazawa, K., Ohori, Y., Izawa, O., Kakegawa, K. and Ul, M. (2003). In vitro metabolism of the glycosidic sweeteners, stevia mixture and enzymatically modified stevia in human intestinal microflora. *Food and Chemical Toxicology*., 41(3):359-374.

Kroyer, G. 2010. Stevioside and Stevia-sweetener in food: application, stability and interaction with food ingredients. *Journal für Verbraucherschutz und Lebensmittelsicherheit*, 5:225-229.

Laribi, B., Rouatbi, N., Kouki, K. and Bettaieb, T. 2012. In vitro propagation of Stevia rebaudiana (Bert.)-A non caloric sweetener and antidiabetic medicinal plant. *International Journal of Medicinal and Aromatic plants*, 2(2):333-339.

Lemus-Mondaca, R., Vega-Gálvez, A., Zura-Bravo, L. and Ah-Hen, K. 2012. Stevia rebaudiana Bertoni, source of a high-potency natural sweetener: A comprehensive review on the biochemical, nutritional and functional aspects. *Food Chemistry*, 132(3):1121-32.

Madan, S., Ahmad, S., Singh, G.N., Kohli, K., Kumar, Y., Singh, R., and et al. 2010. Stevia rebaudiana (Bert.) Bertoni-a review. *Indian Journal of Natural Product and Resources*, 1(3):267-286.

Manisha, G., Soumya, C. and Indrani, D. 2012. Studies on interaction between stevioside, liquid sorbitol, hydrocolloids and emulsifiers for replacement of sugar in cakes. *Food Hydrocolloids*, 29:363-373.

Mogra, R. and Dashora, V. (2009). Exploring the Use of Stevia rebaudiana as a Sweetener in Comparison with Other Sweeteners. *Journal of Human Ecology*, 25(2):117-120.

Nasiri, Sh., Razavi, H. and Hojjatoleslami, M. 2013. Effect of replacementCMC gum and Stevia instead of sugar on the physical properties - chemical, rheological and sensory simple Malt beverages. *Twenty-first National Congress of Food Science and Technology*, Shiraz, Shiraz University, Iran. *http://www.civilica.com/Paper-NCFOODI21-NCFOODI21_664.html.*

Omidvar, S., Keramat, J., Hojjatoleslami, M., Ghabousi, S. H. H., Ghandehari Yazdi, A. P. and Shariati, M. A. 2014. The Investigation of Saccharose Replacing by Adding Maltodextrin-Stevioside Mixture on the Rehological and Sensory Properties of Hlava Masghati Lari (an Iranian Confectionary). *International Journal of Scientific Research Engineering & Technology*,3(4):748-754.

Rad, A. H., Delshadian, Z., Arefhosseini, S. R., Alipour, B. and Jafaabadi, M. A. 2012. Effect of Inulin and Stevia on Some Physical Properties of Chocolate Milk. *Health promotion perspectives*., 2:42.

Reddy, V., Urooj, A. and Kumar, A. 2005. Evaluation of antioxidant activity of some plant extracts and their application in biscuits. *Food Chemistry*, 90: 317-321.

Shah, A. B., Jones, G. P. and Vasiljevic, T. 2010. Sucrose-free chocolate sweetened with Stevia rebaudiana extract and containing different bulking agents-effects on physicochemical and sensory properties. *International journal of food science & technology*, 45:1426-1435.

Shokouhi Toroghi, F. 2013. Effect of Stevia as a natural sweetener plant in sugar-free products powder *Twenty-first National Congress of Food Science and Technology*, Shiraz, Shiraz University, Iran. *http://www.civilica.com/Paper-NCFOODI21-NCFOODI21_1009.html.*

Shourudeh, M., Taslimi, A., Azizi Tabrizzad, M. H., Mohammadifar, M. A. and Mashayekh, M. 2010. Effects of D-tagatose and inulin of some physicochemical, rheological and sensory properties of dark chocolate. *Journal of Nutrition Sciences & food technology*, 5(3): 29-38.

Thomas, J. E. and Glade, M. J., (2010). Stevia: Its not just about calories. Benefits. *The Open obesity Journal.*, 101-109.

Torres, M. D., Raymundo, A. and Sousa, I. (2013). Effect of sucrose, stevia and xylitol on rheological properties of gels from blends of chestnut and rice flours. *Carbohydrate polymers*, 98**:** 249-256.

Vatankhah, M., Yaghbani, M., Elhamirad, A.H. and Nadian, N. 2013. Investigate the color of Naneghandi, production is based on natural sweetener Stevioside by using image processing. *Twenty-first National Congress of Food Science and Technology, Shiraz, Shiraz University, Iran. http://www.civilica.com/Paper-NCFOODI21-NCFOODI21_1405.html.*

Vatankhah, M., Yaghbani, M., Elhamirad, A. H. and Nadian, N. 2013a. evaluation physical characteristics of Naneghandi production based on natural sweetener Stevioside. *National Congress of Food Science and Technology, Shiraz, Shiraz University, Iran. http://www.civilica.com/Paper-NCFOODI21-NCFOODI21_1669.html.*

Vatankhah, M., Garavand, F., Elhamirad, A. and Yaghbani, M. 2014. Influence of sugar replacement by stevioside on physicochemical and sensory properties of biscuit. *Quality Assurance and Safety of Crops & Foods,* 1-8.

Wheeler, A., Boileau, A., C. Winkler, P. C., Compton, J. C., Prakash, I., Jiang, X. and Mandarino, D. A. 2008. Pharmacokinetics of rebaudioside A and stevioside after single oral doses in healthy men. *Food and chemical toxicology*, 46**:**S54-S60.

Yosefi Asl, M., Goli, S. A. H., Kadivar, M. and Zaeim, D. 2012. Changes in physicochemical and sensory characteristics of low-calorie jam during storage. *Twenty-first National Congress of Food Science and Technology*, Shiraz, Shiraz University*, Iran. http://www.civilica.com/Paper-NCFOODI21-NCFOODI21_237.html.*

Yosefi Asl, M., Goli, S. A. H. and Kadivar, M. 2012a. Optimization of Low-CalorieI Quince jam production with stevioside sweetener. *Journal of food research*, 22(2): 155-164.

Regional variations of antioxidant capacity and phenolic properties in the Iranian jujube collection

Ali Azizi*, Maryam Pirbodaghi

Department of Horticultural Sciences, Faculty of Agriculture, Bu-Ali Sina University, Hamedan, Iran;
***Email:** azizi@basu.ac.ir*

ARTICLE INFO

***Topic:** Medicinal Plants*

Key words:
- ✓ *Iranian jujube collection*
- ✓ *Total phenol*
- ✓ *Flavonoid*
- ✓ *Anthocyanin*
- ✓ *Antioxidant capacity*

ABSTRACT

Background & Aim: Fruits from the jujube plant (*Ziziphus jujuba*) possess health-promoting effects and medicinal properties. Jujube has a long history of usage as a remedy in Iranian traditional medicine and is recommended for the treatment of some diseases. This study investigated the variations in antioxidant capacities (AOX), total phenol (TPH), total flavonoid (TF) and total anthocyanin (TA) contents of fruit extracts among 29 jujube accessions originating from 7 provinces of Iran.
Experimental: The fruits from 29 accessions were extracted with methanol (85%). DPPH assay were performed for determination of antioxidant capacity of each extract. The total phenols were measured by Folin-Ciocalteu method and total flavonoids evaluated using the aluminum chloride colorimetric procedure while total anthocyanins were determined by pH-differential method.
Results & Discussion: The results from the analysis of variance (ANOVA) revealed that the examined accessions of *Z. jujuba* were highly variable in all evaluated phytochemical traits ($P < 0.01$). Principal component analysis (PCA) based on four phytochemical characters confirmed this broad variation and also identified three distinct group among the accessions. The accessions Hamidabad (Mazandaran), Bayaziyeh (Isfahan) and kuhpayeh2 (Isfahan) can considered by their high values for the TPH, TF, and TA values, respectively. On the other hand, accessions Ardestan (Isfahan), Ghaziolya (Ghom) and Maroon (Ghom) showed high AOX. No correlation was found between total phenol content and antioxidant activity.
Industrial and practical recommendations: These findings suggest the importance of genotype and origin for determining antioxidant potential and phenolic contents of jujube plants. The knowledge of the diversities, found in this study, will allow a better plant exploitation related to pharmaceutical uses and also a better conduction of breeding programs for *Ziziphus jujuba* ecotypes.

1. Introduction

The protective effects of some fruits against coronary heart disease and cancer have been attributed to the presence of phenolic compounds such as flavonoids including flavonols, flavonones and anthocyanins (Steinmetz and Potter, 1996). Phenolic phytochemicals, a specific group of secondary metabolites, have potentially beneficial effects on health including antimicrobial, anti-inflammatory, antioxidant and anti-mutagenic activity (Liu, 2003). Antioxidant capacity is defined as the ability to reduce free radical formation and scavenge reactive oxygen species (ROS) (Narayana *et al.*, 2001). It has been shown that the phenolic components and the antioxidant activity of fruits vary considerably. Differences gauged between plant accessions and cultivars may be explained by genotype (Howard *et al.*, 2003; Scalzo *et al.*, 2005) and environmental factors (Wang *et al.*, 2008).

The jujube (*Ziziphus jujuba* Mill.) is one of the world's major fruit crops and is cultivated in the Middle East, Russia, southern Europe, India and especially China (Outlaw *et al.*, 2002). The jujube is one of many species of the genus, *Ziziphus* belonging to the family *Rhamnaceae,* used as a remarkable nutritional and medicinal plant (Mahajan and Chopda, 2009). To date, more than 700 cultivars of jujube have been bred and found in China and this country is the only land known to be exporting jujube fruits (Gao *et al.* 2013). Food and Agriculture Organization of the United Nations (FAO) does not maintain statistics on this crop. International Centre for Underutilized Crops has identified jujube as a crop with substantial growth potential (Azam-Ali *et al.*, 2006).

The seeds of *Ziziphus jujuba* var. spinosa (Bunge) are also used as a traditional Chinese medicine (Li *et al.*, 2005b). Recent studies on jujubes, describe potential anticancer (Huang *et al.*, 2007), immunological (Zhao *et al.* 2006), anti-inflammatory (Yu *et al.*, 2012), Antioxidant (Xue *et al.*, 2009), neuro-protective (Yoo *et al.*, 2010) and antiepileptic (Pahuja *et al.*, 2011) effects of fruit extracts in model animals and humans. Previous studies have also revealed that jujube contains various chemical constituents including triterpene acids, amino acids, polysaccharides, cerebrosides, phenolic acids and flavonoids (Mahajan and Chopda, 2009; Gao *et al.* 2013). Consequently, the biological activity of extracts from fruits, seeds (Peng et al., 2000) and even leaves (Zhang *et al.*, 2014) causes a high pharmaceutical and industrial interest in *Ziziphus jujuba*.

In Flora Iranica, 5 species were identified and reported for the genus *Ziziphus* namely *Z. spina-christi*, *Z. nummularia*, *Z. jujuba*, *Z. oxyphylla* and *Z. aucheri* (Rechinger, 1977). Common jujube (*Z. jujuba*) is widely distributed in Iran and cultivated especially in Birjand, South Khorasan province (Ghollassi Mood, 2008). The ripe edible fruits of *Z. jujuba* have, for a long time, been used in Iranian folk medicine. Fruit extracts of jujubes, originated from Iran, have recently been reported to have antimicrobial activity (Daneshmand *et al.*, 2013), antioxidant ability (Memarpoor-Yazdi *et al.*, 2013) and profound effects on Alzheimer's disease (Zare-Zardini *et al.*, 2013). The objective of this investigation was to evaluate phytochemical variations among Iranian accessions of Jujube with respect to antioxidant capacity as well as total phenol, flavonoid and anthocyanin contents.

2. Materials and Methods

2.1. Plant Material

A total of 29 Iranian accessions of *Ziziphus jujuba* were investigated (Table 1). All accessions were sampled from collection of Badieii research station located in western part of Qom, Iran (Natural resources & Agriculture research centre in Qom). The plant materials were originated from 7 provinces of Iran. All accessions in the collection have been planted in 1999. This study was conducted in 2014. Three trees (replicates) of each accession and five fruits for each tree were analysed. Fully ripened fruits were randomly selected and harvested from all experimental plants.

2.2. Extraction procedure

The fruits of each jujube tree were thoroughly homogenized in a blender. Two grams of homogenized fruit samples were extracted through maceration (48 h) in 10 ml of methanol 85% (v/v) at 40° C and avoiding light. The homogenate was then centrifuged for 15 min at 10,000g. The supernatant was then concentrated at 40° C and stored at -20° C. The concentrated sample was used as a sample extract for the estimation of TPH, TF, TA and AOX. The estimations were carried out in triplicate and the results were averaged.

2.3. Determination of total phenols (TPH)

The contents of total phenols were measured according to the method described by McDonald et al., (2001) with some modification. Folin-Ciocalteu reagent was used for the determination of TPH. First, a calibration curve was plotted for the quantification purpose using Gallic acid as a standard. The standard curve obtained from measuring the absorbance of known concentrations (0, 50, 100, 150, 200, 250 mg/l) of Gallic acid. The absorbance of standard solutions was measured at 765 nm using a UV/Vis spectrophotometer (Varian CARY 100, USA). A diluted fruit extract of each plant (300µl of 1:100g/ml) was mixed with 1500µl of Folin-Ciocalteu reagent (previously diluted to tenfold with distilled water). After 5 min, 1200µl of sodium carbonate solution (7%) was added to the mixture. Subsequently, the mixture was shaken mechanically for 2h at room temperature and absorbance was then measured at 765 nm. Total phenol values were expressed as mg of Gallic acid equivalents per g dry weight.

Table 1. Sources and origin of the investigated Jujube accessions

Accession	source	Province of origin
1 Ardestan	Qom research centre	Isfahan
2 Ghaziolya	Qom research centre	Qom
3 Maroon	Qom research centre	Qom
4 Nudan-1	Qom research centre	Fars
5 Nudan-2	Qom research centre	Fars
6 Dahane-Larim	Qom research centre	Mazandaran
7 Kalaghneshin-1	Qom research centre	Qom
8 Pudeh-1	Qom research centre	Isfahan
9 Pudeh-2	Qom research centre	Isfahan
10 Shahreza	Qom research centre	Isfahan
11 Kouhpayeh-1	Qom research centre	Isfahan
12 Nahalestan	Qom research centre	Qom
13 Kamchenar	Qom research centre	Qom
14 Kasva	Qom research centre	Qom
15 Kolaleh	Qom research centre	Golestan
16 Kalaghneshin-2	Qom research centre	Qom
17 Magham-Sari	Qom research centre	Mazandaran
18 Hamvarelak	Qom research centre	Qom
19 Dolatabad	Qom research centre	Qom
20 Gelyan-Birjand	Qom research centre	South Khorasan
21 Alghoo-Birjand	Qom research centre	South Khorasan
22 Niyasar	Qom research centre	Isfahan
23 Bayaziyeh	Qom research centre	Isfahan
24 Larim	Qom research centre	Mazandaran
25 Natanz	Qom research centre	Isfahan
26 Dashte bayaz	Qom research centre	South Khorasan
27 Hamidabad-Sari	Qom research centre	Mazandaran
28 Kouhpayeh-2	Qom research centre	Isfahan
29 Hamedan	Qom research centre	Hamedan

2.4. Determination of total flavonoids (TF)

TF contents of fruit samples were determined based on the aluminium chloride colorimetric procedure adapted from Chang *et al.* (2002), with some modifications. Methanol extract (0.5 mL), 10% aluminium chloride (0.1 mL), 1M potassium acetate (0.1 mL) and dd-H_2O (2.8 mL) were mixed in a 10mL test tube. After incubation at room temperature for 30 min, the absorbance was measured at 415 nm. Quercetin was used to make the calibration curve. The flavonoid content was expressed as mg quercetin equivalent per g dry weight.

2.5. Determination of total anthocyanins (TA)

The total anthocyanins were detected according to the pH-differential method of Lee et al. (2005). Acidified methanol (1% HCL) extracts of fruits were filtered through Whatman No.1 paper and then used for TA evaluation. An aliquot of clear extract (1 ml) was prepared with pH 1.0 buffer. Another 1 ml of extract was also provided with pH 4.5 buffer. The absorbance of solutions was measured at 510 and 700 nm. Cyanidin 3-glucoside was used to make the calibration curve. The concentration of total anthocyanins was calculated using the following equation:

$$\text{Total anthocyanins (mg/l)} = A \times MW \times DF \times 1000/(e \times L)$$

Where A is the absorbance = $(A_{510\ nm} - A_{700\ nm})$ pH 1.0 - $(A_{510\ nm} - A_{700\ nm})$ pH 4.5, MW is the molecular weight of cyanidin-3-glucoside (433.2), DF is a dilution factor (10), e is the extinction coefficient for cyanidin 3-glucoside of 31,600 and L is the cell path length (1 cm). Finally, total anthocyanins (TA) were expressed as mg cyanidin 3-glucoside equivalents/ g dry weight.

2.6. Evaluation of antioxidant capacity (AOX)

The antioxidant capacity of extracts was measured by DPPH (2,2'-diphenyl-1-picrylhydrazyl) free radical scavenging assay using the method described by Brand-Williams et al. (1995) with some modifications (Brand-Williams *et al.*, 1995). This method is based on the ability of the antioxidant to scavenge the DPPH caution radical. Briefly, 75 µl of each methanol extract was added to 2925 µl of DPPH reagent (0.1 mM in methanol) and vortexed vigorously. The mixture was incubated in dark for 30 min at room temperature. The absorbance of the sample extract was measured at 517 against a methanol blank. The percentage of DPPH radical scavenging ability was calculated according to the following equation:

$$\text{DPPH scavenging effect (\%)} = ((A_0 - A_1)/A_0)) \times 100$$

Where A_0 is the absorbance of control DPPH solution at 0 min and A_1 is the absorbance in the presence of test sample at 30 min.

2.7. Statistical Analysis and Principal Component Analysis (PCA)

Data represent the mean of three replicate analyses. To assess the trait variability and the significant differences between the accessions, analysis of variance (ANOVA) was performed using the general linear model (GLM) in the Statistical Analysis System (SAS). Data are reported as means ± standard deviation of the mean. Mean values were compared by Duncan's multiple range test at 0.01 probability level. To provide an overall distance measure between the accessions based on four phytochemical traits, a PCA (Principal Component Analysis) was conducted on the accession means for each observed character using the MINITAB software, version 14 (Minitab Inc., State College, PA, USA). The first two principal components were extracted, and the scatter plot obtained by plotting the scores of PC-1 versus PC-2.

3. Results and discussion

The results from the analysis of variance (ANOVA) revealed that the examined accessions of *Z. jujuba* were significantly variable ($p<0.01$) in all evaluated phytochemical characters including TPH, TF, TA and AOX (Table 2). This study showed the important role played by genetic background for determining the antioxidant potential and phenolic properties of jujube plants. These aspects had not been deeply investigated previously in the Iranian jujube collection.

Table 2. Analysis of variance with mean squares for TPH, TF, TA and AOX of the jujubes as affected by ecotype (accession).

Parameter	Source	df	Mean squares	CV	P-value
Total Phenols (TPH)	Ecotype	28	0.01226437	2.12	< 0.01
	Error	58	0.00017833		
Total Flavonoids (TF)	Ecotype	28	0.00105113	4.53	< 0.01
	Error	58	0.00001345		
Total Anthocyanins (TA)	Ecotype	28	5.3245223	5.77	< 0.01
	Error	58	0.0103299		
Antioxidant Capacity (AOX)	Ecotype	28	61.179937	1.45	< 0.01
	Error	58	1.642789		

3.1. Total phenol content

A significant variation in total phenol content was found among the 29 accessions of jujube studied and the values ranged from a low of 5.80 mg GAE/g DW to a high of 9.24 mg GAE/ g FW reflecting a 1.6-fold difference (Figure 1). This was not surprising considering that the genotype-dependent phenol content variations have previously been observed for many other fruits (Howard *et al.*, 2003; Scalzo *et al.*, 2005). The range of TPH content in jujubes found in our study was similar to those (5.18–8.53 mg GAE/g DW) reported by Li et al. (2005a) in Chinese jujube and was relatively higher than the values (1.70–5.70 mg GAE/g DW) obtained by Gao et al. (2011) in some other cultivars of Chinese jujube, but much lower than the values (25–43 mg GAE/g DW) reported by Kamiloglu et al. (2009) in jujube genotypes selected from Turkey.

As shown in Figure 1, the highest level of TPH content was observed in Hamidabad-Sari accession. It is previously found that phenolic compounds contribute to fruit quality by modifying colour, taste, aroma, and flavour, and also by improving medicinal properties. These compounds also play a role in plant defensive mechanisms by counteracting reactive oxygen species (ROS), thus minimizing molecular damage due to biotic and abiotic plant stress (Mittler, 2002).

3.2. Total flavonoid content

Total flavonoids content of the jujube fruits was determined by the colorimetric method and was expressed as mg quercetin equivalent per g dry weight (mg QE/g DW). Based on results (Table 2), the fruits from different regions showed significant variations in their total flavonoid contents ($p < 0.01$). As it can be seen in Figure 2, TF content of 29 accessions of jujube ranged from a low of 0.054 mg QE/g DW in two accessions, Hamidabad-Sari and Dahane-Larim, to a high of 0.140 mg QE/g DW in Bayaziyeh, reflecting a 2.6-fold difference. Our results are consistent and similar with those of Choi et al. (2011) who reported TF contents of several jujube plants grown in Korea. They obtained the quantitative amounts of flavonoids (0.072- 0.180 mg QE/g DW) with a 2.5-fold difference. The mean values of TF content in jujube found in our study was somewhat lower than the records by Li et al. (2005a) in Chinese jujube (0.159-0.230 mg QE/g DW) and also much lower than the values reported in Italian fruits of jujube measured by HPLC (Pawlowska *et al.*, 2009).

Flavonoids are natural phenolic compounds and have been proven to display a wide range of physiological and pharmacological properties (Di Carlo *et al.*, 1999). The reported levels of total flavonoid content for jujube plants are very low in some literature (Hudina *et al.* 2008; San and Yildirim, 2010) which might be partially due to genotype, agronomic practices, harvesting time, climatic conditions and altitude of the local area.

3.3. Total anthocyanin content

Figure 3 shows the values recorded for total anthocyanins of 29 investigated jujube accessions. The values of TA was expressed as mg Cyanidin 3-glucoside equivalent per g dry weight (mg CE/g DW). Anthocyanins are mainly responsible for the red, blue and purple colours of fruits, and cyanidin-3-glucoside is the most common anthocyanin (Mazza and Miniati, 1993).

Our results shows that the accession Kouhpayeh-2 from Isfahan province had the highest TA content (4.71 mg CE/g DW) followed by Gelyan-Birjand accession from South Khorasan province which had a TA content of 4.42 mg CE/g DW. The lowest TA content (0.26 mg CE/g DW) was found in Dahane-Larim accession from Mazandaran province. Therefore, a very high difference (18-fold) was observed in TA contents among the evaluated accessions. The levels of TA content for jujube plants obtained in our work are relatively lower than the values (2.51–7.98 mg CE/g DW) reported by Sun et al. (2011) in *Z. jujuba* Mill. var. *spinosa* (Bunge). Previous studies have reported UV radiation in high altitude increased the accumulation of anthocyanins and other UV-absorbing compounds, flavonoids and total polyphenols in plants (Mazza and Miniati, 1993).

3.4. Antioxidant capacity

The model of scavenging the stable DPPH radical is a widely used procedure to evaluate antioxidant capacity of natural compounds and plant extracts in a relatively short time compared with other methods. Alcoholic solutions of DPPH have a characteristic absorption maximum at 517 nm. The radical-scavenging activity in the presence of a hydrogen-donating antioxidant can be monitored as a decrease in absorbance of DPPH solution.

Antioxidant capacities of the analysed jujube accessions are shown in Figure 4. The highest value of AOX was obtained for Ardestan accession from Isfahan province (93.93% inhibition) followed by two accessions from Qom province including Maroon and Ghaziolya (93.42 and 93.06 % inhibition, respectively). The lowest AOX was recorded for Hamedan accession from Hamedan province (70.69% inhibition). Therefore the investigated extracts demonstrated very different radical-scavenging activities. The range of AOX in jujubes found in our study was similar to those (80–99% inhibition) reported by Kamiloglu et al. (2009) in jujube genotypes selected from Turkey and was much higher than the values (27–53% inhibition) obtained by Li et al. (2005a) in Chinese jujube.

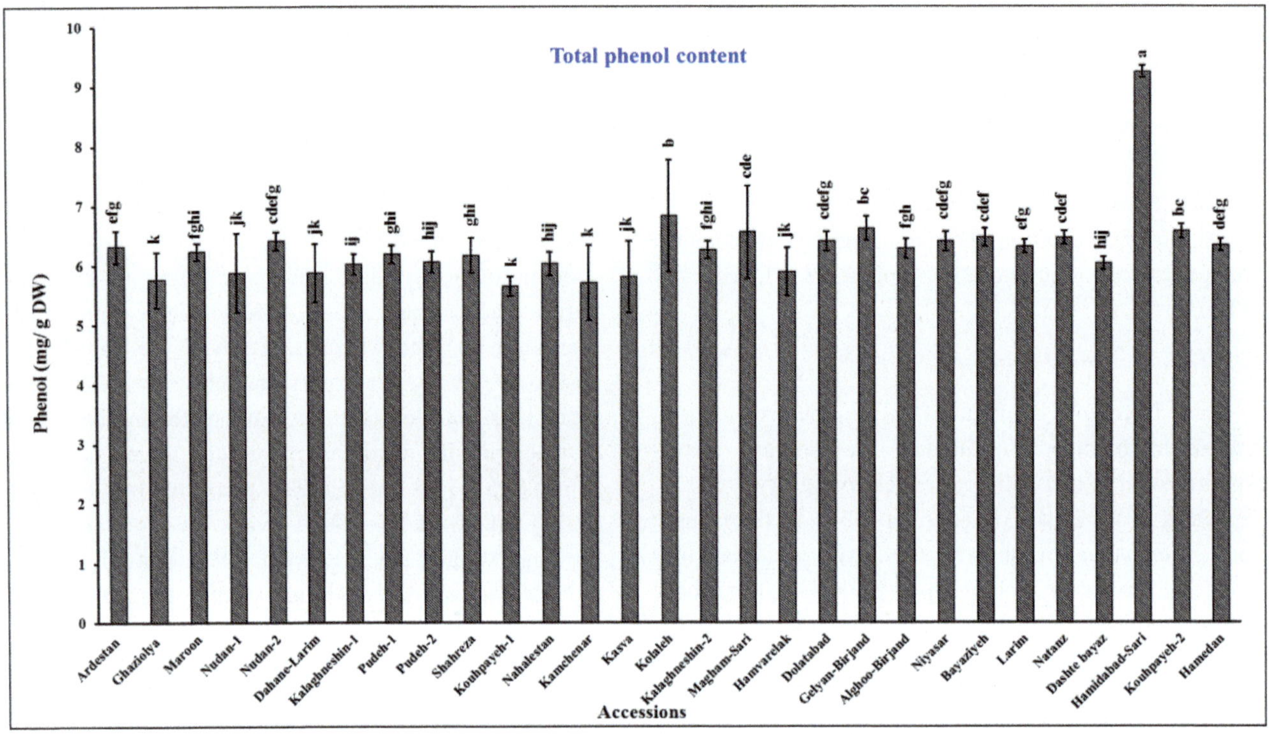

Fig 1. Differences in TPH contents of 29 tested accessions of jujube. Values represent means ± S.D. of triplicate measurements. Significant differences between accessions were measured by Duncan's multiple range tests at $P < 0.01$ and indicated by different letters.

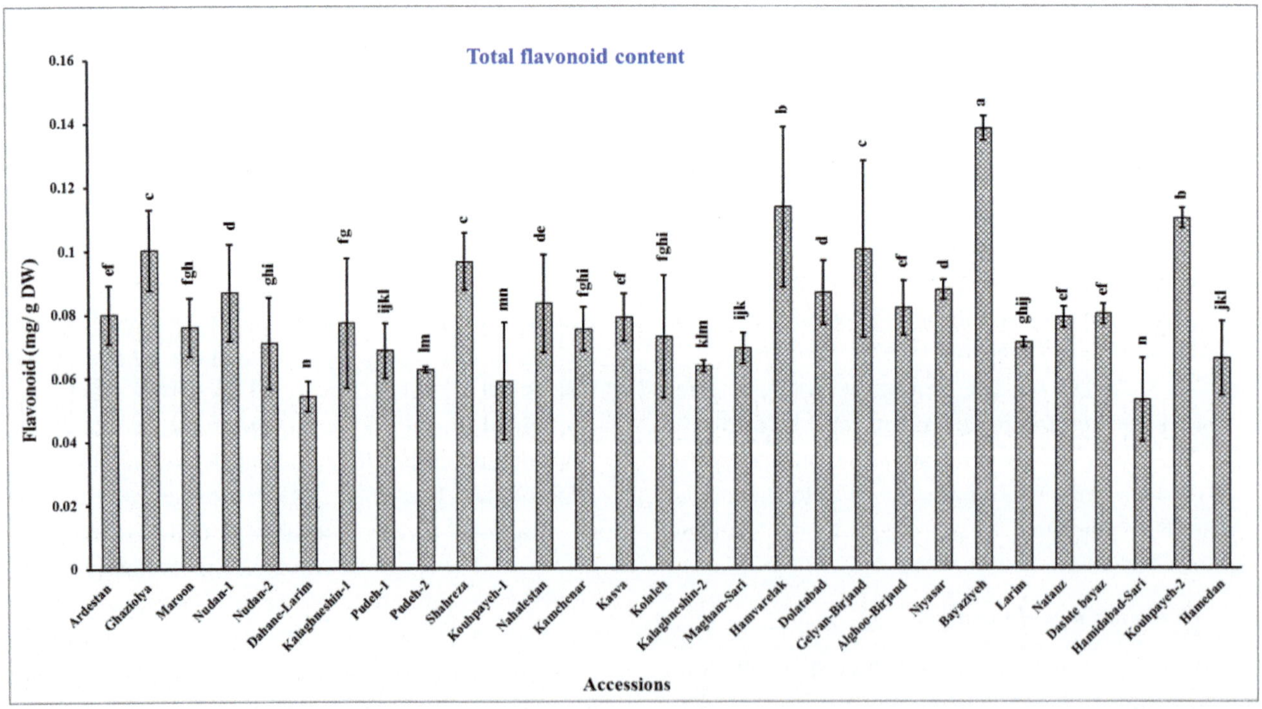

Fig 2. Differences in TF contents of 29 tested accessions of jujube. Values represent means ± S.D. of triplicate measurements. Significant differences between accessions were measured by Duncan's multiple range tests at $P < 0.01$ and indicated by different letters.

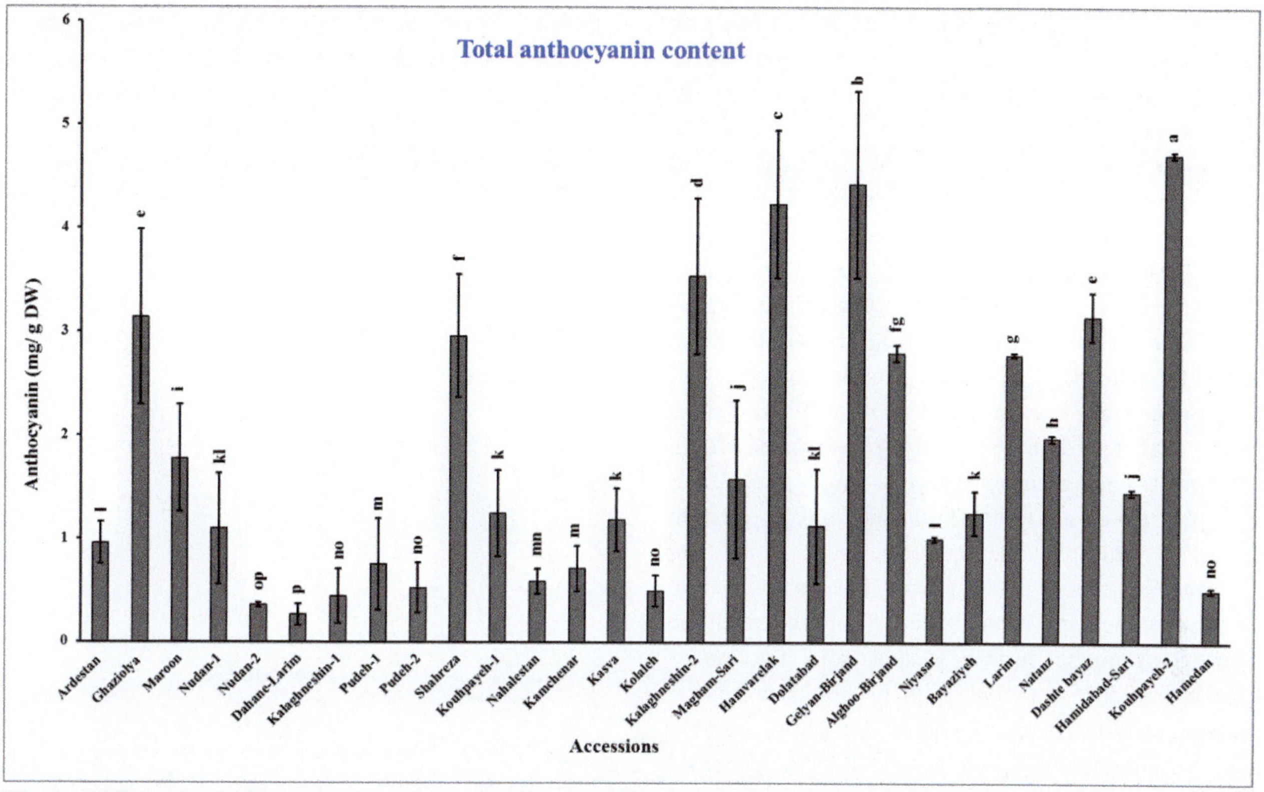

Fig 3. Differences in TA contents of 29 tested accessions of jujube. Values represent means ± S.D. of triplicate measurements. Significant differences between accessions were measured by Duncan's multiple range tests at P < 0.01 and indicated by different letters.

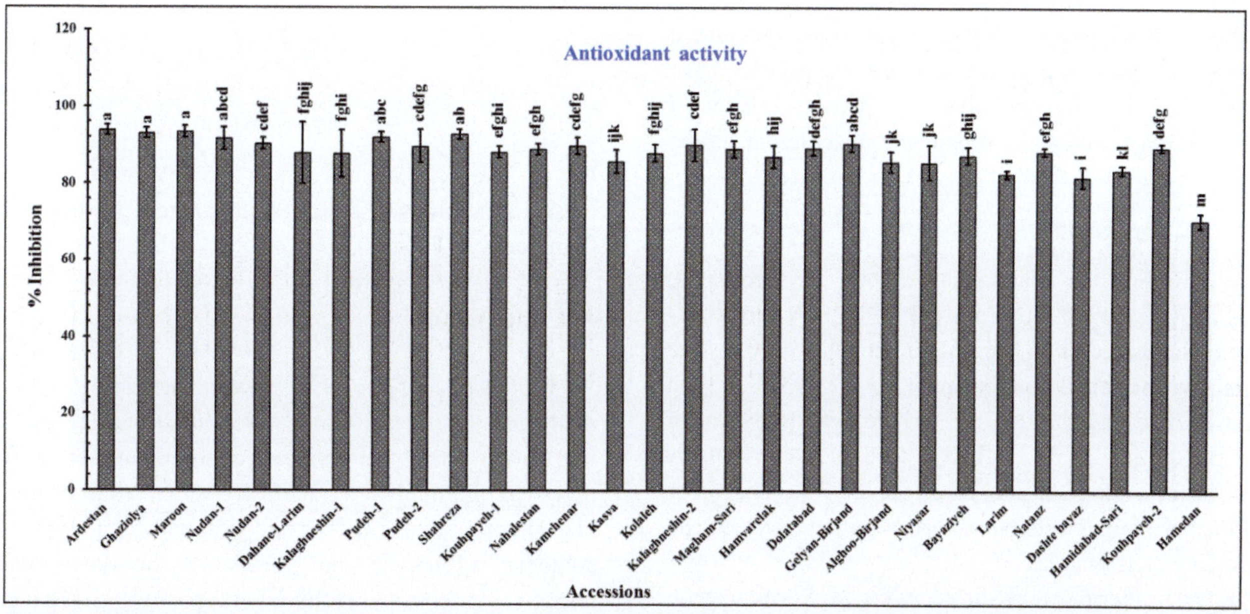

Fig 4. Differences in AOX of 29 tested accessions of jujube. Values represent means ± S.D. of triplicate measurements. Significant differences between accessions were measured by Duncan's multiple range tests at P < 0.01 and indicated by different letters.

It has long been recognized that naturally occurring substances in some medicinal plants have antioxidant activity. Among those substances, the phenolic compounds, widely distributed in fruits, have the ability to scavenge free radicals, superoxide and hydroxyl radicals by single-electron transfer.

Interestingly, the accession Ghaziolya had a low total phenol content compared with other accessions (Figure 1), whereas its antioxidant capacity was higher than other investigated jujubes (Figure 4). Therefore, no correlation between total phenolic contents and antioxidant capacities of extracts from 29 accessions jujube was found in this study. Our results are in agreement with many other reports on *Z. jujuba*. For example, Li et al. (2005a) obtained no correlation between total phenolic contents and antioxidant activities in Chinese jujube fruits. They stated that the antioxidant activity is not solely from the phenolic contents of jujube. Instead, a substantial fraction of total antioxidant activity is likely also due to the presence of other natural compounds such as ascorbic acid, tocopherol and pigments, as well as the presence of synergistic effects among compounds that contribute to the total antioxidant activity.

Also, Kamiloglu et al. (2009) found no significant relationships between total phenolic content and antioxidant activity (in all three methods used) of extracts from fruits of the fifteen selected jujube genotypes from Turkey. Although some studies have demonstrated the positive correlations between phenolic contents and antioxidant capacities in jujube (Xue *et al.*, 2009; Choi *et al.*, 2011; Gao *et al.*, 2011)

3.5. PCA of the samples

To define the relationships among 29 accessions, the main values of four traits (TPH, TF, TA and AOX) were elaborated as the variables to conduct a PCA. The first two principal components (PC-1 and PC-2) with more than 67.9% of the whole variances were extracted for analysis. PC-1 accounted for 40.2% variances and PC-2 accounted for 27.7%. The other principal components which had a minor effect on the model were discarded.

The scatter plot was shown in Figure 5, where each sample (accession) was represented as an observed marker. It was noticeable that the samples were clearly clustered into three domains. Accessions 27(Hamidabad-Sari) and 29 (Hamedan) were in domain I, accessions 2,10,18,20,23 and 28 were in domain III, and the others were in domain II. Actually, these results supported the viewpoints of Guo et al. (2009) who suggested that the presented method may be helpful for discrimination jujube accessions and cultivars from each other in chemotaxonomy.

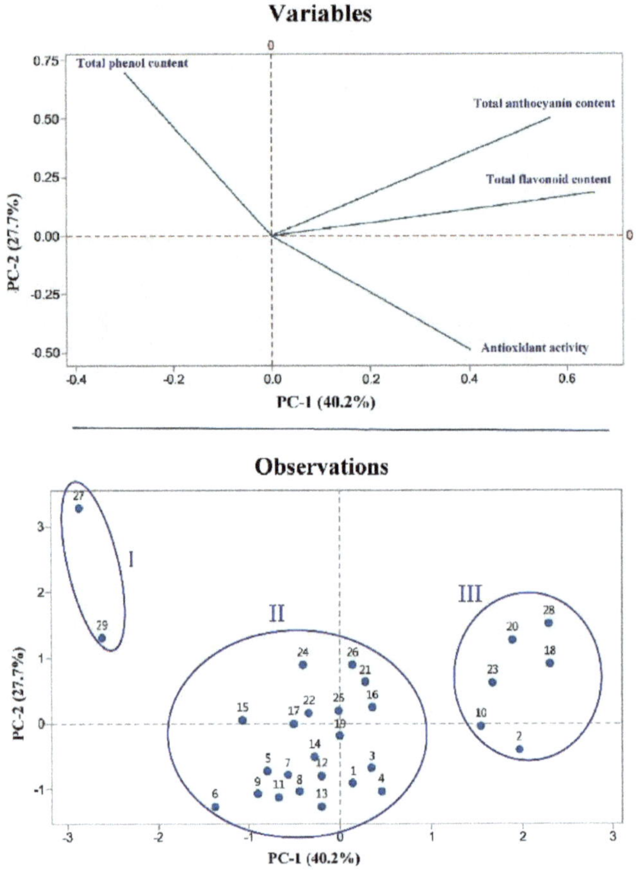

Fig 5. The scatter plot obtained by PCA of the 29 Iranian accessions of *Ziziphus jujuba* from 7 provinces (numbered in Table 1).

4. Conclusion

The results of the present work indicate that the methanol extracts from 29 jujube accessions originating from 7 provinces of Iran had different levels of antioxidant capacities (AOX), total phenol (TPH), total flavonoid (TF) and total anthocyanin (TA) contents. Moreover, no correlation between total phenolic contents and antioxidant capacities of extracts was found. On the basis of the results of this study, it is also indicated that *Zizyphus jujuba* from Iran can be used as accessible source of natural antioxidants and as a possible food supplement or in medical and pharmaceutical industries. It is suggested that further work could be performed on the isolation and identification of the antioxidant components. Since commercial jujube cultivars in large scale do not exist in Iran, these results could be important for determining which of these genotypes to use as breeding materials for future traditional breeding strategies or advanced biotechnological studies.

5. Acknowledgements

Financial support by Bu-Ali Sina University through a M.Sc. program is gratefully acknowledged. The authors are also thankful to Mr. Reza Shahhoseini for providing some necessary facilities to carry out the work.

6. References

Azam-Ali, S., Bonkoungou, E., Bowe, C., de Kock, C., Godara, A., Williams, J.T. 2006. Fruits for the future 2: Ber and other jujubes; International Centre for Underutilized Crops: Southampton, U.K., p 289.

Brand-Williams, W., Cuvelier, M.E., Berset, C. 1995. Use of a free radical method to evaluate antioxidant activity. *LWT-Food Science and Technology*, 28(1): 25–30.

Chang, C.,Yang, M., Wen, H., Chern, J. 2002. Estimation of total flavonoid content in propolis by two complementary colorimetric methods. *Journal of food and drug analysis*, 10:178–182

Choi, S.H., Ahn, J.B., Kozukue, N., Levin, C.E., & Friedman, M. 2011. Distribution of free amino acids, flavonoids, total phenolics, and antioxidative activities of jujube (*Ziziphus jujuba*) fruits and seeds harvested from plants grown in Korea. *Journal Agriculture and Food Chemistry*, 59(12): 6594–6604.

Daneshmand, F., Zare-Zardini, H., Ebrahimi, L. 2013. Investigation of the antimicrobial activities of Snakin-Z, a new cationic peptide derived from *Zizyphus jujuba* fruits. *Natural Products Researches*, 27: 2292–2296.

Di Carlo, G., Mascolo, N., Izzo, A.A., Capasso, F. 1999. Flavonoids: old and new aspects of a class of natural therapeutic drugs. *Life sciences*, 65(4): 337-353.

Gao, Q.H., Wu, P.T., Liu, J.R., Wu, C.S., Parry, J.W., Wang, M. 2011. Physico-chemical properties and antioxidant capacity of different jujube (*Ziziphus jujuba* Mill.) cultivars grown in loess plateau of China. *Scientia Horticulture*, 130(1): 67–72.

Gao, Q.H., Wu, C.S., Wang, M. 2013. The Jujube (*Ziziphus Jujuba* Mill.) Fruit: A review of current knowledge of fruit composition and health benefits. *Journal Agriculture and Food Chemistry*, 61: 3351–3363.

Ghollassi Mood, S. 2008. A contribution to some ethnobotanical aspects of Birjand flora (Iran). *Pakistan Journal of Botany*, 40(4): 1783–1791.

Guo, S., Duan, J.a., Tang, Y., Su, S., Shang, E., Ni, S., Qian, D. 2009. High-performance liquid chromatography—Two wavelength detection of triterpenoid acids from the fruits of Ziziphus jujuba containing various cultivars in different regions and classification using chemometric analysis. *Journal of Pharmaceutical and Biomedical Analysis*, 49(5): 1296-1302.

Howard, L.R., Clark, J.R., Brownmiller, C. 2003. Antioxidant capacity and phenolic content in blueberries as affected by genotype and growing season. *Journal of the Science of Food and Agriculture*, 83:1238–47.

Huang, X., Kojima-Yuasa, A., Norikura, T., Kennedy, D.O., Hasuma, T., Matsui-Yuasa, I. 2007. Mechanism of the Anti-Cancer Activity of *Zizyphus jujuba* in HepG2 Cells. *The American Journal of Chinese Medicine*, 35(3): 517–532

Hudina, M., Liu, M., Veberic, R., Stampar, F., Colaric, M. 2008. Phenolic compounds in the fruit of di fferent varieties of Chinese jujube (*Ziziphus jujuba* Mill.). *Journal of Horticultural Science and Biotechnology*, 83: 305–308.

Kamiloglu, Ö., Ercisli, S., Sengül, M., Toplu, C., Serçe, S. 2009. Total phenolics and antioxidant activity of jujube (*Zizyphus jujube* Mill.) genotypes selected from Turkey. *African Journal of Biotechnology*, 8(2): 303–307.

Lee, J., Durst, R.W., Wrolstad, R.E. 2005. Determination of total monomeric anthocyanin pigment content of fruit juices, beverages, natural colorants, and wines by the pH differential method: collaborative study. *Journal of AOAC International*, 88: 1269–1278.

Li, J.w., Ding, S.d., Ding, X.l. 2005a. Comparison of antioxidant capacities of extracts from five cultivars of Chinese jujube. *Process Biochemistry*, 40(11): 3607–3613.

Li, L.M., Liao, X., Peng, S.L., Ding, L.S. 2005b. Chemical Constituents from the Seeds of *Ziziphus jujube* var. spinosa (Bunge) Hu. *Journal of Integrative Plant Biology*, 47 (4): 494−498

Liu, R.H. 2003. Health benefits of fruit and vegetables are from additive and synergistic combinations of phytochemicals. *American Journal of Clinical Nutrition*, 78: 517–520.

Mahajan, R.T., Chopda, M.Z. 2009. Phyto-Pharmacology of *Ziziphus jujuba* Mill, A plant review. *Pharmacognosy Reviews*, 3: 320–329.

Mazza, G., Miniati, E. 1993. Anthocyanins in fruits, vegetables, and grains. CRC Press, Boca Raton, FL, USA.

McDonald, S., Prenzler, P.D., Antolovich, M., Robards, K. 2001. Phenolic content and antioxidant activity of olive extracts. *Food Chemistry*, 73(1): 73–84.

Memarpoor-Yazdi, M., Mahaki, H., Zare-Zardini, H. 2013. Antioxidant activity of protein hydrolysates and purified peptides from *Zizyphus jujuba* fruits. *Journal of Functional Foods*, 5: 62–70.

Mittler, R. 2002. Oxidative stress, antioxidants and stress tolerance. *Trends in Plant Sciences*, 7(9): 405-410.

Narayana, K.R., Reddy, M.S., Chaluvadi, M.R., Krishna, D.R. 2001. Bioflavonoids classification, pharmacological, biochemical effects and therapeutic potential. *Indian Journal of Pharmacology*, 33: 2–16.

Outlaw Jr, W.H., Zhang, S., Riddle, K.A., Womble, A.K., Anderson, L.C., Outlaw, W.M., Outlaw, N.N., Outlaw, E.C., Thistle, A.B. 2002. The Jujube (*Ziziphus jujuba* Mill.), a multipurpose plant. *Economic Botany*, 56(2): 198–200.

Pahuja, M., Mehla, J., Reeta, KH., Joshi, S., Gupta, Y.K. 2011. Hydroalcoholic extract of *Zizyphus jujuba* ameliorates seizures, oxidative stress, and cognitive impairment in experimental models of epilepsy in rats. *Epilepsy Behavior*, 21: 356−363.

Pawlowska, A.M., Camangi, F., Bader, A., Braca, A. 2009. Flavonoids of *Zizyphus jujuba* L. and *Zizyphus spina-christi* (L.) Willd (Rhamnaceae) fruits. *Food Chemistry*, 112: 858 –862.

Peng, W.H., Hsieh, M.T., Lee, Y.S., Lin, Y.C., Liao, J. 2000. Anxiolytic effect of seed of *Ziziphus jujuba* in mouse models of anxiety. *Journal of Ethnopharmacology*, 72(3): 435–444.

Rechinger, K. 1977. Plants of the Touran protected area, *Iranian Journal of Botany*, 1: 155–180.

San, B., Yildirim, A.N. 2010. Phenolic, alpha-tocopherol, beta-carotene and fatty acid composition of four promising jujube (*Ziziphus jujuba* Miller) selections. *Journal of Food Composition and Analysis*, 23:706–710.

Scalzo, J., Politi, A., Pellegrini, N., Mezzetti, B., Battino, M. 2005. Plant genotype affects total antioxidant capacity and phenolic contents in fruit. *Nutrition*, 21: 207–213.

Steinmetz, K.A., Potter, J.D. 1996. Vegetables, fruit, and cancer prevention: a review. *Journal of the American Dietetic Association*, 96(10): 1027–1039.

Sun, Y.F., Liang, Z.S., Shan, C.J., Viernstein, H., Unger, F. 2011. Comprehensive evaluation of natural antioxidants and antioxidant potentials in *Ziziphus jujuba* Mill. var. spinosa (Bunge) Hu ex HF Chou fruits based on geographical origin by TOPSIS method. *Food Chemistry*, 124(4): 1612–1619.

Wang, S.Y., Chen, C.T., Ciarappa, W.S., Wang, C.H., Camp M.J. 2008. Fruit quality, antioxidant capacity, and flavonoid content of organically and conventionally grown blueberries. *Journal Agriculture and Food Chemistry*, 56: 5788–5794.

Xue, Z.P., Feng, W.H., Cao, J.K., Cao, D.D., Jiang, W.B. 2009. Antioxidant activity and total phenolic contents in peel and pulp of Chinese jujube (*Ziziphus jujuba* Mill.) fruits. *Journal of Food Biochemistry*, 33: 613 −629.

Yoo, K.Y., Li, H., Hwang, I.K., Choi, J.H., Lee, C.H., Kwon, D.Y., Ryu, S.Y., Kim, Y.S., Kang, I.J., Shin, H.C., Won, M.H. 2010. *Zizyphus* attenuates ischemic damage in the gerbil hippocampus via its antioxidant effect. *Journal of Medicinal Food*, 13: 557−563.

Yu, L., Jiang, B.P., Luo, D., Shen, X.C., Guo, S., Duan, J.A., Tang, Y.P. 2012. Bioactive components in the fruits of *Ziziphus jujuba* Mill. against the inflammatory irritant action of Euphorbia plants. *Phytomedicine*, 19:239–244.

Zare-Zardini, H., Tolueinia, B., Hashemi, A., Ebrahimi, L., Fesahat, F. 2013. Antioxidant and cholinesterase inhibitory activity of a new peptide from *Ziziphus jujuba* fruits. *American Journal of Alzheimer's Diseases*, 28(7): 702–709.

Zhang, R., Chen, J., Shi, Q., Li, Z., Peng, Z., Zheng, L., Wang, X. 2014. Phytochemical analysis of Chinese commercial *Ziziphus jujube* leaf tea using high performance liquid chromatography–electrospray ionization-time off light mass spectrometry. *Food Research International*, 56: 47–54.

Zhao, Z.H., Li, J., Wu, X.M., Dai, H., Gao, X.M., Liu, M.J., Tu, P.F. 2006. Structures and immunological activities of two pectic polysaccharides from the fruits of *Ziziphus jujuba* Mill. cv. Jinsixiaozao Hort. *Food Research International*, 39: 917– 923.

Recognition of Sulfur Compounds in Tissue Culture Different Organs of Persian Shallot (*Allium hirtifolium* Boiss) by GC/MS

Mahtab Esfahanizadeh Hoseinpoor[1*], Forough Mortazaeinezhad[2]

[1] *Young Researcher and Elit Club, Isfahan (khorasgan) Branch, Islamic Azad University, Isfahan, Iran;*
[*] **Email:** ***mahtab.esfahanizadeh@gmail.com***

[2] *Department of Horticultural Sciences, Isfahan (khorasgan) Branch, Islamic Azad University, Isfahan, Iran;*

ARTICLE INFO

Topic: *Medicinal Plants*

Key words:

- ✓ *Headspace*
- ✓ *in vitro culture*
- ✓ *Medicinal plant*
- ✓ *Stem-disc bulb*

ABSTRACT

Background & Aim: Persian shallot (*Allium hirtifolium* Boiss) with common name of "Musir" is one of the endemic medicinal plants in Iran. Leaves and bulbs with antibacterial, antifungal, anticancer, anti-diabetes and anti-obesity effects are edible parts of this plant. The tissue culture is an influential method to multiply plant productions in order to meet demands of pharmacy and food industries. Therefore this article will focus on levels and structures of sulfur compounds in seeds, grassland bulbs and compare them with those of leaves, roots, bulbs and callus obtained from the tissue culture using the headspace- Gas chromatography-Mass Spectrophotometry (GC/MS) method.

Experimental: At the first of the study, seeds and stem-discs of grassland bulbs were cultured in MS media. After 90 days seeds, grassland bulbs, seed-leaves, seed-bulbs, leaves and roots of seed-bulbs, stem-disc bulbs, and callus of stem-discs analyzed by GC/MS-headspace method.

Results & Discussion: The results of analysis showed the highest variety of sulfur compounds was in seed bulb roots, while lowest levels were found in seeds, seed bulb leaves and callus. And also the highest level of sulfur compounds was discovered in stem-disc bulbs (28.31%), seed bulb roots (18.61%) and grassland bulbs (6.23%).

Industrial and practical recommendations: Our findings has been shown Persian shallot sulfur compounds have mono, di and tri sulfur in structures and the best source for these metabolites were roots and stem-disc bulbs producing by *in vitro* culture method.

1. Introduction

Alliums with more than 800 species are the biggest monocotyledon genus (Li *et al.*, 2010). This genus has hundreds medicinal plants specie, and it is one of the necessary medicinal and life supporting drugs resources (Gaitant *et al.*, 2010). Allium plants have antibacterial, antifungal, antiviral effects and are used in remedies of diabetes, stress, arthritis, hemorrhoid, colds and flu (Azadi *et al.*, 2008; Taran *et al.*, 2006). *Allium hirtifolium* Boiss belongs to Alliaceae family and is one of the important endemic Alliums that grows wildly in cold mountains of Iran (Ebrahimi *et al.*, 2009). This plant are propagated by seeds and bulbs (Etemadi *et al.*, 2011; Mohammadi *et al.*, 2010). The storage tissue of Persian shallot is usually a single main bulb like, yellow with oval white skinned (Ebrahimi *et al.,* 2009). The shallot is a perennial, herbaceous and aromatic plant which is in danger of extinction (Asili *et al.,* 2010). It is a valuable vegetable to provide dry products such as shallot powder. Moreover, Persian shallot has linoleic acid, linolenic acid and other important elements including Potassium(k), Iron(Fe), Copper(Cu), Zinc(Zn) and Manganese (Mn) (Diaz *et al.,* 2011). This herb with reducing polymerization microtubules protein has a crucial role in treated HeLa (cervival cancer) and Mcf-7 (human, caucasion, breast, and enocarcinoma) (Azadi *et al.,* 2009). In addition, by affecting activity of glycosynase enzyme, hidroalcholic extract of Persian shallot is useful for delaying the development and disorders of diabetes (Hoseini *et al.,* 2011). Mousavi et al. (2013) reported that *Allium hirtifolium* Boiss have more beneficial effects on the treatment of atherosclerosis. Also Ismail et al. (2013) mentioned Persian shallot hydro methanolic extract is effective against some pathogenic bacteria such as *Staphylococous aureus*, *Streptococous peneumoniae*, *Escherichia coli* and *Salmonella typhimunium*. The tissue culture technique is being used for producing primary and secondary metabolites as early as 1950's (Saxena and Roy, 2007). Some of the secondary components are important to medicinal properties of plants and the tissue culture is an effective method for increasing secondary metabolites in different organs of plants. Persian shallot with (-SH) groups of sulfur compounds can oxidize the lipid synthesizing enzymes and this activity may lead to the reduction or even inhibition of lipid synthesis (Nasim *et al.,* 2009). Since there is insufficient data to investigate the effects of tissue culture on sulfur compounds of Persian shallot, this study aims to examine levels and structures of sulfur compounds in seeds, grassland bulbs and compare them with those in leaves, roots, bulbs and callus obtained from the tissue culture by Gas Chromatography-Mass Spectrophotometry (GC/MS) with the headspace method.

2. Materials and Methods

2.1. Seed Culture

Seeds of Persian shallot were surface sterilized with 70% ethanol for 1 min and 25% (v/v) Sodium hypochlorite solution with two drops of Tween 20 for 15 min. Then the seeds were washed three times by sterile distilled water in side an aseptically flow cabinet. The seeds were cultured in half Murashig and Skoog (MS) (1962) with 2 mg/l N6-benzyl adenine (BA) medium and placed at 4°C temperature. After generation all cultures were transferred to a growth chamber at 22°Ctemperature and 16/8h photoperiod.

2.2. Stem-disc Culture

Bulbs of Persian shallot, coming from the grassland were stored at 4°C for 5 months. For internal disinfection roots and outer peels were removed from bulbs which were washed with tap water and then put in hot water (45°C) for one hour. The bulbs were surface sterilized with 70% ethanol for 1 min and sodium hypochlorite 25% (v/v) with two drops of Tween20 for 25 mins. After rinsing three or four times with sterile distilled water stem-discs were cut into 0.5mm diameter and cultured in Murashig and Skoog (1962) medium without hormones. All cultures were incubated in a growth chamber with white light, 16/8h photoperiod and 22°C temperature.

2.3. GC/MS Analysis Preparation

After 90 days seeds produced bulbs with leaves and roots and, callus and bulbs were generated from stem disc explants (Fig 1).

For Gas chromatography-Mass Spectrophotometry (GC/MS) analysis seeds, grassland bulbs, seed-leaves, seed-bulbs, leaves and roots of seed bulbs, stem-disc bulbs, and callus of stem-discs were dried at the room temperature (25°C) with sterile conditions. In the end the volatile compounds of 0.1 g of each sample were evaluated using the headspace method.

2.4. GC/MS Injection Condition

Qualitative analysis of the samples was performed by an Agilent model 6890 GC interfaced to a 5975 mass selective detector. The separation was achieved using 30 m Hp-5MS capillary column with inner diameter of 0.25 mm and 0.25 μm tick stationary phase film. Oven temperature was programmed to initiate at 40 °C for 5 minutes, then the temperature was raised to 270 °C at rate of 5 °C min^{-1}, and finally increased up to 280 °C and held there for 5 °C. The total run time was about 60 minutes.

3. Results and discussion

After GC/MS separation sulfur compounds were confirmed by kovats index calculated with help of standard carbons peaks that had been injected to GC/MS and match quality factors of Wiley library (Table 1). Dry matters of seeds and grassland bulbs of *Allium hirtifolium* Boiss were analyzed using the GC/MS headspace. The GC/mass showed that the grassland bulbs had four sulfur compounds (6.23% grassland bulb) comprising Disulfide dimethyl, Dimethyl trisulfide, 2,3,5-trithiahexane and N-butyl-Benzene sulfonamide and seeds only have one (0.1% seed) sulfur component namely N-butyl-Benzenesulfonamide (Fig. 2). Study of tissue culture samples only identified N-butyl-Benzene sulfonamide in the seed bulb leaves (2.58%) and callus (1.82%) (Fig. 3).

Table 1. Names and chemical information of sulfur compounds

Compounds name	Molecular Formula	Kovats index (KI)	Retention time (RT)
Disulfide, dimethyl	$C_2H_6S_2$	722	3.299
Dimethyl trisulfide	$C_2H_6S_3$	962	11.175
2,3,5-trithiahexane	$C_3H_8S_3$	1119	17.217
Chloromethyl methyl sulfide	$C_3H_8S_2$	1120	17.218
4-Mercaptopyridine	C_5H_5NS		23.348
2,4-Dithiapentane	$C_3H_8S_2$	1506	26.606
N-butyl-Benzene sulfonamide	$C_{10}H_{15}NO_2S$	1774	31.669

Also we found three other sulfur compounds including N-butyl-Benzene sulfonamide (1.98%), Chloromethyl methyl sulfide (1.70%) and Disulfide dimethyl (1.53%) in dry matter of seed bulbs. Analysis of seed bulb roots and stem-disc bulbs driven from the tissue culture method showed both samples had Disulfide dimethyl, Dimethyl trisulfide and 2,3,5-trithiahexane and seed bulbs roots contained N-butyl-Benzene sulfonamide and 4-Mercaptopyridine. Examination of sulfur compounds samples revealed a large variety of sulfur compounds in seed bulb roots, grassland bulb and stem-disc bulbs. In grassland bulb, in addition to 4-Mercaptopyridin, there are the same sulfur compounds as there are in roots (Table 2).

Seed bulb leaves, callus and seeds with 2.58%, 1.82%, and 1.11% respectively of N-butyl-Benzene sulfonamide have less variety and levels of sulfur compounds. Results showed maximum amount of sulfur compounds in stem-disc bulbs (35.67%), seed bulb roots (18.61%) and grassland bulb (6.23%) (Table 3).

Furthermore among sulfur compounds, Dimethyl disulfidein grassland bulbs and seed bulb roots with 64.55% and 11.91% respectively and 2,3,5-trithiahexane in stem-disc had the highest levels. Generally sulfur compounds of Persian shallot obtained from the headspace method were mono, di and tri sulfide in in vivo and in vitro samples (Table 2).

Many Allium species have different types of sulfur compounds such as Allin, a non-protein sulfur amino acid and etc. (Benkeblia and Lanzotti, 2007). Sulfur is required for the synthesis of other compounds such as secondary sulfur compounds (glocosinolates, phytochelatins, allins), thiol (glutathione) and sulpholipids, which play important roles in the physiology, adaptation and protection of plants against pests and stress. Proteins have sulfur; cysteine and methionine residues which are highly significant in the conformation, function and structure of proteins are good illustrations (Durenkamp and Kok, 2004). Organosulfur compounds are known for anticancer, anti HIV and antifungal properties, so diets that are generally rich in plants from family of Alliaceae have beneficial health effects (Haq and Ali, 2003).

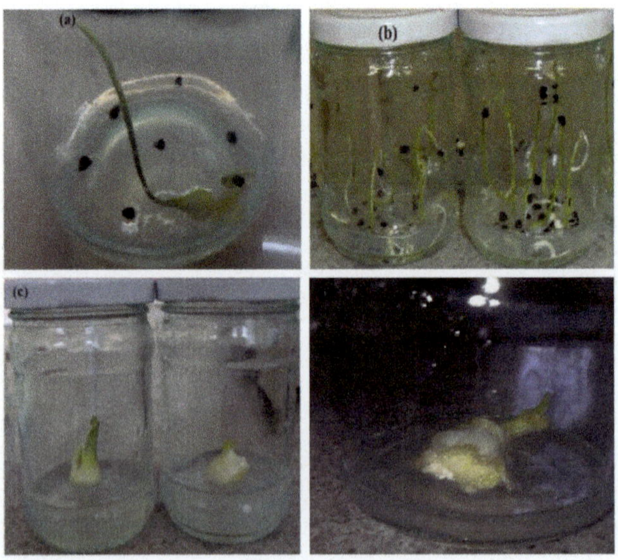

Fig 1. (a) Seed bulb; Seed leaves (b); Stem-disc bulbs(c); Callus induction(d)

The volatile compounds of Allium genus mainly represented by thiosulfinate are very unstable. Depending on the species and under different conditions, thiosulfinates of Allium species can be decomposed to additional sulfur constituents including methyallyl, diallyl, diethyl mono,di-, tri-, tetra-, penta and hexasulfieds (Shams, 2003). Cell suspentions, callus and other tissue cultures have been used successfully for study of allin (s-allyl-L cysteien) synthesis in garlics and isoallin in onions (Hughes *et al,* 2005). The result in this paper argued that the tissue culture had very important effects on sulfur components of Persian shallot because the highest level of sulfur compounds are found in seed bulb roots growing in Murashig and Skoog medium with five different compounds such as Disulfide, dimethyl, Dimethyl trisulfide, 2,3,5-trithiahexane, N-butyl-Benzene sulfonamide and 4 –Mercapto pyridine that constitute 35.67% of total volatile.

Table 2. Sulfur compounds of samples; Seeds(A), Grassland bulbs(B), Stem-disc bulb(C), Seed bulb(D), Seed leaves(E),Seed bulb leaves(F), Seed bulb roots(G), Callus(H).

Sulfur compounds name	Samples							
	A	B	C	D	E	F	G	H
Disulfide, dimethyl	-	+	+	+	+	-	+	-
Dimethyl trisulfide	-	+	+	-	-	-	+	-
2,3,5-trithiahexane	-	+	+	-	-	-	+	-
Chloromethyl methyl sulfide	-	-	-	-	+	-	-	-
N-butyl-Benzenesulfonamide	+	+	-	+	+	+	+	+
2,4-Dithiapentane	-	-	+	-	-	-	-	-
4-Mercaptopyridine	-	-	-	-	-	-	+	-

Table 3. Data analysis of different sample; Disulfide, dimethyl(DD), Dimethyl trisulfide(DT), 2,3,5-trithiahexane(TTH), Chloromethyl methyl sulfide(CMS), N-butyl-Benzenesulfonamide(NBS), 2,4-Dithiapentane(DP), 4-Mercaptopyridine(MP).

		Mean Square						
Fd		DD	DT	TTH	CMS	NBS	DP	MP
Seed	7	0.00^{f}	0.00^{d}	0.00^{d}	0.00^{b}	0.09^{d}	0.00^{b}	0.00^{b}
Grassland bulb	7	4.87^{c}	0.95^{c}	0.49^{c}	0.00^{b}	0.02^{d}	0.00^{b}	0.00^{b}
Stem-disc bulb	7	8.09^{b}	3.01^{a}	19.47^{a}	0.00^{b}	0.00^{d}	3.88^{a}	0.00^{b}
Seed bulb	7	0.92^{e}	0.00^{d}	0.00^{d}	1.07^{a}	1.41^{c}	0.00^{b}	0.00^{b}
Leaf seed	7	2.20^{d}	0.00^{d}	0.00^{d}	0.00^{b}	2.40^{a}	0.00^{b}	0.00^{b}
Leaf seed bulb	7	0.00^{f}	0.00^{d}	0.00^{d}	0.00^{b}	2.58^{a}	0.00^{b}	0.00^{b}
Root	7	12.00^{a}	2.66^{b}	0.98^{b}	0.00^{b}	1.85^{b}	0.00^{b}	1.43^{a}
Callus	7	0.00^{f}	0.00^{d}	0.00^{d}	0.00^{b}	1.89^{b}	0.00^{b}	0.00^{b}
Error	16							
Total	23							

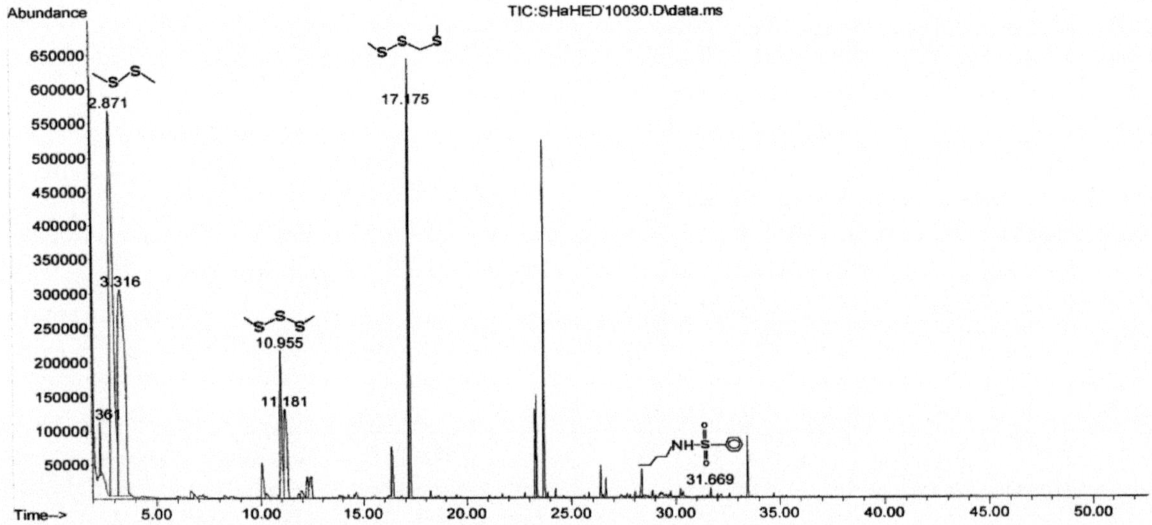

Fig 2. GC/MS peak of Grassland bulb sulfur compounds.

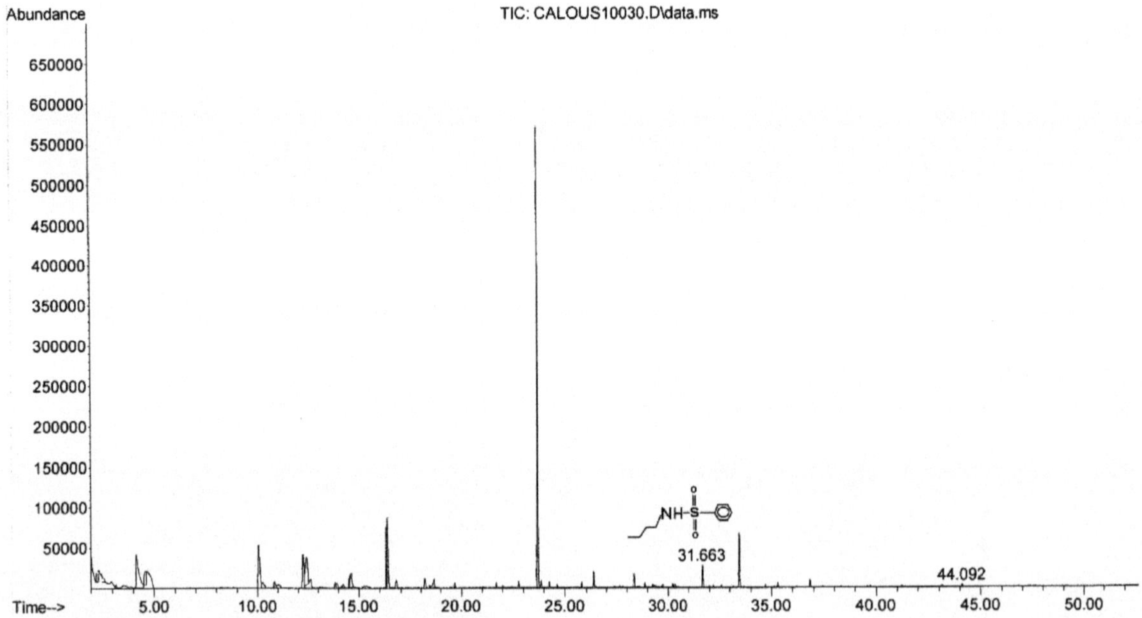

Fig 3. GC/MS peak of Callus sulfur compounds.

The active volatiles compounds in *Allium resoum* identified by Gas Choromatography Mass Spectophotometery with the headspace sampling include dimethyl disulfide, disulfide allyl dimethyl, trisulfide dimethyl, sulfide dimethyl, disulfide diallyl, trisulfideallyl dimetyl, trisulfideallyl methyl, trisulfidediallyl 2-perpenyl and tetrasulfideallyl dimethyl (Najja *et al.,* 2011). Our findingshave showed N-butyl-Benzenesulfonamide was the only sulfur compound which was found in all samples except the control sample where 2,4-Dithiapentane was observed. The major sulfur compounds of chive flowers and onions were 3,4-dimethyl thiaphene, methyl n-propyl disulfide and dimethyl trisulfide (Grzeszczuk *et al.,* 2011) .

Volatile analysis of chive by GC/MS with the headspace method indicated this plant had di and trisulfur compounds (Mann *et al,* 2011). Melluki *et al.*

(1994) reported that the essential oil of callus sulfur compounds of chives (*Allium schoenoparsum* L.) were less than that of leaves. Allin (s-allyl-L-cysteineSulfoxide) is one of the sulfur compounds in lily family (Melluki *et al.,* 1994). Nasim *et al.* (2009) demonstrated that the most amount of Allin was in leaves between different organs of garlics such as leaves, roots, embryos, and callus. Allin, Isoallin, s-methyl- and s-propyl-L-systeine-s-oxide are commonly present in Allium plants that can decompose to other sulfur compounds with allinase enzymes (Benkeblia and Lanzotti, 2007). In this study sulfur compounds of callus (1.825%) were less than those of seed leaves (4.47%) and seed bulb leaves (2.58%). Also the most important compounds of grassland bulbs in other sections of Persian shallot were 2,3,5-trithiahexane (Roshan *et al.,* 2012) and trisulfid dimethyl (Sham, 2003). Diaz *et al.* (2011) reported essential oil of Leaves and roots of *Allium schoeoprasum* L. analyzed by GC/MS, consisted of bis-(2-sulfhydryethyl-) disulfide with the major components in both samples (72.06% leaves, 56.47% roots)(Diaz *et al.,* 2011). Also they found 2,4,5-trithiahexan in leaves (5.54%) and roots (15.90%) (Ebrahimi *et al.*, 2008). *Allium ascalonicum* L. growing in Thailand and *Allium tuberosum* Rottlerin China had diallyl mono, di, tri. In this study, the chemical analysis has identified sulfur compounds obtained from GC/MS were mono, di and tri sulfide. The thiosulfinate can break down to disulfide and trisulfide that are toxic to insect herbivores (Mohammadi *et al.,* 2010).

4. Conclusion

Our findings by Gas chromatography-Mass Spectrophotometry with headspace method has been shown Persian shallot (Musir) sulfur compounds has mono, di and tri sulfur in structures and the best source for these metabolites were roots and stem-disc bulbs producing by invitro culture method. Significantly, the data obtained from the present study suggests that the tissue culture is an effective method of increasing sulfur compounds in *Allium hirtifolium* Boiss.

5. Acknowledgment

We would like to acknowledge chemistry faculty, Islamic Azad University of Isfahan (Khorasgan) for help us with the GC/MS analysis.

6. References

Asili, J., Behravan, M.R., Naghavi and Asili, J. 2010. Genetic diversity of Persian shallot (Allium hirtifolium) ecotypes based on morphological traits, allicin content and RAPD markers. *Journal of Medicinal Aromatic Plants*, 1: 1-6.

Azadi, H.G., Riazi, G.H., Ghaffari, S.M., Ahmadian S. and Khalife, T.J. 2009. Effects of Allium hirtifolium (Iranian shallot) and its allicin on microtubule and cancer cell lines. *African Journal of Biotechnology*., 8: 5030-5037.

Azadi, H.G., Ghaffari, S.M., Riazi, G.H., Ahmadian, S. and Vahedi, F. 2008. Antiproliferative activity of chloroformic extract of Persian Shallot, Allium hirtifolium, on tumor cell lines. *Cytotechnology*, 56: 179-185.

Benkeblia, N. and Lanzotti,V. 2007. Allium thiosulfinates: Chemistry, biological properties and their potential utilization in food preservation. *Food*, 1: 193-201.

Diaz, A.B., Vera, J.R., Fermin, L.R., Mendez, A.M., Zambrano, R.A. and Contreras, L.R. 2011. Composition of the essential oil of leaves and roots of Allium schoenoprasum L. (Alliaceae). *Boletin Latinoamericano Caribe Planta Medicinales Aromaticas*, 10: 218-221.

Durenkamp, M. and de Kok, L.J. 2004. Impact of pedospheric and atmospheric sulphur nutrition on sulphur metabolism of Allium cepa L., a species with a potential sink capacity for secondary sulphur compounds. *Journal of Experimental Botany*, 55: 1821-1830.

Ebrahimi, R., Zamani, Z. and Kashi, A. 2009. Genetic diversity evaluation of wild Persian shallot (Allium hirtifolium Boiss.) using morphological and RAPD markers. *Scientific Horticulture*., 119: 345-351.

Ebrahimi, R., Zamani, Z., Kashi, A. and Jabbari, A. 2008. Comparison of fatty acids, mineral elements of 17 Iranian shallot landraces (Allium hirtifolium Boiss.). *JFST*, 5: 61-68.

Etemadi, N., Maryam H. and Zamani, N. 2011. Optimizing seed germination threatened endemic species of the Persian shallot (Allium hirtifolium Boiss.). *African Journal of Agriculture Research*, 6: 5133-5138.

Gantait, S., Mandal, N. and Das, P.K. 2010. An overview on in vitro culture of genus Allium.

American Journal of Plant Physiologyl., 5: 325-337.

Grzeszczuk, M., Wesolowska, A. Jadczak, D. and Jakubowska, B. 2011. Nutritional value of chive edible flowers. *Acta Scientiarum Polonorum. Hortorum Cultus*, 10: 85-94.

Haq, K. and Ali, M. 2003. Biologically Active Sulphur Compounds of Plant Origin. In: Sulphur in Plants, Abrol, Y.P. and A. Ahmad (Eds.). Kluwer Academic Publishers, Dordrecht, Netherlands, pp: 375-386.

Hoseini, J., Hoseinizijuvand, M., Mohamadi, M., Hashemi, M., Arsalande, F. and Zeinivand, M. 2011. Hydro alcoholic extract of Persian shallot *Allium hirtifolium* increased activity of glycokinaze enzyme in liver of diabetic mouse. Proceedings of the 1st National Congress of Biotechnology Students, December 15-17, 2011, Tehran, Iran.

Hughes, J., Tregova, A., Tomsett, A.B., Jones, M.G., Cosstick, R. and Collin, H.A. 2005. Synthesis of the flavour precursor, alliin, in garlic tissue cultures. *Phytochemistry*, 66: 187-194.

Ismail, S., Jalilian, F.A., Talebpour, A.H., Zargar, M., Shameli, K., Sekawi, Z. and Jahanshiri, F. 2013. Chemical composition and antibacterial and cytotoxic activities of *Allium hirtifolium Boiss. BioMed Research International*, 1-8.

Li, Q.Q., Zhou, S.D., He, X.J., Yu, Y., Zhang, Y.C. and Wei, X.Q. 2010. Phylogeny and biogeography of Allium (Amaryllidaceae: Allieae) based on nuclear ribosomal internal transcribed spacer and chloroplast. Rps 16 sequences, focusing on the inclusion of species endemic to China. *Annals of Botany*, 106: 709-733.

Mann, R.S., Rouseff, R.L., Smoot, J.M., Castle, W.S. and Stelinski, L.L. 2011. Sulfur volatiles from Allium spp. affect Asian citrus psyllid, Diaphorina citri Kuwayama (Hemiptera: Psyllidae), response to citrus volatiles. *Bulletin of Entomological Research*, 101: 89-97.

Melluki, F., Vannrean, A., Auger, J., Marcotte, J.L. and Cosson, L. 1994. Flavor prodaction in tissue cultures of chive *(Allium schoenopasum* L.*)*: Callus structure and flavor production. *Plant Science*, 95: 165-173.

Mohammadi, J., Olfati-Chirani, J.A., Khasmakhi-Sabet, S.A., Golshani, M., Mortazavi, S.N. and Jafari, F. 2010. Effect of incubation temperature, seed age and scarification on germination and emergence of Persian Shallot. *Pakistanian Journal of Agriculture Science*, 47: 317-319.

Mousavi, S.A., Chitsaz, A., Rahimi, S., Ghanadian, M., Askari, G. and Khorvash, F. 2013. A placebo control double blind study of effects of *atorvastatin + allium hirtifollium* on carotid intima media thickness. *Pakistanian Journal of Medicine Science*, 29: 269-301.

Murashige, T. and Skoog, F. 1962. A revised medium for rapid growth and bioassays with tobacco tissue cultures. *Physiologia Plantarum*. 15: 473–497.

Najja, H., Fattouch, S., Ammar, E. and Neffati, M. 2011. Antimicrobial Potentials of *Allium roseum*: Recent Advances and Trends. In: Science against Microbial Pathogens: Communicating Current Research and Technological Advances, Mendez-Vilas, A. (Ed.). Vol. 2, Formatex Research Center, USA. pp: 1025-1210.

Nasim, S.A., Mujib, A., Rashmi, K., Samar, F. and Junaid, A. 2009. Improved alliin yield in somatic embryos of *Allium sativum* L. (cv. Yamuna safed) as analyzed by HPTLC. *Acta Biologica Hungarica*, 60: 441-454.

Roshan, V., Azad, N.M., and Bahmanzadegan, A. 2012. Evaluation of volatile component of fresh, salted and dried corm of Persian shallot *(Allium hirtifolium* Boiss.*)* using headspace/ GC-MS. Proceedings of the National Congress on Medicinal Plants, May 16-17, Kish Island.

Saxena, K.K. and Roy, S. 2007. Isolation and identification of trigonelline from the tissue culture of *Allium sativum* Linn. *Asian Journal Experimantal Sciences*, 21: 277-280.

Shams, M. 2003. Investigation of compound in Hamedan moosir and compression to Isfahan moosir. Ph.D. Thesis, University of Tehran, Tehran, Iran.

Taran, M., Rezaeian, M. and Izaddoost, M. 2006. In vitro antitrichomonas activity of *Allium hirtifloium* (Persian Shallot) in comparison with metronidazole. *Iranian Journal of Public Health*, 35: 92-94.

The ethnopharmacological review of medicinal plants in uses hypertension treatment in Iranian complementary medicine

Hamidreza Ardalani

Department of Horticultural Sciences, Science and Research Branch, Islamic Azad University, Tehran, Iran;
***Email:** hrardalani@srbiau.ac.ir*

ARTICLE INFO

***Topic:** Medicinal Plants*

Key words:
✓ *Ethnopharmacology*
✓ *Hypertension*
✓ *Medicinal Plants*
✓ *Traditional Medicine*
✓ *Blood Pressure*
✓ *Iran*

ABSTRACT

Background & Aim: One of the most common diseases in the world, especially among Iranian people, is high blood pressure which can cause many cardiovascular disorders such as heart attack. The disease is often associated with other diseases such as diabetes and hyperlipidemia. Methyldopa and captopril are the most common drugs among several medications used to control blood pressure in Iran. Nowadays, herbal medicines are very prevalent because medicinal plants have least of the side effects. Various herbals are used in the Iranian traditional medicine to improve hypertension, but among them, barberry, olive leaf, garlic, celery, sumac and hibiscus are the most prevalent.

Experimental: In this paper, the most herbs in uses in treatment of hypertension were studied and these effects of natural products on these plants were clarified.

Results & Discussion: The results indicate that these plants and their phenolic compounds can be used as an alternative or supplement to chemical medicines used to control blood pressure.

Industrial and practical recommendations: There is suggestion for pharmaceuticals and food industrials to use of these herbs for improve new methodology in herbal drugs production.

1. Introduction

Arterial hypertension is most important diseases in developing countries. This common and asymptomatic disease is curable and can be easily diagnosed, but it may have fatal consequences if left untreated (Leng *et al.*, 1996). Hypertension in adults refers to an increase in systolic blood pressure equal to or more than 140 mm/hg as well as diastolic blood pressure equal to or more than 90mm/Hg separately or together (Lloyd-Jones *et al.*, 2005). Some studies show that a great number of factors contribute to the raised blood pressure in hypertensive patients, and their relative roles may differ between individuals. Among the factors that have been intensively studied are salt intake, obesity and insulin resistance, the renin-angiotensin system, and the sympathetic nervous system (Beevers *et al.*, 2001). Studies have shown that if hypertension disorder is left untreated, it can cause problems such as heart failure, coronary artery disease, angina, myocardial infarction, development of thrombosis, and cerebral hemorrhage (MacMahon *et al.*, 1990). Hypertension management consists of two main approaches: lifestyle modifications and pharmacological treatment .lower intake of salt and fat, regular exercise and limited alcohols intake are the most important lifestyle factors (Appel *et al.*, 2003). There are some mechanisms for lowering blood pressure: decreasing blood volume and Na, decreasing peripheral resistance, restrain heart activity, peripheral vasodilation by interfering NO and angiotensin suppression. There are several groups of antihypertensive drugs, including diuretics, anti-adrenergic receptor, a vascular dilator and angiotensin-converting enzyme inhibitors (ACEI) (Collaboration, 2000). Nowadays, the need for multiple drug therapy especially for whom with resistant hypertension and rising number of patients suffering from adverse effects and side effects of synthetic drugs have led to the popularity of herbal medicines. Growing use of medicinal plants highlights the need for more research on medicinal plants and their effects on clinical trials. Many medicinal plants in traditional medicine in Iran are used to control blood pressure for their relatively high effectiveness, slight side effects, being natural, and lower prices compared to expensive drugs. In this review, several plants are used to treat hypertension which is studied clinically and in laboratory conditions focused on Iranian complementary medicine. In many reference books such as Canon written by Ibn Sina many of these plants are mentioned (Tekol, 2007).

Berberis Vulgaris

A shrub 1 to 5 meters in length with small red fruits that, fruit of this plant contains alkaloids such as Berberine , Jatrorrhizine , Chloramine , Palmatine , Oxycodone , this is fluorine Eyes and Magnoflorine which have antibiotic effects and help lower blood pressure (Imanshahidi and Hosseinzadeh, 2008). There is plenty of evidence that barberry fruit improve blood pressure and this characteristic is attributed to alkaloid berberine (Fatehi-Hassanabad *et al.*, 2005). In experimental intravenous administration of aqueous extract of barberry to rats suffering from high blood pressure it was shown that the reduced blood pressure was significant at the probability level of P <0.01. In this experiment blood pressure was caused by sodium chloride in the drinking water of rats, then, blood pressure was significantly reduced by injecting the aqueous extract of barberry (Hong *et al.*, 2002). In another experiment, aqueous extract of barberry in the form of 200 mg capsules was administered to 60 patients three times a day and for two weeks. At the end, the average systolic blood pressure was reduced from 169.05 to 145.08 and diastolic blood pressure was reduced from 99.8 to 83.75 and the reduction was significant at P <0.01 (Cicero and Ertek, 2009).

Alium sativum

Garlic is an herbaceous perennial plant consisting of 10 to 50 cubes. The uses of garlic to treat various diseases back to thousands years ago. However, there is little scientific support for medicinal properties of garlic (Koch and Lawson, 1996). But in the past decade, the protective properties of garlic against cancer was proved by epidemiological studies and animal experiments (Thomson and Ali, 2003; Wargovich, 1987). Garlic contains the various compounds such as organosulfur compounds, amino acids, vitamins and minerals. It is possible that some sulfur compounds, including allicin, ojeone, allyl cystein, diallyl thiosulfinate are responsible for the health benefits of garlic (Kimbaris et al., 2006). Animal studies showed that garlic extract reduces plasma lipids and cholesterol (Ali *et al.*, 2000; Eidi *et al.,* 2006). In an experiment the effect of garlic pill on the patients with high blood pressure was examined and the results indicated that the garlic pill significantly reduced blood sugar, blood lipid and systolic blood pressure (Reinhart *et al.,* 2008).

Apium graveolens

Celery is a plant of Apiaceous family, which has different chemical compounds including glycosides, sugars, pectin and ether essence (Momin and Nair, 2001). Apigenin as the importance flavonoid in celery is a potent antiplatelet agent and this vascular relaxant effect in animals has been demonstrated (Zhang *et al.,* 2011). In another study, the effects of the celery seed tea bag were examined clinically in 37 patients with hypertension (Moghadam *et al.*, 2013). Before the experiment, the mean systolic and diastolic blood pressure was 171.35 and 94.3, respectively and after the treatment, they were measured 154.3 and 89.6, respectively. This difference was significant at the probability level of 0.05. This effect is probably produced by opening vascular effects of diuresis (Fazal and Singla, 2012). In the other study it was shown that aqueous celery extract significantly reduced fat in the blood serum of mice (Mansi *et al.*, 2009).

Olea europae

Olive is a plant which belongs to the Oleaceae family and the scientific name of the fruit is *Olea europae*. Its leaf and fruit are used in traditional medicine. Olive leaf has a bitter taste with diuretic and astringent properties, that it also improving blood pressure. Olive leaf reduces blood pressure by opening ducts of surface vessels without affecting heart (Perrinjaquet-Moccetti *et al.*, 2008). Olive leaf contains a substance called oleuropein whose relaxant effects on the isolated arteries walls of animals were demonstrated (Huang and Sumpio, 2008). Another study conducted by Fehri *et al* (1993) demonstrated that aqueous olive leaf extract reduces blood pressure, blood sugar and uric acid levels in the rodent (Fehri *et al.,* 1993). In another study conducted on mice, aqueous extract of olive leaf significantly reduced systolic blood pressure compared to placebo (Susalit *et al.*, 2011).

Hibiscus Sabdariffa

An annual plant with 2 to 3 m high bush which has 3-5 faceted yellowish green leaves and red flowers with green sepals which go red the fruit ripens. This plant has a very sour taste because of containing high citric acid level. Its effectiveness on reducing blood pressure has been demonstrated in several article which in most cases consider anthocyanin as the main factor for hypertension improving (Faraji and Tarkhani, 1999; Mozaffari-Khosravi *et al.*, 2009). In several countries the aqueous extract of sour tea has been used to treat digestive disorders, hypercholesterolemia, and diuretic, diaphoretic [causing sweating] and anti- hypertensive for many years. The experimental values of 500 mg / kg and 1000 mg / kg body weight calyx of hibiscus tea infusion in hypertensive and normotensive wistar-kyoto rats, significantly reduced the systolic and diastolic (Onyenekwe *et al.*, 1999). In an experiment conducted by Whabi *et al.* (2010), the blood pressure-lowering property of this plant in diabetic patients has been demonstrated (Wahabi *et al.*, 2010). In another experiment to compare the effects of anti- hypertensive and tolerability of a standardized extract from hibiscus tea with captopril, a randomized controlled clinical trial, patients 30 to 80 years of age were diagnosed with hypertension and were not treated for at least one month prior to study. One group of subjects drank the infusion made from 10 g sepal of hibiscus tea dried flower in half a liter of water [containing 9.6 g anthocyanin] before breakfast and the other group used 25 mg captopril twice a day. The results showed that the hibiscus tea reduced the systolic blood pressure from 139.05 to 123.73 mmHg and diastolic blood pressure from 90.81 to 79.52 mmHg. At the end of the study, no significant difference was observed in blood pressure measured in two treatment groups (Herrera-Arellano *et al.,* 2004). In the other study, the tolerance for both treatment groups was 100%. A natriuretic effect was observed in hibiscus tea. The obtained data showed that in terms of hypotensive, and anti-hypertensive effectiveness as well as tolerance there was no significant difference between Hibiscus tea extract standardized on 6.9 mg of anthocyanin's and 50 mg of captopril (Ajiboye *et al.*, 2011).

2. References

Ajiboye, T.O., Salawu, N.A., Yakubu, M.T., Oladiji, A.T., Akanji, M.A., Okogun, J.I. 2011. Antioxidant and drug detoxification potentials of Hibiscus sabdariffa anthocyanin extract. *Drug and chemical toxicology,* 34: 109-115.

Ali, M., Al-Qattan, K., Al-Enezi, F., Khanafer, R., Mustafa, T. 2000. Effect of allicin from garlic powder on serum lipids and blood pressure in rats fed with a high cholesterol diet. *Prostaglandins, leukotrienes and essential fatty acids*, 62: 253-259.

Appel, L.J., Champagne, C.M., Harsha, D.W., Cooper, L.S., Obarzanek, E., Elmer, P.J., Stevens, V.J., Vollmer, W.M., Lin, P.-H., Svetkey, L.P. 2003. Effects of comprehensive lifestyle modification on blood pressure control: main results of the PREMIER clinical trial. *Journal of the American Medical Association.*

Beevers, G., Lip, G.Y., O'Brien, E. 2001. ABC of hypertension: Blood pressure measurement: Part II—Conventional sphygmomanometry: technique of auscultatory blood pressure measurement. *British Medical Journal*, 322: 1043.

Cicero, A.F., Ertek, S. 2009. Metabolic and cardiovascular effects of berberine: from preclinical evidences to clinical trial results. *Clinical Lipidology*, 4: 553-563.

Collaboration, B.P.L.T.T. 2000. Effects of ACE inhibitors, calcium antagonists, and other blood-pressure-lowering drugs: results of prospectively designed overviews of randomised trials. *The Lancet,* 356: 1955-1964.

Eidi, A., Eidi, M., Esmaeili, E. 2006. Antidiabetic effect of garlic (Allium sativum L.) in normal and streptozotocin-induced diabetic rats. *Phytomedicine*, 13: 624-629.

Faraji, M.H., Tarkhani, A.H. 1999. The effect of sour tea (Hibiscus sabdariffa) on essential hypertension. *Journal of Ethnopharmacology,* 65: 231-236.

Fatehi-Hassanabad, Z., Jafarzadeh, M., Tarhini, A., Fatehi, M. 2005. The antihypertensive and vasodilator effects of aqueous extract from Berberis vulgaris fruit on hypertensive rats. Phytotherapy Research, 19: 222-225.

Fazal, S.S., Singla, R.K. 2012. Review on the pharmacognostical & pharmacological characterization of Apium graveolens Linn. *Indo Global Journal of Pharmaceutical Sciences,* 2: 36-42.

Fehri, B., Aiache, J., Memmi, A., Korbi, S., Yacoubi, M., Mrad, S., Lamaison, J., 1993. [Hypotension, hypoglycemia and hypouricemia recorded after repeated administration of aqueous leaf extract of Olea europaea L.]. *Journal de pharmacie de Belgique*, 49: 101-108.

Herrera-Arellano, A., Flores-Romero, S., Chavez-Soto, M., Tortoriello, J. 2004. Effectiveness and tolerability of a standardized extract from Hibiscus sabdariffa in patients with mild to moderate hypertension: a controlled and randomized clinical trial. *Phytomedicine*, 11: 375-382.

Hong, Y., Hui, S.-C., Chan, T.-Y., Hou, J.-Y. 2002. Effect of berberine on regression of pressure-overload induced cardiac hypertrophy in rats. *The American journal of Chinese medicine,* 30: 589-599.

Huang, C.L., Sumpio, B.E. 2008. Olive oil, the mediterranean diet, and cardiovascular health. *Journal of the American College of Surgeons*, 207: 407-416.

Imanshahidi, M., Hosseinzadeh, H. 2008. Pharmacological and therapeutic effects of Berberis vulgaris and its active constituent, berberine. *Phytotherapy research*, 22: 999-1012.

Kimbaris, A.C., Siatis, N.G., Daferera, D.J., Tarantilis, P.A., Pappas, C.S., Polissiou, M.G. 2006. Comparison of distillation and ultrasound-assisted extraction methods for the isolation of sensitive aroma compounds from garlic (Allium sativum). *Ultrasonics sonochemistry,* 13: 54-60.

Koch, H.P., Lawson, L.D. 1996. Garlic: the science and therapeutic application of Allium sativum L. and related species. baltimore, Maryland: Williams & Wilkins xv, 329p. ISBN.

Leng, G.C., Lee, A.J., FOWKERS, F.G.R., WHITEMAN, M., Dunbar, J., Housley, E., Ruckley, C.V. 1996. Incidence, natural history and cardiovascular events in symptomatic and asymptomatic peripheral arterial disease in the general population. *International journal of epidemiology*, 25: 1172-1181.

Lloyd-Jones, D.M., Evans, J.C., Levy, D., 2005. Hypertension in adults across the age spectrum: current outcomes and control in the community. *Journal of the American Medical Association*, 294: 466-472.

MacMahon, S., Peto, R., Collins, R., Godwin, J., Cutler, J., Sorlie, P., Abbott, R., Neaton, J., Dyer, A., Stamler, J. 1990. Blood pressure, stroke, and coronary heart disease: part 1, prolonged differences in blood pressure: prospective observational studies corrected for the regression dilution bias. *The Lancet*, 335: 765-774.

Mansi, K., Abushoffa, A.M., Disi, A., Aburjai, T. 2009. Hypolipidemic effects of seed extract of celery (Apium graveolens) in rats. Pharmacognosy magazine, 5: 301.

Moghadam, M.H., Imenshahidi, M., Mohajeri, S.A. 2013. Antihypertensive effect of celery seed on rat blood pressure in chronic administration. Journal of medicinal food, 16: 558-563.

Momin, R.A., Nair, M.G. 2001. Mosquitocidal, nematicidal, and antifungal compounds from Apium graveolens L. seeds. Journal of agricultural and food chemistry, 49: 142-145.

Mozaffari-Khosravi, H., Jalali-Khanabadi, B., Afkhami-Ardekani, M., Fatehi, F., Noori-Shadkam, M. 2009. The effects of sour tea (Hibiscus sabdariffa) on hypertension in patients with type II diabetes. *Journal of human hypertension*, 23: 48-54.

Onyenekwe, P., Ajani, E., Ameh, D., Gamaniel, K. 1999. Antihypertensive effect of roselle (Hibiscus sabdariffa) calyx infusion in spontaneously hypertensive rats and a comparison of its toxicity with that in Wistar rats. *Cell Biochemistry and Function*, 17: 199-206.

Perrinjaquet-Moccetti, T., Busjahn, A., Schmidlin, C., Schmidt, A., Bradl, B., Aydogan, C. 2008. Food supplementation with an olive (Olea europaea L.) leaf extract reduces blood pressure in borderline hypertensive monozygotic twins. *Phytotherapy Research,* 22: 1239-1242.

Reinhart, K.M., Coleman, C.I., Teevan, C., Vachhani, P., White, C.M. 2008. Effects of garlic on blood pressure in patients with and without systolic hypertension: a meta-analysis. *Annals of Pharmacotherapy*, 42: 1766-1771.

Susalit, E., Agus, N., Effendi, I., Tjandrawinata, R.R., Nofiarny, D., Perrinjaquet-Moccetti, T., Verbruggen, M. 2011. Olive (Olea europaea) leaf extract effective in patients with stage-1 hypertension: comparison with Captopril. *Phytomedicine*, 18: 251-258.

Tekol, Y., 2007. The medieval physician Avicenna used an herbal calcium channel blocker, Taxus baccata L. *Phytotherapy Research*, 21: 701-702.

Thomson, M., Ali, M. 2003. Garlic [Allium sativum]: a review of its potential use as an anti-cancer agent. *Current cancer drug targets,* 3: 67-81.

Wahabi, H., Alansary, L., Al-Sabban, A., Glasziuo, P. 2010. The effectiveness of Hibiscus sabdariffa in the treatment of hypertension: a systematic review. *Phytomedicine*, 17: 83-86.

Wargovich, M.J., 1987. Diallyl sulfide, a flavor component of garlic (Allium sativum), inhibits dimethyihydrazine-induced colon cancer. *Carcinogenesis*, 8: 487-489.

Zhang, Q., Zhou, M.M., Chen, P.L., Cao, Y.Y., Tan, X.L., 2011. Optimization of Ultrasonic-Assisted Enzymatic Hydrolysis for the Extraction of Luteolin and Apigenin from Celery. *Journal of food science*, 76: C680-C685.

Rheological properties of the gum fractions from psyllium (*Plantago psyllium* L.)

Mohammad Hojjatoleslamy[1*], Fatemeh Raisi[1], Masoumeh Asadi[1], Mehran Mohammadian[2], Narges Samanian[3]

[1]*Department of Food Science and Technology, Faculty of Agriculture, Islamic Azad University, Shahrekord Branch, Shahrekord, Iran;*
Email:** ***mohojjat@iaushk.ac.ir

[2]*Laboratory of Vice-chancellor for Drug and Food Organization, Shahrekord, Iran;*

[3]*Department of Food Engineering, Ferdowsi University, Mashhad, Iran;*

ARTICLE INFO

Topic: *Food Technology*

Key words:
- *Psyllium* (Plantago psyllium)
- *Rheology*
- *Temperature*

ABSTRACT

Background & Aim: Psyllium (*Plantago psyllium* L.) is a native plant that grows widely in India and Iran. Different cases of using psyllium gum for its suitable rheological properties in a wide range of food products exist in nature.
Experimental: In this study, different fractions of psyllium gum were extracted by water and alkali treatments. Rheological properties of these fractions were measured by Brookfield rheometer (RV DVIII). The obtained data was fitted by Herschel-bulkly model in three temperatures 30, 60 and 80°C.
Results & Discussion: Results indicated that fractions show different behaviours during heating treatment.
Recommended applications/industries: According to results of present study, the largest variations were observed in $AEG_{0.5}$ fraction.

1. Introduction

Psyllium gum (*Plantago psyllium* L.) is known as psyllium gum in Iran. *Plantago psyllium* is an annual herb which belongs to the family Plantaginaceace (Ghasemi Pirbalouti, 2010). Though it is found all around the world, its abundance can be seen generally in India, Pinjab, Pakistan, Iran and Canary islands. India, selling 39000 tons annually, is one of the most prominent exporters of the seed. The plant is diversely outspread in different provinces of Iran due to the different climate. It has also been long used in Iranians traditional medicine (Guo, 2009).

The term "Psyllium" is used for the crust, seed and the whole plant (Theuissen, 2008). It is considered as a good source for soluble and insoluble fiber. Its soluble content is almost eight times more than that of oat's bran. The diet fibers extracted from the plant possess pharmaceutical properties and can be used in producing low calorie food (Theuissen, 2008). The studies have revealed the beneficial uses of psyllium such as its reducing effect on blood fat and sugar that are considered as the main risk factor of cardiovascular diseases (Yu , 2003; Theuissen , 2008).

Psyllium can also be used as a laxative and its crust as an dietetic fiber can augment the healthy environment of the colons (Singh, 2007). Some of the impacts can be due to its bioactive components, namely phenolic compounds such as Acetoside and Isoacetoside. Antidotal and antioxidant activities beside being painkillers are among their biological functions (Li, 2005). The so called properties have made psyllium a suitable functional dietetic fiber to use in some food products. It can be used as a bioactive oligosaccharide with probiotic properties (Askari, 2008). Investigating the chemical properties of seed, crust and the psyllium produced -mucilage shows that, they contain 6.05, 6.24, and 6.13% moisture respectively. The total protein content of the seed exceeds the one of the crust and the mucilage and the crust and the mucilage output is 28%. About 90% of the seed, crust and mucilage are made of the carbohydrates and xylose and arabinose are the most important of all.

The suitable gelling properties of the psyllium polysaccharides make it a suitable choice in many fields (Ghasemi Pirbalouti, 2010). For instance, it can be used as a binding agent in pharmaceutical industry or lubricating agent for soil in petroleum usages. It can also be a good alternative in sewage separation. As data on gelling properties of the psyllium gum is scarce and the mechanism of gel construction is not completely known yet, the possibility of performing more research in this field to reach a suitable understanding of how to use it efficiently in food industry still exists (Guo, 2009). The usage of the psyllium fiber has been noticed in several studies. In a research done in 1988, the use of psyllium and mucilage was studied. Some of these usages such as instant drinks, pies, dietetic bakery products, soft gel puddings, sauces and in particular meat sauces, soups and confectionary products have been pointed to.

Frust et al. (1989) proposed psyllium to produce a water dispersible component that can be used as a dietetic bulking agent. Due to the findings of a study which was carried out in 1998, psyllium mucilage is a natural dietetic fiber which can be used to decrease the caloric value of the puffed cereal products. This component may modify the dough texture while cutting, drying and puffing (Frust, 1989).

The products obtained from psyllium crust can be used to prevent ice crystal formation. They can substitute mono and disaccharides in ice cream (Nikoozadeh 2008). Park et al. (1997) used a mixture of wheat fiber and psyllium crust (7:3). Their study showed a loaf of bread containing fiber and antioxidant, in a single portion (268 g) would provide 1.2 g or 8% of the daily requirement of the dietetic fiber which exists in 30% soluble form and its calorie value is 16% less than white bread (Park, 1997).

The hydrophobicity of the psyllium seed hydrocolloid was also investigated. All the solutions showed non Newtonian shear thinning behaviour in different concentrations and pH. The viscosity of the psyllium crust solution is temperature, pH, concentration and shear rate dependent (Farahnaki, 2010). About 90% of the whole seed, crust and mucilage are made of carbohydrates and specially, xylose and arabinose are among the 3 major components of the polysaccharides extracted from psyllium crust namely, WE, $AEG_{0.5}$, $AES_{0.5}$. The arabinose / xylose ratio the 3 major parts of the psyllium crust are WE = 1:4.2, $AES_{0.5}$ = 1:3.1 and $AEG_{0.5}$ = 1:2.3 (Fischer, 2004). Studies have revealed that xylose existing in psyllium gum is extensively in the form Pyranosyl ring, while the only structure of arabinose is furanosyl. The output of these 3 polysaccharide parts is about 99% and among them the major part with 60% of the whole output belongs to $AEG_{0.5}$.

Significant amounts of Uronic acid (around 15%) exists in $AES_{0.5}$, WE, while $AEG_{0.5}$ lacks Uronic acid. Investigating the 3 polysaccharide component shows WE has the simplest side branches and the highest stability in alkali condition is related to $AEG_{0.5}$ (Guo, 2008). The so called components also differ in water solubility. As WE is water soluble, $AES_{0.5}$ can also be solved in water, and can be extracted with alkali solution. $AEG_{0.5}$ is also extractable with alkalis (Guo, 2008).

2. Materials and Methods

In this work, to study the effect of psyllium gum fractions on its rheological properties, at first 5 grams of psyllium crust powder (purchased from Rose Darvak corporations) was mixed with 1000 ml distilled water and the obtained gel was heated while mixing at 80 °C. The extraction operation was carried out with some modifications based on Guo et al. (2008) (Fig 1).

This gel was named 'gel-1' and contained all main (WE, $AES_{0.5}$, and $AEG_{0.5}$) and sub fractions ($AES_{1.2}$, and $AES_{2.0}$). Rheological properties of gel-1 were determined using a Brookfield Rheometer, RV DVIII and small sample adapter at 30, 60 and 80 °C. In the next stage, gel-1 was centrifuged for 1 h at 21000*g*. During this stage, gel-2 and its supernatant were formed. The supernatant contained a main fraction called WE. Then, gel-2 lacks the water soluble WE fraction. The rheological properties of gel-2 were studied likewise.

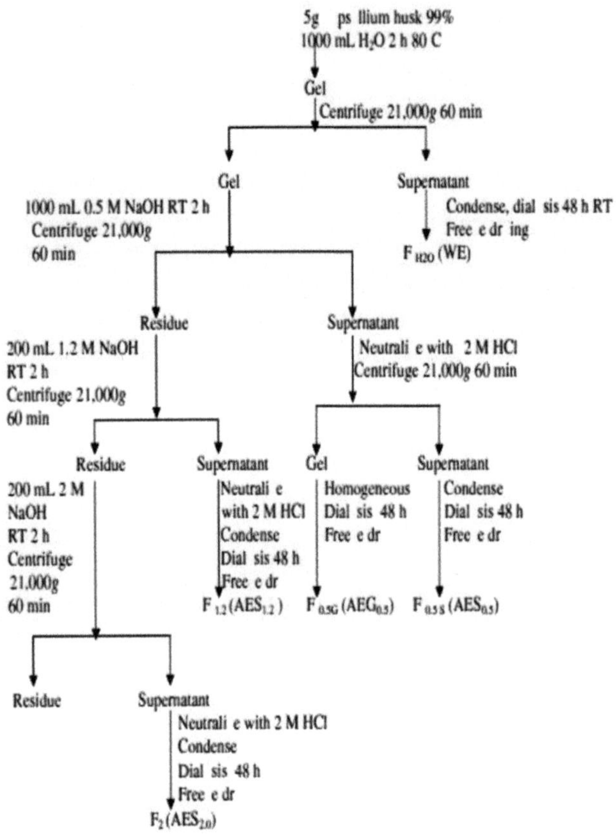

Fig1. Extraction path for psyllium gum (Guo, 2008)

The psyllium crusts present in gel-2 was precipitated using 1000 ml of sodium hydroxide (0.5 M). The resulted sediment contained $AES_{1.2}$, $AES_{2.0}$, and psyllium crusts. The sediment was separated and then centrifuged for 1 h at 21000g and then was neutralized using a 2 M hydrochloric acid and then the supernatant was again neutralized using 2 M hydrochloric acid and was centrifuged again at 21000*g*, thus gel-3 with its supernatant was obtained. This stage's supernatant contained the soluble fraction of $AES_{0.5}$, which is another main fraction. It is clear then, that it lacks the main fractions $AES_{0.5}$, WE and sub fractions $AES_{1.2}$, AES_2 and only contains $AEG_{0.5}$ (the extraction path is shown in Fig 1.). The rheological properties of gel-3 were also determined using the rheometer and then was fitted with a Hercshel- Bulky model using a Rheocalc $_{\text{(version 3.2)}}$ software (Eq. 1).

Eq.1

$$\sigma = k\gamma^n + \sigma_0$$

Where:

σ: shear rate(D/cm^2)

γ: shear rate(1/s)

σ_0: yield stress (D/cm^2)

k: consistency index (Poise)

n: flow constant (Steffe, 1996)

Smaller than one amounts for n, indicate a shear thinning behaviour while when it exceeds 1, the flow is shear thickening.

3. Results and discussion

Considering the explanation above, and Fig. 1, the extracted gels contain components as below:

Gel-1: ($WE+AES_{0.5}+AEG_{0.5}$) + ($AES_{2.0}+AES_{1.2}$)

Gel-2: ($AES_{0.5}+AEG_{0.5}$) + ($AES_{2.0}+AES_{1.2}$)

Gel-3: $AEG_{0.5}$

WE: is one of the main fractions, which is completely water soluble and has the highest stability in alkali condition.

$AES_{0.5}$: one of the main fractions, completely water soluble and extractable by alkali solution.

$AEG_{0.5}$: completely soluble in alkali solution- this fraction is extractable through using alkali solutions- among all fraction this is the only one that can form a gel and exists in all the gels 1, 2 and 3. This fraction lacks Uronic acid while WE and $AES_{0.5}$ contain Uronic acid. After analyzing the obtained graphs, the rheological properties were reported in Table 1 using Rheocalc 3.2 software. As it can be seen in Table 1, the yield stress for all treatments and all temperatures is zero; it means that, no fraction needs an initial stress for starting to flow. Thus all the graphs originate in zero and can be interpreted by the power law model. (Eq. 2)

Eq. 2 $$\sigma = k\gamma^n$$

Gel-1 indicates a shear thickening behavior in all temperatures. In this gel the flow index decreases by increasing the temperature and approximates a Newtonian behavior, while consistency index, which is an indicator of the apparent viscosity, shows an increase with temperatures.

Table 1. Rheological properties of the extracted gels from psyllium

temperature		Gel1	Gel2	Gel3
	K	0.109	0.930	5.125
30	n	1.400	1.257	0.946
	σ_0	0.000	0.000	0.000
60	K	0.290	0.094	10.900
	n	1.294	1.143	0.599
	σ_0	0.000	0.000	0.000
80	K	0.463	0.062	2.270
	n	1.198	1.140	0.599
	σ_0	0.000	0.000	0.000

As it was mentioned before, this fraction has large amounts of WE, and $AES_{0.5}$ that both are among the main fractions of psyllium and are high in Uronic acid. In lower temperatures, the ionization constant of the acid agent is low and therefore its molecular elongation and hydrodynamic radius are smaller. This shows how with increase in temperature, the amount of ionization and gel consistency raises. Some other probable reasons may be the intermolecular interactions which happens because of the electric charge of the carboxyl groups in the fractions and weakens the effect of temperature in decreasing the consistency and viscosity.

In gel-2, WE is one of the main gel forming Uronic acid containing component- exits, decreasing consistency with temperature would follow a reasonable behaviour. Considering the partition of WE from the other fraction, the hypothesis of the charged carboxyl group and intermolecular interaction intensifies. This gel also shows a shear thickening behaviour.

As it was mentioned before gel-3 lacks Uronic acid and it's the only fraction that is able to form a firm gel. It can be seen in Table 3 that this gel shows a shear thinning behaviour ($n<1$) in all temperatures, and as temperature raises n shows a decreasing procedure. This gel has got a large consistency index in compare with the other 2 gels. This amount increases at 60 °C and decreases again at 80 °C. To understand the real cause of this phenomenon, it is required to measure the molecular radius precisely in future studies. The changes in rheological properties (shear stress, shear rate) have been depicted in figures 1, 2, and 3. As it can be seen, Fig 2 verifies the information done in Table 2. It can be seen that rheological properties of this gels are completely different from each other and they show different behaviour toward temperature changes.

Regarding to Fig 2, it can be perceived that, to provide desirable consistency at lower temperatures, gels 2 and 3 are more suitable while in higher temperatures gel 1 is the better choice. Thus the presence of the fraction WE which is high in Uronic acid effects the temperature behavior of the psyllium gum dramatically. Due to the works of Askari et al. (2008) who described the psyllium gel as shear thinning and the results shown in Table 1 and Fig 2, it seems that the properties of gel-3, is more effective on the gel which is resulted from the whole fractions, and can affect the overall properties of the gel. The fraction 1 and 2 of the gel that are shear thinning, are less effective than fraction 3.

4. Conclusion

A large number of researches have been performed on rheological properties of psyllium gel have been performed, but due to the manifold of its fractions and because of the different properties of the food products, only one fraction may be effective on rheological attributes of the final product, thus to gain a better perception of functions the psyllium gel, separating its fractions is inevitable. Therefore, the necessity of the future studies on its technological properties seems quite clear.

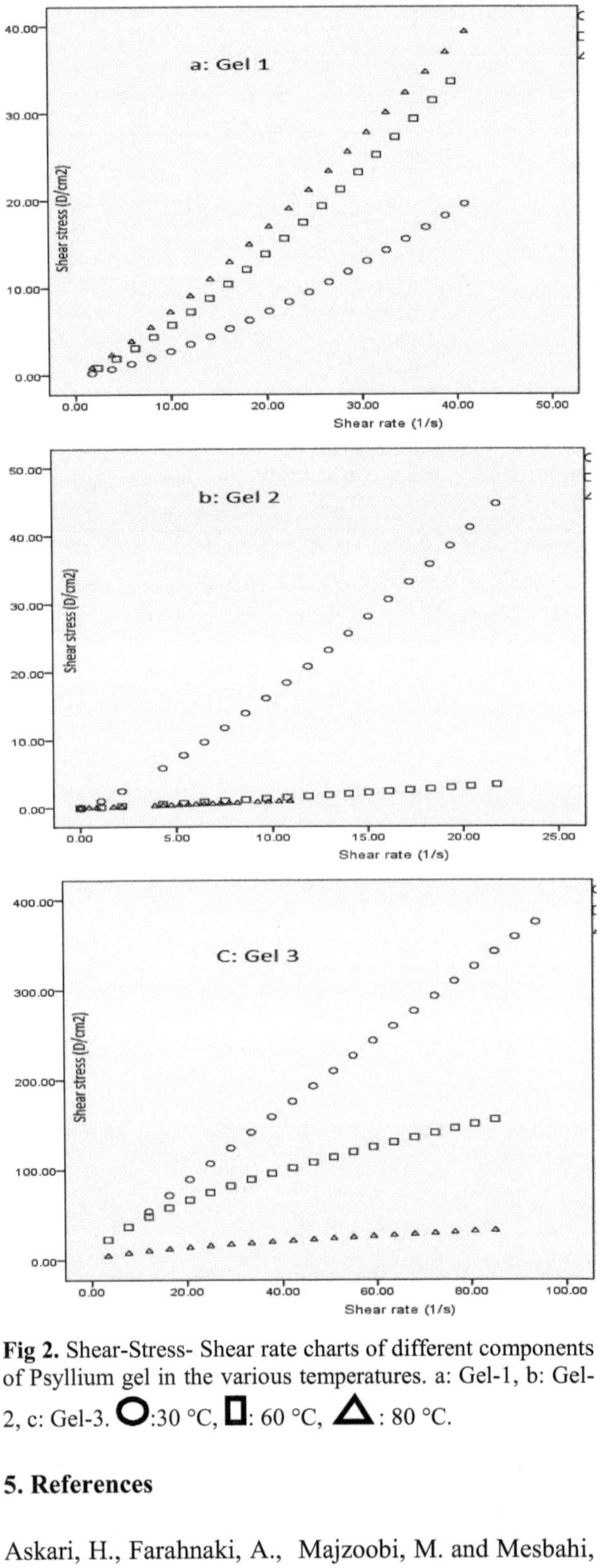

Fig 2. Shear-Stress- Shear rate charts of different components of Psyllium gel in the various temperatures. a: Gel-1, b: Gel-2, c: Gel-3. **O**:30 °C, **□**: 60 °C, **△**: 80 °C.

5. References

Askari, H., Farahnaki, A., Majzoobi, M. and Mesbahi, Gh. 2008. Hydrocolloid extraction from Psyllium husk and investigation on its rheological properties. 18th, National Iranian food science and technology conference.

Farahnaki, A., Askari, H., Majzoobi, M. and Mesbahi, G.H. 2010. The impact of concentration, temperature and pH on dynamic rheology of Psyllium gels. *Journal of Food Engineering*., 1-8.

Fischer, M. H., Yu, N., Gray, G. R., Ralph, J., Anderson, L. and Marlette, J. 2004. The gel forming polysaccharide of Psyllium husk (*Plantago ovata* Fork). *Carbohydrate Research*., 339: 2009-20017.

Dennis, E., Allen Peter, C., Altamore, Gene, A., Furst 1989. Water-dispersible compound containing psyllium powder as a dietary bulking agent. US. 4: 828-842.

Guo, Q. W., Cuit, S. W., Wang, Q. and Young, J. C. 2008. "Fravtion and polysaccharide characterization of Psyllium gum." *Carbohydrate Polymers*., 73: 35-43.

Guo, Q. W., Cuit, S. W., Wang, Q. Goffa, H. D. and Smith, A. 2009. "Microstructure and rheological properties of Psyllium polysaccharide gel." *Food Hydrocolloids*., 23: 1542-1547.

Li, L., Tsao, R., liu, S., Yang, J. C., Zhu, H., deng, Z., Xie, M. and Fu, Z. 2005. Isolation and purification of acetoside and isoacetoside from Plantago Psyllium L. by high speed counter current chromatography. *Journal of Chromatography.,* 1063: 161-169.

Nikoozadeh, H., Taslimi, A. and Azizi, M. 2008. The effect of Psyllium husk addition on rheological properties of dough and quality of Sangak bread. 18th, *National Iranian Food Science and Technology Conference.*

Park, H., P. A. Seib. and Chung. 1997. Fortifying bread with a mixture of wheat fiber and psyllium husk fiber plus three antioxidants. *Cereal Chemistry*., 74(3): 207-211

Singh, B. 2007. Psyllium as therapeutic and drug delivery agent. Int. *Journal of Pharmaceutics*., 334: 1-14.

Steffe, J. 1996. Rheological methods in food process engineering. East Lasting, Freeman Press.

Theuissen, E. a. M., R. P. 2008. Water soluble dietary fibers and cardiovascular disease. *Physiology and Behavior*., 94: 285-292.

Yu, L. a. P. 2003. Effect of solid-state enzyme treatments on the water absorbing and gelling properties of Psyllium. *LWT - Food Science and Technology*., 36: 203-208.

Investigating effect of chamomile hydroalcoholic extract on movement disorders in the animal model of Parkinson's disease

Shahrbanoo Alami Rostami[1*], Maryam Rafieirad[2]

[1]*Department of Biology, Islamic Azad Univercity ,Gomishan center, Gorgan Branch,Gorgan Iran;*
***Email: sh_alemi_r@yahoo.com**

[2]*Department of Biology, faculty of Sciences, Islamic Azad University, Izeh branch, Izeh-Iran;*

ARTICLE INFO

Topic: *Medicinal Plants*

Key words:
- ✓ *Chamomile extract*
- ✓ *Parkinson's disease (PD)*
- ✓ *Movement disorder*
- ✓ *Rats*

ABSTRACT

Background & Aim: Parkinson's disease (PD) is a kind of disorder in the nervous system, which is characterized with multiple movement disorders. Factors such as oxidative stress are the most important causes for the degeneration of dopaminergic neurons in the substantia nigra and occurrence of Parkinson's disease. Thus, medications that have antioxidant functions could be an interesting target for treating the movement disorders caused by Parkinson's disease. Chamomile is the natural source of antioxidants.
Experimental: In this study, 50 adult male Wistar rats were randomly divided into control and Parkinson's groups with 10 rats along with 3 Parkinson's groups, which received chamomile extract by gastric gavage method and doses of 5, 10, and 50 mg/kg once per day for 14 days. Also, 8 μg of 6-hydroxydopamine (6-OHDA) neurotoxin in 2 μl saline containing 1% ascorbic acid was injected into medial forebrain bundle (MFB) of the left hemisphere of the brain of the rats to induce Parkinson's disease. Results were presented as mean ± SD, one-way analysis of variance, and Tukey's post-hoc test.
Results: Following subcutaneous injection 2.5 mg/kg apomorphine 14 days after injury with 6-OHDA in MFB of left brain, animals were rotated 360 degrees to the right by 10 <rpm. Moreover, these rats showed a significant difference in movement tests (balancing, immobility, and step length) compared with the control group. Treatment of the Parkinson's animals using different doses of chamomile extract compared with the untreated group resulted in significant improvement in motor activities and the doses of 10 and 50 mg/kg had maximum therapeutic effects.
Recommended applications/industries: Probably because of its strong antioxidant effect and interference with the activity of movement pathway receptors, chamomile extract can be used to improve and reduce the movement disorders of Parkinson's disease in addition to pharmacotherapy.

1. Introduction

Parkinson's disease (PD) is a neurodegenerative disease which is caused by the gradual loss of dopamine nerve cells in the substantia nigra nucleus of the midbrain (Rosenthal, 1998). The loss of these cells causes a spectrum of movement disorders such as clinical disorders, resting tremor, muscle rigidity, and slow motion (Philippens *et al.*, 2010). The cause of dopamine cell death in the substantia nigra nucleus has not been fully understood (Shrivastava *et al.*, 2013). Axon of dopaminergic neurons in the pars compacta of the substantia nigra moves along the middle frontal brain

(MFB) and ends in the striatum (Da Cunha *et al.*, 2002). In fact, inputs to the striatum's GABAergic neurons are destroyed in PD (Kleppner and Tobin, 2001). Unilateral injection of 6-OHDA into the MFB in rats is conventionally used to develop an animal model for PD (Sun *et al.*, 2010). The formation of free radicals and oxidative stress may play an important role in the pathogenesis of PD and the central nervous system shows a very high degree of vulnerability to reactive oxygen species (ROS) (Ebadi *et al.*, 1996). Unbalanced and excessive production of ROSs may lead to increased oxidative stress, which can induce many neurological injuries and, eventually, lead to the death of neurons by apoptosis and necrosis (Abou-Sleiman *et al.,* 2006). Healthy cells have a number of mechanisms to resist damage caused by free radicals (Yeh *et al.,* 2009). Antioxidants are considered one of the most important mechanisms for protecting the brain and rapidly prevent the generation of induced ROS (Tanaka *et al.,* 2006). Chamomile with the scientific name of *Matricaria chamomilla* belongs to *Asteraceae* family (Singh *et al.*, 2011). Today, chamomile is used worldwide to treat many diseases, including skin inflammation and tumors (Singh *et al.*, 2011). In the traditional medicine, chamomile is commonly used for relieving pain, acting as antispasmodic and anti-inflammatory agents, treating skin diseases (psoriasis and eczema), curing bronchitis, cold, cough, and fever, healing wounds, and treating gastrointestinal problems (Golparvar *et al.*, 2011; Singh *et al.*, 2011). Chamomile extract is composed of 120 kinds of chemical compounds, which include chamazulenes, flavonoids, and coumarins. Its most active constituent is chamazulene, apigenin, and bisabolol (McKay and Blumberg, 2006). According to the pervious scientific research, the compounds contained in chamomile extract have anti-inflammatory, antibacterial, and antioxidant effects(Golparvar *et al.*, 2011). Chamomile is rich in flavonoids, which are effective antioxidants for neutralizing oxygenated radicals (Srivastava *et al.*, 2010). Considering the antioxidant properties of chamomile, in this study, the effect of its different doses on movement disorders was investigated in a PD animal model.

2. Materials and Methods

In this study, 50 Wistar rats with the weight range of 200-250 g (prepared from Ahvaz Jundishapur University of Medical Sciences) were used. The animals were kept in individual cages in 12 h light and 12 h dark conditions, temperature of 21±2°C, and access to enough food and water ad libitum. Then, they were randomly divided into the following groups:

1- Control group to which no lesion was induced.
2- Rats with PD which received 2 µl of 8 µg 6-hydroxydopamine neurotoxin in the MFB.
3- Three treated Parkinson's groups: which were similar to the Parkinson's group and received intragastric gavage of chamomile extract 7 days after the recovery (5, 10, and 50 mg/kg) for 14 days. On the 15th day, the behavioral tests were performed (Gholami Z and M, 2014).

2.1. *Stereotaxic surgery method*

First, the rats were weighed and anesthetized by intraperitoneal (IP) injection of 90 mg/kg of ketamine hydrochloride and 10 mg/kg of xylazine per kg of body weight (both drugs were produced by Alosfan Company in the Netherlands). Afterwards, the animals were placed in the stereotaxic device, on which they were fixed using a mouthpiece and intramedullary rods. The hair at the dorsal skull was also shaved. The head skin was disinfected using a piece of soft cotton and a longitudinal incision was made through the back of the head between the two eyes up to the middle dorsal point of the ears. Connective tissues on the skull surface were removed and the bregma point was made visible. Bregma and lambda points were placed at an equal level, on which the device indicator was set. Then, according to the coordinates extracted from Atlas of Neurosurgical Techniques: Brain, the MFB coordinate (with coordinates of -4.8; a relative to Bregma point ±1.6, ML, -8.2; DV) was determined (Sarkaki et al., 2013). In this study, to make a PD animal model, the unilateral injection of 6-OHDA into the MFB was used.

2.2. *Preparing 6-hydroxy-dopamine dissolution*

6-hydroxy-dopamine (Sigma Company) was prepared with the concentration of 8 µg in 2 ml of normal saline containing 0.01% ascorbic acid (Sarkaki *et al.*, 2013).

2.3. *Preparing apomorphine dissolution*

(Sigma Corporation of America): This drug was dissolved in the normal saline containing 0.02% ascorbic acid.

2.4. *Preparing chamomile extract*

Chamomile flowers were collected from around Ize, Khuzestan Province, early in May. The flowering branches were maintained for two weeks in a dark and dry environment in order to dry. After powdering and grinding the plant, 250 g was weighed and reached the volume using 1,000 ml of 70% alcohol. After keeping the plant for 3 days in the laboratory environment and mixing (to isolate all the plant constituents in water and alcohol), they were scattered on the tray to dry. Purity degree of the extract was 25%. After drying, the powdered plant was collected and kept for making different doses of the extract (Seifi Zangeneh *et al.*, 2015).

2.5. Apomorphine-induced rotation test

The rotational behavior of the rats was tested by injecting 2.5 mg/kg of apomorphine hydrochloride. Complete rotations (in a cylindrical chamber) were measured for 60 min in 10 min intervals (Sarkaki *et al.*, 2013).

2.6. Catalepsy test (horizontal bar)

Both hands of the animals were placed on a bar with the height of 9 cm; while their legs were on the bottom of a wooden box, the period of time it takes for the animal to remove the hands was recorded (Dekundy *et al,*. 2006).

2.7. Rotarod test (motor coordination test)

This test is performed to measure motor performance and coordination. For this purpose, the animals were placed on the Rota rod with variable speed. The initial rotation speed of the rod was 5 rpm, which was later gradually increased to 25 rpm within 300 sec (5 min). The main criterion for the balance in all the groups was 25 rpm. The animals were formerly familiarized with this test. Then, each rat was tested 3 times per day with 45 min interval between the sessions. Also, the mean time was calculated (Sarkaki *et al.*, 2012).

2.8. Stride length test

This device consisted of a dark wooden box with a sliding door and dimensions of 10×17×20 cm, to which a narrow tunnel with the dimensions of 4.5×10×45 was connected. The end of the tunnel was open. The boundary between the square part and the tunnel was separated by a guillotine blade. There was a plastic square box with the ink-stained floor at the open end of the tunnel, the floor of which was coated with a white paper tape with the width of 4.3 cm. Then, motor organs of the rats with its tail were placed in the inky box and directed toward the tunnel; once the rats entered the dark box, guillotine blade was released and they were confined inside the dark box to prevent returning and walk on the paper inside floor of the tunnel. Then, the paper tape was removed from the tunnel floor to dry the fingerprints. In this manner, paces were recorded on the paper. It is necessary to note that the animal got familiar with the box before the test (Sarkaki *et al.*, 2012).

3. Results and discussion

3.1. Apomorphine rotation test

Apomorphine was injected subcutaneously into the control group and, 2 weeks after the surgery, into the rats with PD after the MFB lesion. It caused a significant contralateral rotation in the lesioned rats (P <0.001). Intragastric administration of chamomile extract to the rats suffering from PD at the doses of 10 and 50 mg/kg significantly reduced the rotations (P <0.001) compared with the Parkinson's group (Figure 1).

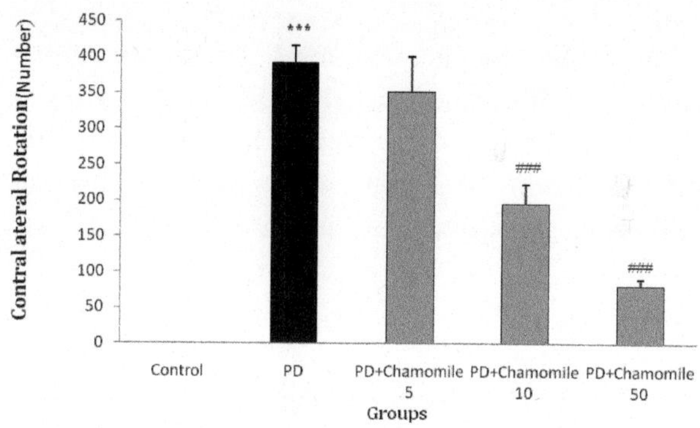

Fig. 1. Effect of 14-day intragastric gavage of 5, 10, and 50 mg/kg of chamomile extract on rotation in the PD animal model. Results were presented as mean ± SD, one-way analysis of variance, and Tukey's post-hoc test (n=10 per group). * and # on the columns show the significant difference from the control and PD groups, respectively.***= (P <0.001) and ### =(P <0.001)

3.2. Immobility test (catalepsy)

In this test, immobility disorder rate in the PD group was significantly increased compared with the control group (P <0.001) and treatment with chamomile extract (10 and 50 mg/kg) significantly reduced the catalepsy level (P <0.01) and (P <0.001) compared with the Parkinson's group. However, 5 mg/kg of the chamomile extract had no therapeutic effect on immobility (catalepsy) caused in the PD rats (Figure 2).

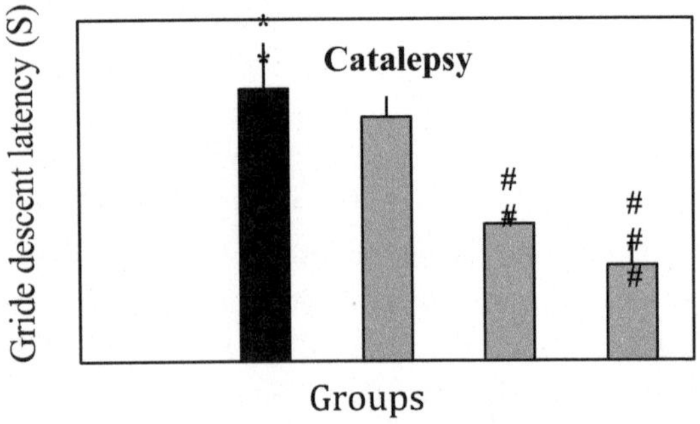

Fig. 2. Effect of 14-day intragastric gavage of 5, 10, and 50 mg/kg of chamomile extract on the immobility (catalepsy) in the PD animal model. Results were presented as mean ± SD, one-way analysis of variance, and Tukey's post-hoc test (n=10 per group). * and # on the columns show the significant difference from the control and PD groups, respectively.***= (P <0.001) and ### =(P <0.001),## =(P <0.01).

3.3. Motor coordination

The motor coordination level in the PD group showed a significant decrease (P <0.001) compared with the control group and the treatment with chamomile extract (50 mg/kg) could significantly increase the motor coordination compared with the PD group (P <0.001) (Figure 3).

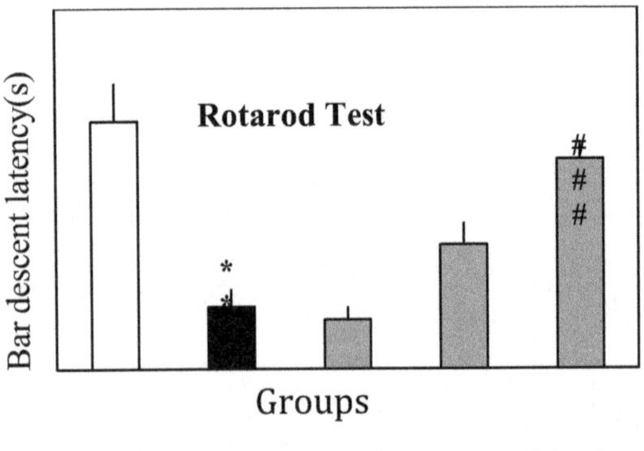

Fig. 3. Effect of 14-day intragastric gavage of 5, 10, and 50 mg/kg of chamomile extract on the motor coordination (rotarod) in the PD animal model. Results were presented as mean ± SD, one-way analysis of variance, and Tukey's post-hoc test (n=10 per group). * and # on the columns show the significant difference from the control and PD groups, respectively.***= (P <0.001) and ### =(P <0.001).

3.4. Stride length test

In measuring the step length, a significant decrease was observed in the PD group compared with the control one (P <0.001). Treatment with chamomile extract (10 and 50 mg/kg) compared with the PD group could significantly increase the step length (P <0.01 and P <0.001, respectively) (Figure 4).

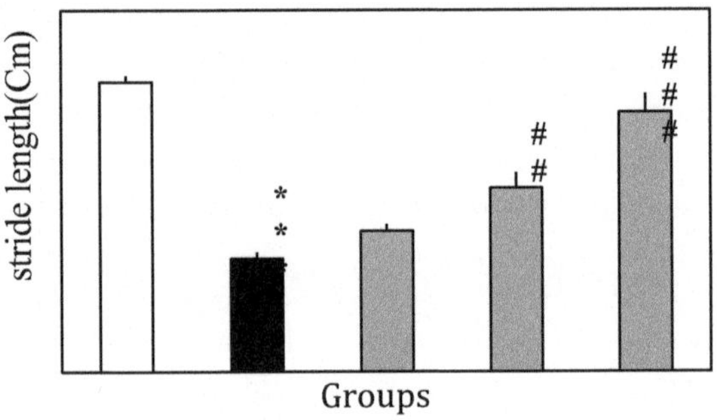

Fig.4. Effect of 14-day intragastric gavage of 5, 10, and 50 mg/kg of chamomile extract on the step length in the PD animal model; Results were presented as mean ± SEM, one-way analysis of variance, and Tukey's post-hoc test (n=10 per group). *and # on the columns show the significant difference from the control and PD groups, respectively.***= (P <0.001) and ### =(P <0.001),## =(P <0.01).

Our findings suggested that dose-dependent chamomile extract could reduce apomorphine- induced rotation and, thereby, reduce the destructive effects of 6-OHDA toxin, which could be probably due to the protective effect on dopamine neurons. Further, treatment with different doses of chamomile extract significantly improved 6-OHDA-induced movement disorders, including catalepsy, step length, and motor coordination, compared with the untreated group. However, this effect was not the same at all doses, among which 10 and 50 mg/kg had a greater effect on the treatment of movement disorders. Many studies have shown that 6-OHDA can lead to dysfunctions in the performance of those parts of the brain responsible for the motor coordination via generating free radicals. It seems that chamomile extract could reverse the above movement disorders and push them toward normal conditions through the elimination of free radicals. In physiological conditions, 6-OHDA toxin is quickly oxidized and converted into hydrogen peroxide, and into hydroxyl radicals during a reaction, which are the most destructive free radicals for living cells (Orallo *et al.*, 2002; Berghauzen-Maciejewska *et al.*, 2016).

Immobility or akinesia that occurs in Parkinson's disease is often because, following a decrease in dopamine secretion in the basal ganglia, its limbic system secretion may be decreased, which may drastically reduce the neural stimulation for physical activity, as a result of which akinesia occurs (Jankovic, 2008). On the other hand, since motor plans need to be continuously changed between excitation and inhibition modes, lack of the inhibitory effect of dopamine prevents the initiation and progression of successive plans requiring inhibitory steps in addition to stimulatory steps, which is exactly what happens in akinesia (Braak *et al.*, 2006). The imbalance process between the free radical production and antioxidant defense system is toward the antioxidants which cause more damage and plays a central role in the pathogenesis of neurological and neurodegenerative diseases such as Parkinson's, trauma, Alzheimer's, and stroke (Tarawneh and Galvin, 2010). Results of Garcia *et al.*'s (2006) study suggested that short-term consumption of juices rich in phenolic compounds improved the body's antioxidant status (Javier *et al.*, 2006). Chamomile essence and extract are considered the natural sources of antioxidant. The active and main chemical elements in chamomile flowers mainly include flavonoids and their oxides (*Zick et al., 2011*). Further, in Bob et al.'s (2003) study, the consumption of fruit juices containing phenolic compounds was shown to reduce oxidative damage to DNA and improve the immune system function (Bub *et al.*, 2003). Polyphenols have protective effects against neurodegenerative diseases (Ebrahimi and Schluesener, 2012). Flavonoids are easily absorbed through the gastrointestinal tract (Ahmad, 2012). The protective effect of flavonoids depends on their hydrogenation ability or scavaging of free radicals (Rice-Evans *et al.*, 1996). Polyphenols have protective effects on dopaminergic neurons in the substantia nigra (Blanchet *et al.*, 2008), which is associated with the activity inhibition of microglials (Li *et al.*, 2006). It has been well proven that the shortage of GABA neurotransmitters is accompanied by several neural disorders such as Huntington's sphere, Parkinson's, Alzheimer's, and other mental disorders such as anxiety, depression, pain, panic, or mania. In recent years, increasing interest has been seen in the synthesis of new drugs derived from GABA derivatives or the drugs with similar effects, which can be used as strong medications for treating neurological disorders (Gajcy *et al.,* 2010). Any drug that can increase the production and release GABA binding to its receptors is effective for the treatment of degenerative brain diseases such as seizures, Parkinson's, epilepsy. Polyphenols are mainly the ligands for receptors in the central nervous system (Marder, 2002). Among these receptors, some specific reference has been made to GABA receptors, to which polyphenols act as benzodiazepine-like molecules (Kahnberg *et al.*, 2002). Chamomile's action mechanism is not exactly known. This mechanism may take place by binding to GABA receptors (Sarris *et al.*, 2011). Chamomile is also effective for the activity of monoamine neurotransmitter system (noradrenaline, dopamine, and serotonin) (Amsterdam *et al.,* 2009). Considering the foregoing discussion and the results of this research, it can be concluded that chamomile extract not only removes free radicals by its antioxidant activity and prevents more neuronal injury and its development, but also improves movements in the PD animal model via affecting GABA receptors, which requires more biochemical and molecular research.

4. Acknowledgment

The author wishes to appreciate Vice Chancellor for Research of Islamic Azad University, Gorgan Branch, for its assistance in the implementation of this project.

5. References

Amsterdam J.D., Li Y., Soeller I., Rockwell K., Mao J.J. and Shults J. 2009. A randomized, double-blind, placebo-controlled trial of oral Matricaria recutita chamomile. extract therapy for generalized anxiety disorder. *Journal of Clinical Psychopharmacol* 29, 378-82.

Berghauzen-Maciejewska K., Wardas J., Kosmowska B., Domin H., Smialowska M., Glowacka U. and Ossowska K. 2016. Adaptive down-regulation of the serotonin transporter in the 6-hydroxydopamine-induced rat model of preclinical stages of Parkinson's disease and after chronic pramipexole treatment. *Neuroscience* 314, 22-34.

Blanchet J., Longpre F., Bureau G., Morissette M., DiPaolo T., Bronchti G. and Martinoli M.G. 2008. Resveratrol, a red wine polyphenol, protects dopaminergic neurons in MPTP-treated mice. *Progress in Neuro-Psychopharmacology and Biological Psychiatry* 32, 1243-50.

Braak H., Rub U., Schultz C. and Del Tredici K. 2006. Vulnerability of cortical neurons to Alzheimer's and Parkinson's diseases. *Journal of Alzheimers Dis* 9, 35-44.

Bub A., Watzl B., Blockhaus M., Briviba K., Liegibel U., Muller H., Pool-Zobel B.L. and Rechkemmer G. 2003. Fruit juice consumption modulates antioxidative status, immune status and DNA damage. *The Journal of Nutritional Biochemistry*
14, 90-8.

Da Cunha C, Angelucci ME, Canteras NS, Wonnacott S and RN T. 2002. The lesion of the rat substantia nigra pars compacta dopaminergic neurons as a model for Parkinson's disease memory disabilities. *Cellular and molecular neurobiology* 22, 227-37.

Dekundy A., Pietraszek M., Schaefer D., Cenci M.A. and Danysz W. 2006. Effects of group I metabotropic glutamate receptors blockade in experimental models of Parkinson's disease. *Brain Research Bull* 69, 318-26.

Ebadi M., Srinivasan S.K. and Baxi M.D. 1996. Oxidative stress and antioxidant therapy in Parkinson's disease. *Progress Neurobiol* 48, 1-19.

Ebrahimi A. and Schluesener H. 2012. Natural polyphenols against neurodegenerative disorders: potentials and pitfalls. *Ageing Research Reviwe* 11, 329-45.

Gajcy K., Lochynski S. and Librowski T. 2010. A role of GABA analogues in the treatment of neurological diseases. *Current Medicinal Chemistry*
17, 2338-47.

gholami Z and M a. 2014. Antinociceptive effects of matricaria chamomilla L. ethanolic extract in mice. *journal of ilam university of medical sciences* 21, 312-7.

Golparvar AR, A G.P. and M. K. 2011. Determination of the effective traits on essence percent and dry flower yield in German chamomile Matricaria chamomilla L.. populations. *Journal of Medicinal Plant Research*
5, 3242 - 6.

Jankovic J. 2008. Parkinson's disease: clinical features and diagnosis. *Journal Neurol Neurosurg Psychiatry* 79, 368-76.

Javier G.A , Gaspar R , Luisa V.G.M and P. J. 2006. Acute intake of phenolic-rich juice improves antioxidant status in healthy subjects. *Nutrition research.* 27, 330-9.

Kahnberg P., Lager E., Rosenberg C., Schougaard J., Camet L., Sterner O., Ostergaard Nielsen E., Nielsen M. and Liljefors T. 2002. Refinement and evaluation of a pharmacophore model for flavone derivatives binding to the benzodiazepine site of the GABAA. receptor. *Journal of Medicinal Chemistry,* 45, 4188-201.

Kleppner S.R. and Tobin A.J. 2001. GABA signalling: therapeutic targets for epilepsy, Parkinson's disease and Huntington's disease. *Expert Opin Ther Targets* 5, 219-39.

Li R., Peng N., Du F., Li X.P. and Le W.D. 2006. Epigallocatechin gallate protects dopaminergic neurons against 1-methyl-4- phenyl-1,2,3,6-tetrahydropyridine-induced neurotoxicity by inhibiting microglial cell activation. *Nan Fang Yi Ke Da Xue Xue Bao* 26, 376-80.

Marder M and P A. 2002. GABAA-receptor ligands of flavonoid structure. *Current Topics in Medicinal Chemistry*, 2, 853-67.

McKay D.L. and Blumberg J.B. 2006. A review of the bioactivity and potential health benefits of chamomile tea Matricaria recutita L. *Phytother Research* 20, 519-30.

Motevalizadekakhky A. 2012. Antimicrobial activity and chemical composition of essential oils of chamomile from Neyshabur, Iran. *Journal Medical Plants Research* 6, 820-4.

Abou-Sleiman P.M., Muqit M.M. and Wood N.W. 2006. Expanding insights of mitochondrial dysfunction in Parkinson's disease. *Nature Reviews Neuroscience*7, 207-19.

Orallo F., Alvarez E., Camina M., Leiro J.M., Gomez E. and Fernandez P. 2002. The possible implication of trans-Resveratrol in the cardioprotective effects of long-term moderate wine consumption. *Molecular Pharmacology,* 61, 294-302.

Philippens I.H., t Hart B.A. and Torres G. 2010. The MPTP marmoset model of parkinsonism: a multi-purpose non-human primate model for neurodegenerative diseases. *Drug Discovery Today* 15, 985-90.

Rice-Evans C.A., Miller N.J. and Paganga G. 1996. Structure-antioxidant activity relationships of flavonoids and phenolic acids. *Free Radical Biology and Medicine,* 20, 933-56.

Rosenthal A. 1998. Specification and survival of dopaminergic neurons in the mammalian midbrain. *Advance Pharmacol,* 42, 908-11.

Sarkaki A, Norooz Zare F, Farbood Y and P A.A. 2013. Impaired movements in 6-OHDA induced Parkinson's rat model improves by pomegranate seed hydroalcoholic extract. *HealthMED journal* 7, 348-58.

Sarkaki A., Eidypour Z., Motamedi F., Keramati K. and Farbood Y. 2012. Motor disturbances and thalamic electrical power of frequency bands' improve by grape seed extract in animal model of Parkinson's disease. *Avicenna Journal Phytomedicin,* 2, 222-32.

Sarris J., Panossian A., Schweitzer I., Stough C. and Scholey A. 2011. Herbal medicine for depression, anxiety and insomnia: a review of psychopharmacology and clinical evidence. *European Neuropsychopharmacol,* 21, 841-60.

Seifi Zangeneh M, Rafieirad M and H. S. 2015. The effect of Kardeh Biarum Bovei. Hydro-alcoholic extract on pain threshold in STZ induced diabetic rats *Journal of Herbal Drugs,* 6, 137-42.

Shrivastava P., Vaibhav K., Tabassum R., Khan A., Ishrat T., Khan M.M., Ahmad A., Islam F., Safhi M.M. and Islam F. 2013. Anti-apoptotic and anti-inflammatory effect of Piperine on 6-OHDA induced Parkinson's rat model. *The Journal of Nutritional Biochemistry* 24, 680-7.

Singh O., Khanam Z., Misra N. and Srivastava M.K. 2011. Chamomile Matricaria chamomilla L. An overview. *Pharmacogn Rev*iew, 5, 82-95.

Srivastava J.K., Shankar E. and Gupta S. 2010. Chamomile: A herbal medicine of the past with bright future. *Molecular Medicine Reports*. 3, 895-901.

Sultan Ahmad, M and Yadav, R. 2012. Evaluation of Antigenotoxic Potential of Ellagic Acid against Aflatoxin B1-Induced Genotoxicity. *Indian Journal of Fundamental and Applied Life Sciences* 2, 177-84.

Sun W., Sugiyama K., Fang X., Yamaguchi H., Akamine S., Magata Y. and Namba H. 2010. Different striatal D2-like receptor function in an early stage after unilateral striatal lesion and medial forebrain bundle lesion in rats. *Brain Res*earch 1317, 227-35.

Tanaka K., Ogawa N. and Asanuma M. 2006. Molecular basis of 6-hydroxydopamine-induced caspase activations due to increases in oxidative stress in the mouse striatum. *Neuroscince Lett*ers 410, 85-9.

Tarawneh R. and Galvin J.E. 2010. Potential future neuroprotective therapies for neurodegenerative disorders and stroke. *Clinical Geriatr Med icin* 26, 125-47.

Yeh C.T., Ching L.C. and Yen G.C. 2009. Inducing gene expression of cardiac antioxidant enzymes by dietary phenolic acids in rats. *The Journal of Nutritional Biochemistry* 20, 163-71.

Zick SM, Wright BD, Sen A and JT. A. 2011. Preliminary examination of the efficacy and safety of a standardized chamomile extract for chronic primary insomnia: a randomized placebo-controlled pilot study. *BMC Complementary and Alternative Medicine Journal* 11: 78.

Assessment of secondary metabolites: *in vitro* antiarthritic and antihemolytic potential of various extracts of garlic

Sonia Johri*, Nasir Khan, Sarita Tiwari, Lovie Shakyawar

Department of Life Sciences, ITM University, Gwalior;
***Email:** soniajohari@itmuniversity.ac.in

ARTICLE INFO

Topic: *Medicinal Plants*

Key words:
- ✓ *Allium sativum*
- ✓ *FTIR*
- ✓ *Antiarthritic*
- ✓ *Antihemolytic*
- ✓ *In vitro*
- ✓ *Secondary metabolites*

ABSTRACT

Background & Aim: *Allium sativum* commonly known as garlic is an herb used over years to prevent from various ailments such as cardiovascular diseases, cognitive disorders and also enhances the immune system. The aim of the present study is to study the *in vitro* antiarthritic and antihemolytic potential of garlic in aqueous and methanolic extracts. Fourier transform infrared spectroscopy was performed to study the presence of functional groups.

Experimental: The study involved detection of primary and secondary metabolites in *allium sativum* i.e garlic. *In vitro* antiarthritic and heat induced haemolytic assay was evaluated so that it could be used against haemolytic diseases such as malaria, swine flu etc. FTIR spectra were performed to detect the presence of functional groups.

Results: Natural products due to their immense bioactivity, finds applications against various diseases without having side effects.

Recommended applications/industrie: This herb is very easily accessible and is edible it can be used as a pharmaceutical agent. Bioactive constituents can be isolated and explored for further activity.

1. Introduction

Herbal medicines are used as prophylactic and therapeutic agents against hepatic, renal, cardiovascular as well as inflammatory diseases, by modulating risk factors such as hypertension, high blood cholesterol, thrombosis, and preventing other chronic diseases associated with ageing (Rahman 2001, Tanaka *et al.*, 2006, Rahman, 2003, Neil *et al.,* 1994).

Secondary plant metabolites play a very important role and has bioapplications. Garlic (*Allium sativum*) which plays a very important dietary and medicinal role for centuries finds therapeutic uses which include beneficial effects as antibiotic, anticancer, anti-inflammatory, hypoglycemic, and hormone-like agents. Garlic extracts have been used to treat infections for thousands of years. It's typical pungent odour and antibacterial activity is due to active principle allicin, which is produced by enzymatic (alliin lyase) hydrolysis of alliin after cutting and crushing of the cloves. Pharmacological effects of garlic are attributed to the presence of pharmacologically active sulfur compounds including diallyl sulfide, diallyl disulfide, allicin, and dipropyl sulfide. These compounds have been known to increase the activity of enzymes involved in the metabolism of carcinogens (Fisher *et al.*, 2007), as well as anti-inflammatory effects *in vitro* and *in vivo (*Sabayan *et al.*, 2007; Murugavel and Pari, 2007; Park *et al.,* 2005; Lang *et al.,* 2004; Son *et al.*, 2006; Chang *et al.*, 2006). Thiacremonone, a novel and major sulfur compound (0.3%) in garlic, has higher anti-oxidant properties compared with other sulfur compounds. Allicin is an odorless sulfur-containing chemical derived from the amino acid cysteine which is further broken down to a compound called Ajoene that inhibits blockage in blood vessels from clots and atherosclerosis (Hwang *et al.*, 2007).

World Health Organisation (WHO) reported that about 80% of the world's population depend mainly on traditional medicine and the traditional treatment involve mainly the use of plant extracts. Natural antioxidants are the secondary metabolites of the plant and do not have side effects when taken *in vivo* (Chen *et al.*, 1992; Walton and Brown, 1999). Many plants contain wide variety of free radicals scavenging molecule such as phenolic compounds, nitrogen compounds, vitamins, terpenoids, and some other endogenous metabolites Phenolic compounds which are important secondary metabolites have redox properties which neutralizes the free radicals thereby quenching singlet and triplet oxygen decomposing peroxides as an important antioxidant. (Osawa, 1994). Tannins also find applications as a potential agent in variety of disease states (Packer *et al.,* 1999).

2. Materials and Methods

2.1. Plant Collection

Fresh garlic cloves were collected from local market of Gwalior, M.P.

2.2. Preparation of garlic powder

1000g of garlic cloves were peeled and cut in to small pieces and shade dried. The dried garlic was ground to a fine powder.

2.3. Preparation of methanolic extract

50 g of powder was weighed and sequentially extracted with methanol and water respectively in soxhelet apparatus for 72 h. After solvent extraction it was evaporated to obtain a powdered extract for various biochemical analysis (Kumar *et al.*, 2012).

2.4. Preparation of aqueous extract

50g of powder was weighed and extracted with distilled water in soxhelet apparatus for 72 h. After solvent extraction it was evaporated to obtain a powdered extract for various biochemical analysis (Kumar *et al.,* 2012).

2.5. Phytochemical analysis of primary metabolites

Preliminary phytochemical screening of the extract was performed for the presence of basic primary metabolites like carbohydrates, proteins and lipids (Plummer, 1987*)*

2.5.1. Carbohydrates. Extracts were dissolved individually in 5 ml distilled water and filtered. The filtrates were used for Molisch's test and Fehling's test for the presence of carbohydrates and reducing sugars respectively.

2.5.2. Proteins.

Biuret's test: To 1 ml of test extract, 4% of sodium hydroxide solution and few drops of 1% copper sulphate solution were added. Formation of a violet red colour indicated the presence of peptide bond.

Ninhydrin test: To 2 ml of test extract, few drops of 0.25% of ninhydrin in acetone were added and heated in boiling water bath for 10 min. The formation of bluish purple colour indicated the presence of amino acid. (Kumar *et al.,* 2012)

2.6. Phytochemical analysis of secondary metabolites

Preliminary phytochemical screening of the extract were performed for the presence of alkaloids, reducing sugars, proteins, flavonoids, tannins, phenols, phytosterol and saponins using the standard procedures (Kumar *et al.,* 2012)

2.6.1. Alkaloids. Alkaloids were detected by using Wagner's test. To 1 ml of extract, 2-3 drops of Wagner's reagent was added. Appearance of reddish brown precipitate indicated the presence of alkaloids.

2.6.2. Saponins by Froth test. Extracts were diluted to 20 ml with distilled water and shaken in a graduated cylinder for 15 minutes. Formation of 1 cm layer of foam indicated the presence of saponins.

2.6.3. Steroids by Salkowski test. A few milligram of extract, 2 ml of chloroform and 2 ml of conc. sulphuric acid were added. Tubes were shaken and allowed to stand. A golden yellow red colour indicated the presence of phytosterols.

2.6.4. Tannins (ferric chloride test). Extract solutions were treated with 5% ferric chloride solution. Formation of blue colour indicated the presence of hydrolysable tannins and formation of green colour indicated the presence of condensed tannins

2.7. *In-vitro* anti-arthritic activity by inhibition of protein denaturation method

- The test experimental (0.5ml) consist of 0.45ml of Bovine serum albumin (5%w/v aqueous solution) and 0 .05ml of test solution (250 μg/ml).
- Test control solution (0.5ml) consist of 0.45ml of bovine serum albumin (5%w/v aqueous solution) and 0 .05ml of distilled water.
- Product control (0.5ml) consists of 0.45ml of distilled water and 0.05 ml of test solution (250 μg/ml).
- Standard solution (0.5ml) consists of 0.45ml of Bovine serum albumin (5%w/v aqueous solution) and 0.05ml 0f diclofenac sodium (250 μg/ml).

All the above solutions were adjusted to pH 6.3 using HCl (1N). The samples were incubated at 37°C for 20 minutes and the temperature was increased to keep the samples at 57°C for 3minutes. After cooling, 2.5 ml of phosphate buffer was added to the above solutions. The absorbance was measured using UV-Visible spectrophotometer at 416nm (Venkataraman *et al.*, 2013).

The percentage inhibition of protein denaturation can be calculated as:

Percentage Inhibition = [100-(optical density of test solution – optical density of product control) / (optical density of test control)] ×100.

The control represents 100% protein denaturation. The results were compared with standard diclofenac sodium. The percentage inhibition of protein denaturation of different concentration was tabulated.

2.8. Heat induced haemolysis

Reaction mixture (2 ml) consisted of 1 ml test solution and 1 ml. of 10% RBC suspension. Saline was replaced with drug in test solution. Aspirin was taken as a standard drug. The tubes were incubated in a water bath at 56 ^{0}C for 30 min. At the end of the incubation, the tubes were cooled under running tap water. Reaction was centrifuged at 2500 rpm for 5 minutes and OD of supernatant taken at 560 nm with UV- visible spectrophotometer (Okoli *et al.,* 2008).

2.9 **FTIR Spectroscopy**: The FTIR from 4000 to 400 cm^{-1} was recorded on a Perkin Elmer (spectrum 2) spectrometer. FTIR is used as a tool for the characterization and identification of compounds or functional groups (chemical bonds) present in an unknown mixture of plants extract (Eberhardt *et al.*, 2007; Hazra *et al.*, 2007).

3. Results and discussion

Table 1 shows preliminary phytochemical analysis of primary and secondary metabolites. Results revealed that both methanolic and aqueous extract had higher content of alkaloids, flavanoids, saponins, protein and carbohydrates. The garlic cloves extract also had the same content. This was followed by tannins cardiac glycosides, carbohydrates, protein and reducing sugars.

Flavonoid is one of the main group of phenolic compound and widely distributed flavonoid, flavones and flavonols. Many flavonoids and related compound are reported to have strong antioxidative characteristics. Flavonoids and phenolics are the effective scavengers of the free radicals and chain breaking agents due to presence of hydroxyl group. Their presence indicates high analgesic and anti-inflammatory effects as a result of their membrane stabilizing ability against free radicals produced as a result of lipid peroxides and superoxides which causes cell membrane destabilization. They also possess anticancer, anti-diabetic, anti-aging properties and prevention of cardiovascular diseases. Tannins possess antiviral, antibacterial and antiparasitic effects and have the potential to fight against cancer. In the present study the pronounced antioxidant activity of *Allium sativum* was possibly due to its high phenolic and flavanoid content. Polyphenolic and flavanoid compounds contain conjugated ring structures and hydroxyl groups; which aids in providing an antioxidant status in cell free systems by scavenging singlet oxygen, superoxide anion, lipid peroxy radicals, hydroxyl ions, nitric oxide ions, and stabilizing free radicals involved in oxidative processes (Shahidi *et al.*, 1992; Dixon *et al.,* 2005).

Table 1. Preliminary phytochemical screening of extracts

Test	Aqueous extract	Methanol extract	Garlic clove extract
Tannins	+	-	-
Anthraquinone	-	-	-
Phlobatannins	+++	++	+
Cardiac glycosides	+	+	+
Carbohydrates (Molisch's test)	+	+	+
Proteins (Biuret test)	+	+	++
Reducing sugar(Fehling's test)	+	+	++
Alkaloids (Wagner's test)	++	++	++
Saponin (Foam test)	++	++	++
Steroids (Salkowski's test)	++	++	++
Tannins	+	+	+
Flavanoids	++	++	++

Table 2 depicts the *in vitro* antiarthritic activity by inhibition of protein denaturstion. The methanolic extract of garlic exhibited significant activity at 800µg/ml (63%) by inhibition of protein denaturation as compared with standard drug diclofenac sodium. The methanolic extract of garlic powder exhibits significant activity at 2000µg/ml (82.94 %) by inhibition of protein denaturation as opposed to the standard drug diclofenac sodium.

The production of auto antigen (like Rheumatoid Factor) in certain arthritic disease is because of protein denaturation. Hence we can conclude that the methanolic extract of garlic are capable of controlling the production of auto antigen or functional groups (chemical bonds) present in an unknown mixture of plant extracts. (Gupta *et al.,* 2013)

Table 3 explains the antihaemolytic activity of the extract in the presence H_2O_2, where ascorbic acid was taken as a positive control. It was found out that when RBC cell were treated with H_2O_2 along with two different extract, marked reduction in the haemolysis was observed than that of cells treated with the toxicant alone. When cells were treated with the extract alone, no haemolysis was obtained explaining the non-toxic behaviour of the extracts on human RBC. Out of all extract, methanolic extract showed better results.

Table 2. Effect of aqueous and methanolic extract of garlic on protein denaturation.

Treatment	Concentration (µg/ml)	Inhibition(%)
Diclofenac sodium	200	89.20
	300	92.46
	500	92.50
	800	98.67
Methanolic Extract	200	33.00
	300	41.00
	500	50.00
	800	63.00
Aqueous Extract	200	15.00
	300	22.00
	500	28.00
	800	43.00

Table 3. Effect of garlic on heat induced hemolysis.

Treatment	Concentration (µg/ml)	Inhibition (%)
Aspirin	200	89.20
	300	98.67
	500	92.46
	800	92.50
Methanolic Extract	200	53.00
	300	50.00
	500	41.00
	800	33.00
Aqueous Extract	200	43.00
	300	28.00
	500	22.00
	800	15.00

Both methanolic and aqueous extracts demonstrated a significant inhibition of hemolysis *in vitro*. The inhibition effect shown by crude extracts of garlic at comparatively lower concentrations (37.5 µg/ml) was comparable with that of standard anti-hemolysis compounds such as aspirin. This experimental evidence indicates that aqueous and methanolic extracts could have a potential therapeutic efficacy in disease processes causing destabilization of biological membrane. Tissue proteins are denatured causing production of autoantigens an arthritic disesases leading to inflammatory and arthritic diseases.

Table 4. FTIR frequency range and functional group present in the cloves of *Allium sativum*.

Frequency range (cm^{-1})	Functional groups
500-600	Bromo alkanes
600-800	Chloro alkanes
900-1000	Aromatic
900-1000	Alphatic amines
1000-1150	Fluoro alkanes
1500-1383	Nitro compound
2885-3000	Halogen compound

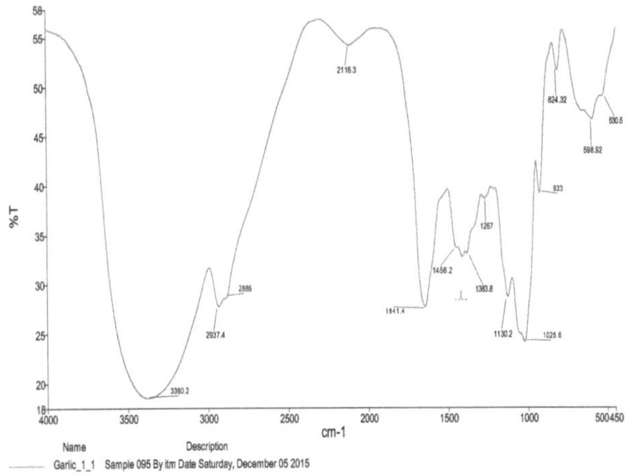

Fig. 1. FTIR spectra for the *Allium sativum* cloves extracts

The mechanism of action may be denaturation of tissue proteins which causes alteration in electrostatic, hydrogen, hydrophobic and disulphide boding. From the result of the present study it can be stated that *Allium sativum* is capable of controlling the production of auto antigens due to *in vivo* denaturation of proteins in rheumatic diseases. Protective effect on heat and hyotonic saline-induced erythrocyte lysis is known to be a very good index of anti- arthritic activity of any agent. Since the membrane of RBC is structurally similar to the lysosomal membrane, the effect of any substance on stabilization of RBC membrane may be extrapolated to the stabilization of lysosomal membrane (Brown and Mackey, 1968).

Table 4 and Figure 1 show the FTIR spectra for the Allium sativum cloves. In the present study FTIR spectroscopy was performed for easy and rapid determination and identification of various functional groups responsible for medicinal properties. IR spectroscopy is basically a vibrational spectrum. Presence of sulphur derivatives, polysaccharides, organic hydrocarbon, haloalkanes, aromatic compounds, aliphatic amines and nitro compounds are responsible for various medicinal properties of garlic.

4. Conclusion

The methanolic extract of garlic was more potential as compared to the aqueous extract. It possessed antiarthritic and antihemolytic potential and can be explored further.

5. Acknowledgment

The authors feel grateful to Department of Life Sciencces, ITM University, Gwalior, M.P., India for providing laboratory facilities. Instrumentation facilities and technical support from P.C. Ray centre for research is highly acknowledged.

6. References

Brown, JH., Mackey, HK. 1968. Inhibition of heat-induced denaturation of serum proteins by mixtures of non- steroidal anti-inflammatory agents and amino acids. *proc soc exp biol med.*, 128:225-28

Chen, C., Pearson, AM., Gray, IJ. 1992. Effects of synthetic antioxidants (BHA, BHT and PG) on the mutagenicity of IQ-like compounds. *Food Chemistry.*, 43: 177-183.

Chiang, Y.H., Jen, L.N., Su, H.Y., Lii, C.K., Sheen, L.Y., Liu, C.T. 2006. Effects of garlic oil and two of its major organosulfur compounds, diallyl disulfide and diallyl trisulfide, on intestinal damage in rats injected with endotoxin. *Toxicol Appl Pharmacol.*, 213:46–54.

Dixon, R.A., Xie, D.Y., Sharma, S.B. 2005. Proanthocyanidins- a final frontier in flavanoid research. *New Phytol.*, 165: 9-28.

Eberhardt, T.L., Li, X., Shupe, T.F., Hse, C.Y. 2007. Chinese Tallow ree (Sapium Sebiferum) utilization: Characterization of extractives and cell-wall chemistry. *Wood Fiber Sci.*, 39: 319–324.

Fisher, C.D., Augustine, L.M., Maher, J.M., Nelson, D.M., Slitt, AL., Klaassen, CD., Lehman-McKeeman, L.D., Cherrington, N.J. 2007. Induction of drug-metabolizing enzymes by garlic and allyl sulfide compounds via activation of car and CAR and Nrf2. *Drug Metab Dispos.*, 35: 995–1000.

Gupta, S.K., Gupta, A., Gupta, A.k., Pakash, D. 2103. *In vitro* anti-arthritic activity of callicarpa macrophylla flower. *Int. Res. J. Pharm.*, 4(3).

Hwang, I.G., Woo, K.S., Kim, D.J., Hong, J.T., Hwang, B.Y., Lee, Y.R., Jeong, H.S. 2007. Isolated and identification of an antioxidant substance from heated garlic (Allium sativum L.). *Food Sci Biotechnol.*, 16: 963–966.

Kumar, S., Sharma, U.K., Sharma, A.k., and Pandey, A.K. 2012. Protective efficancy of *Solanum xanthocarpum* root extracts against free redical damage: Phytochemical analysis and antioxidant effect. *Cell. Mol. Biol.,* 58(1): 174-181.

Lang, A., Lahav, M., Sakhnini, E., Barshack, I., Fidder, H.H., Avidan, B., Bardan, E., Hershkoviz, R., Bar-Meir S., Chowers Y. 2004. *Clin Nutr*, Allicin inhibits spontaneous and TNF-alpha induced secretion of proinflammatory cytokines and chemokines from intestinal epithelial cells. 23:1199-1208.

Murugavel P, Pari L. 2007. Effects of diallyl tetrasulfide on cadmium-induced oxidative damage in the liver of rats. *Hum Exp Toxicol.*, 26: 527–534.

Neil A., Silagy C., 1994. Garlic: its cardiovascular-protective properties. *Curr Opin Lipidol.*, 5: 989S–993S.

Osawa T. Japan: Japan Scientific Societies Press; 1994. Novel natural antioxidants for utilization in food and biological system; pp. 241–51.48

Okoli CO, Akah PA, Onuoha NJ, Okoye TC, Nwoye AC, Nworu CS. 2008. Acanthus montanus: An experimental evaluation of the antimicrobial, anti-inflammatory and immunological properties of a traditional remedy for furuncles. *BMC Complement Altern Med.* 8: 27.

Park EY., Ki SH., Ko MS., Kim CW., Lee MH., Lee YS., Kim SG.,2005. Garlic oil and DDB, comprised in a pharmaceutical composition for the treatment of patients with viral hepatitis, prevents acute liver injuries potentiated by glutathione deficiency in rats. *Chem Biol Interact1.*, 55: 82–96.

Pari L, Murugavel P, Sitasawad SL, Kumar KS.2007. Cytoprotective and antioxidant role of diallyl tetrasulfide on cadmium induced renal injury: an in vivo and in vitro study. *Life Sci.*, 80: 650–658.

Packer L, G. *Rimbach*, and F. Virgili. 1999. Antioxidant activity and biological properties of a procyanidin-rich extract from pine (Pinusmaritima) bark, pycnogel. *Free RadicBiol Med.*, 27: 704-24.

Plummer, D.T., 1987. An Introduction to Practical Biochemistry. Mc Graw Hill Education (India) Private Limited. Third Edition. PP. 157-181

Rahman, K., 2001. Historical perspective on garlic and cardiovascular disease. *J Nutr.*, 131: 977S–979S.

Rahman K. 2003. Garlic and aging: new insights into an old remedy. *Ageing Res Rev.*, 2: 39–56.

Sabayan B., Foroughinia F., Chohedry A. 2007. A postulated role of garlic organosulfur compounds in prevention of valproic acid hepatotoxicity. *Med Hypotheses.*, 68: 512-514.

Son EW., Mo SJ., Rhee DK., Pyo S. 2006. Inhibition of ICAM-1 expression by garlic component, allicin, in gamma-irradiated human vascular endothelial cells via downregulation of the JNK signalling pathway. *Int Immunopharmacol.* 6: 1788-1795.

Shahidi F., Wanasundara P.K.J.P.D., 1992. Phenolic antioxidants. *Food Sci Nutr.*, 32:67-103.

Tanaka S., Haruma K., Yoshihara M., Kajiyama G., Kira K., Amagase H., Chayama K. 2006. Aged garlic extract has potential suppressive effect on colorectal adenomas in humans. *J Nutr.,* 136: 821S–826S.

Venkataraman N.D., W Clement Atlee, T Purushoth Prabhu, , G Surya, R Kannan, I Sheik Nasar, 2013 , Evaluation of *In-vitro* Anti-Arthritic Potential of Aerial Parts of *Ipomoeapes- caprae* (L.) R.Brand Estabilishment of Its Mechanism of Action. *Research Journal of Pharmaceutical, Biological and Chemical Sciences.*, 4(2): 1561-65

Walton N. J. and D. E. Brown. 1999. Chemicals from plants: Perspectives on plant secondary product. London: Imperial College press.

Cytotoxic effect of hydroalcoholic extract from *Thymus daenesis* Celak on MCF-7 cancer cells line

Fatemeh Sadeghi Samani[1], Hossein Sazegar[*1], Abdollah Ghasemi Pirbalouti[2]

[1]*Department of biology, Faculty of Basic Sciences , Shahrekord Branch, Islamic Azad University, Sahrekord, Iran;*

Email:** ***hoseinsazgar@yahoo.com

[2]*Department of Medicinal Plants, Shahrekord Branch, Islamic Azad University, Shahrekord, Iran;*

ARTICLE INFO

Topic: *Medicinal Plants*

Key words:

- *Thymus daenesis* Celak
- *MTT test*
- *Breast cancer*
- *MCF-7*

ABSTRACT

Background & Aim: Breast cancer is the second most common cancer in women after lung cancer. Given that the herbal ingredients are used for centuries to treat cancer, The aim of this study was to determine the cytotoxic effect of hydroalcoholic extract from *Thymus daenesis* Celak on MCF-7 cancer cells line.

Experimental: Breast cancer cells MCF-7 and natural fibroblast cells were cultured in DMEM medium containing fetal bovine serum and antibiotics. The cells were exposed to different doses of hydroalcoholic extract of *Thymus daenesis* Celak (0.156, 0.312, 0.625, 1.25, 2.5mg/ml) and incubated for 24, 48 and 72 hours, respectively. After incubation, the modified MTT colorimetric test was used to determine cytotoxicity.

Results: The results of MTT test showed that hydroalcoholic extract of *Thymus daenesis* Celak has dose- and time-dependent anti-cancer effect on MCF-7 cancer cells, so that by increasing the concentration and 72h incubation, the most cell death was observed ($P<0.05$). Plant extract did not show significant cytotoxicity on natural fibroblast cells. Then, it seems that its compounds can be used in treating cancer through more future research.

Recommended applications/industries: With regard to the increasing use of herbal medicines to treat many diseases, hydroalcoholic extract of *Thymus daenesis* Celak can be used to treat cancer with drug therapy due to having antioxidant properties.

1. Introduction

Cancer is one of the non-communicable chronic diseases which involves broad group of diseases. Like other chronic diseases, this disease is occurred in any person, age groups and all races and is considered as a major hygiene problem which is effective on the heath of society. Cancer is the second most common cause of death after cardiovascular diseases and accidents in less developed countries (Siegel *et al.*, 2011).

Breast cancer is the second most common cancer after lung cancer and the most common type of cancer among women around the world (Hamta & Parvini, 2011). This cancer is responsible for 33 percent of all cancers in women and 20 percent of deaths from cancer, incidence of breast cancer is increasing in developing countries and in many parts of the world, it has become the most common malignancy disease among women (O'Hara *et al.,*1998).

Complementary therapies such as surgery and drug therapy, hormonal, chemotherapy and radio therapy are among the methods of treating breast cancer. These treatments have many limitations and side effects for cancer patients. Today, using herbal drugs is considered in relation to chemical ones duo to their less side effects (Gordanian *et al.,* 2014). Many herbs and spices contain some factors to prevent cancer which can enforce their effects in various steps of growth of cancer cells (Abdullaev, 2001).

The main objective in the prevention of cancer by natural or chemical materials is to slow or inhibit the carcinogenic process. This approach focuses on abnormal intracellular pathways that lead to abnormal cell functions (Aggarwal *et al.,* 2007).

Thymus daenesis with the scientific name *Thymus daenesis* Celakis from mint family Lamiaceae (Golparvar *et al.,* 2012). It is an herbaceous and perennial plant with multiple and thick whose height is up to 25-30cm. Leaves are mutual and small, oval or ovate, sharp and up to1 cm in length. Flowers are purplish- white or violet and integrated along the leaves, a flower bowl is in pipe or Bluebell form whose teeth are about 0.5 mm in the upper part. The plant is growing in some areas of the Chaharmahal & Bakhtiari, Fars, Hamedan, Ilam, Central, Kohkilooye and Boyer Ahmad and Kurdistan (Karimi *et al.,* 2010).

Thymus daenesis Celak contains tannins, flavonoids, glycosides, caffeic acid and rosemaric acid compounds (Ghasemi Pirbalouti *et al.,* 2013). Based on the results obtained by some researchers, thymol, Paracemenu, Gamatripinin, carvacrol and beta-cariofilin are the major compounds of this plant (Barazandeh & Bagherzadeh, 2007).

Brewed and decoction of this plant is used as taster, anti-cough, anti-spasm, mucus, carminative, anti-microbial and anti-fungal. In Iran and other countries, it is used for treating the common cold (Karimi *et al.,* 2010). In several studies, its antimicrobial properties against *Candida albicans* (Ghasemi Pirbalouti *et al.,* 2009), *Staphylococcus aureus*, *Escherichia coli, Pseudomonas aeruginosa, Klebsiella pneumoniae* has been confirmed (Ghasemi Pirbalouti *et al.,* 2010). What has been recently considered by researchers is anti-cancer and anti-carcinogenic properties of thyme plant (Hamta & Ghazaghi, 2014).

Cell culture is one of the modern methods of research and study and its traces are found in almost all scientific disciplines. One of the objectives of cell culture is to study the cells in terms of growth, food needs and cause of stop in their growth. So studying the cell cycle, development of cancer cell growth methods and gene expression modulation require the culture of these cells *in vivo*. (Forouzandeh *et al.,* 2014).

MCF-7 is human breast cancer cell line which first time was separated in 1970 from a malignant cancerous tissue of a 69 year old Caucasian woman who had breast cancer metastasis and thereafter, this cell line is used as useful model for studying cancer (Osborne *et al.,* 1987).

The antioxidant properties *Thymus daenesis* Celak have been demonstrated in previous studies (Sefidkon & Ahmadi, 2000). In this study the cytotoxic effect of hydroalcoholic extract of *Thymus daenesis* Celak on MCF-7 cancer cells line was evaluated.

2. Materials and Methods

2.1. Extraction of hydroalcoholic extract of Thymus daenesis Celak

Aerial organs including leaves and stem of *Thymus daenensis* Celak were collected from Chahrmahal & Bakhtiari and extraction of its hydroalcoholic extract was performed by Rotary. For extraction, the leaves and stems of plants were first dried and powdered by mechanical grinding, then the intended powder was poured into cylindrical casting and solvent was poured on it, the solvent was ethanol 90 % mixed with water, this hydro alcoholic solvent was used to the extent that the plant powder is completely covered. The resulted solution was placed in the oven that was set to 50°C, After 72 hours remaining in the oven, solution was exited of the machine and passed through filter paper, then the filtrated solution was placed in stearic rotary apparatus little by little to concentrate. The resulted extract was used for providing extract in various dosses.

2.2. Cell culture

MCF-7 Cell line of breast cancer and fibroblast cell line were provided from National Center for Genetic Resources of Iran. For culturing MCF-7 cells and fibroblast cells, the culture medium DMEM (Dulbecco's Modified Eagle Medium) Containing 10%

FBS (Fetal bovine serum) and 1% Penicillin-Streptomycin was used. And they were cultured under standard incubation conditions (temperature of 37°Cand 5% $CO_2$and humidity 95%). After three passages, the cells were used for later processing, cell count and the number of living cells were performed by using hemocytometer using Trypan blue.

2.3. MTT (Methyl Tetrazolium) test

To measure the cytotoxic effect of hydroalcoholic extract of *Thymus daenesis* Celak, MTT test was used. In this method, the methyl thiazolyltetrazolium bromide salt or MTT is converted to insoluble and purple formazan through mitochondrial dehydrogenase enzymes of active cells. Light absorption of this compound after dissolving in DMSO (Dimethyl sulfoxide) can be measured by using Eliza reader and in wavelength 492-630 nm (Mosmann, 1983).

2.4. Study the toxicity of hydroalcoholic extract of Thymus daenesis Celak*, by using MTT*

After covering the flask bed with cell, cell layer sticky to flask bottom was separated in enzyme method and by using Trypsin and was centrifuged in 1200 rpm in 5 min after transferring to sterile test tubes. Then cells were suspended by using Pasteur pipette in new culture medium and cell suspension was provided from them. After counting, cells were poured in smooth-floor 96-well plates as 10^4 cells and plates were incubated at 37°Cfor 24 hours. After the required time, the supernatant was removed slowly and carefully and new medium and hydroalcoholic extract of *Thymus daenesis* Celak in concentrations 0.156, 0.312, 0.625, 1.25 and 2.5mg/ml were added to all wells. Serum containing medium without extract was added to control wells. Plates were incubated for 24, 48 and 72 h. After the incubation period, plates were removed from the incubator, supernatant of each well was completely removed by sampler, cells were washed with 100 ml PBS (Phosphate – buffered saline) and then 80 microliter medium and 20 ml yellow MTT solution was added and the plates were incubated for 3 hours, after the required time ,first the supernatant was completely removed and each well was washed with 100 ml PBS and 100ml DMSO was added to dissolve formazan crystals, then the resulted color change was read by device Eliza reader at a wavelength of 492-630 nm.

In order to convert the amount of light absorption (OD) the percentage of live cells, the following formula was used and life percent of cells after 24, 48 and 72 h was computed.

Biological ability percent = OD Control / OD Test ×100

A concentration of tested compound which halved the cell viability was considered as IC_{50} (The half maximal inhibitory concentration).

2.5. Statistical analysis

Data were analyzed using SPSS software via one way ANOVA method and mean comparison was done through Tukey method. The p-values less than 0.05 were considered to be statistically significant.

3. Results and discussion

3.1. Effect of different concentrations of hydroalcoholic extract of Thymus daenesis Celak on bio-viability of MCF-7 cancer cells at different times by using MTT

Statistical analysis showed that in 24-hour incubation time, viability was reduced by increasing the dose of hydroalcoholic extract of *Thymus daenesis*CelakinMCF-7cell line. So that the viability percentage was reduced from 96.79% to in 0.156 mg/ml concentration to 17.39% in concentration 2.5 mg/ml, it was statistically significant ($p<0.05$).

In 48-hour incubation, dose-dependent reduction of viability was observed. So that the percentage of viability was decreased from 90.29% in 0.156 mg/ml concentration to 13.92% in concentration 2.5 mg/ml, it was statistically significant ($p<0.05$).

In 72-hour incubation, the reduction of viability percent was also observed from 79.71 % in concentration 0.156 mg/ml to 11.45% in 2.5 mg, it was statistically significant ($p <0.05$).

Statistical analysis by using ANOVA test and Tukey showed significant difference at all concentration and in all three time in this cell line ($p <0.05$). The most toxicity effect was observed in concentration 2.5 mg/ml and 72 h incubation (Figure 1). 50% cell growth inhibitory concentration (IC_{50}) of *Thymus daenesis* Celak hydroalcoholic extract for MCF-7 cancer cells was 0.625 mg/ml.

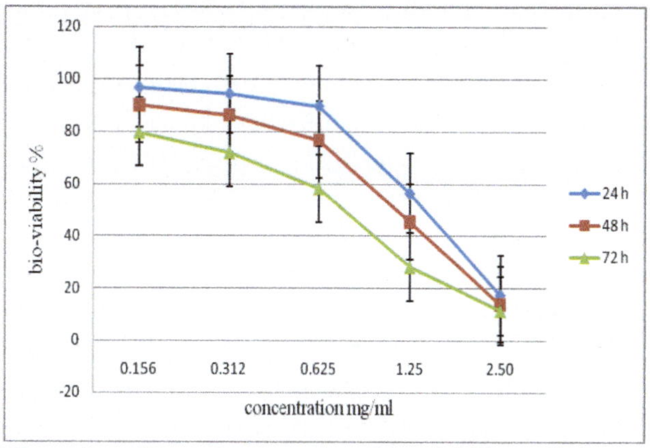

Fig. 1. The changes in bio-viability (%) of hydroalcoholic extract of *Thymus daenesis* Celak on MCF-7 cancer cells in different concentrations (mg/ml) and times by using MTT.

3.2. Effect of different concentrations of hydroalcoholic extract of Thymus daenesis Celak on the bio-viability of natural fibroblast cells at different times by using MTT

Natural fibroblast cells with various concentrations of hydroalcoholic extract of *Thymus daenesis* Celak (0.156, 0.312, 0.625, 1.25, 2.5 mg/ml) were treated for 24, 48 and 72 hours. The results of MTT assay showed that hydroalcoholic extract of *Thymus daenesis* Celak had little effect on fibroblast cells (Figure 2).

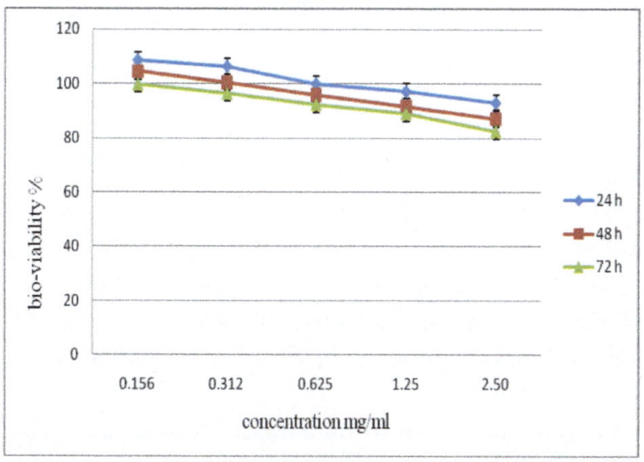

Fig. 2. The changes in bio-viability (%) of hydroalcoholic extract of *Thymus daenesis* Celak on fibroblast cells in different concentrations (mg/ml) and times by using MTT.

MCF-7 cancer cell growth after 72 hours of treatment with hydroalcoholic extract of *Thymus daenesis* Celak at a concentration of 2.5 mg/ml (Figure 3. B) was prevented in comparison to the control group (no treatment with hydroalcoholic extract of *Thymus daenesis* Celak) (Figure 3. A).After exposure to a concentration of 2.5 mg/ml of extract, cells were distorted and their morphology was changed, showing toxicity effect of hydroalcoholic extract of *Thymus daenesis* Celak on these cells.

In the present study, cytotoxic effect of hydroalcoholic extract of *Thymus daenesis* Celak on MCF-7 cancer cell line and natural fibroblast cells was examined. The results of this study showed that the effects of hydroalcoholic extract of *Thymus daenesis* Celak results in death of MCF-7 cancer cells. While it doesn't have any significant toxic effect on natural fibroblast cells.

Many herbs and spices have pharmacological and biochemical properties including antioxidant, anti-inflammatory and anti-cancer property that appears to be involved in anti-mutagenic activity of the cell. Given that tumor progression is closely related with inflammation and oxidative stress, antioxidant compound that has anti-inflammatory properties can be an anti-cancer agent (Afshari *et al.,* 2011).

Thymus daenesis Celakis one of the plants that not only has many applications in traditional medicine, but also has confirmed anti-microbial activity against fungal and bacterial isolates and antioxidant property due to phenolic compounds such as thymol and carvacrol (Sefidkon& Ahmadi, 2000).

Based on the results of various studies, traces of oxidative stress and free radical production in the transformation of the growth and differentiation and carcinogenesis have been demonstrated (Keramati *et al.,* 2011).

Studies have shown that plant extracts rich in phenolic compounds result in protective effect of cells through reducing oxidative stress. Phenolic compounds are a group of aromatic plant secondary metabolites that are widely distributed throughout the plant and have various biological effects including antioxidant and antibacterial activity (Kumaran & Karunakaran, 2006).

The antioxidant activity of phenolic compounds in plants is mostly resulted from their regenerative power and chemical structure, allowing them to neutralize free radicals, form complexes with metal ions and turn off the single and triple oxygen molecules. Phenolic compounds inhibit oxidation reactions through donating electron to free radicals (Shun *et al.,* 2003). Therefore, it is likely that phenolic compounds such as thymol and carvacrol in hydroalcoholic extract of *Thymus daenesis* Celak reduce oxidative stress through scavenging free radicals.

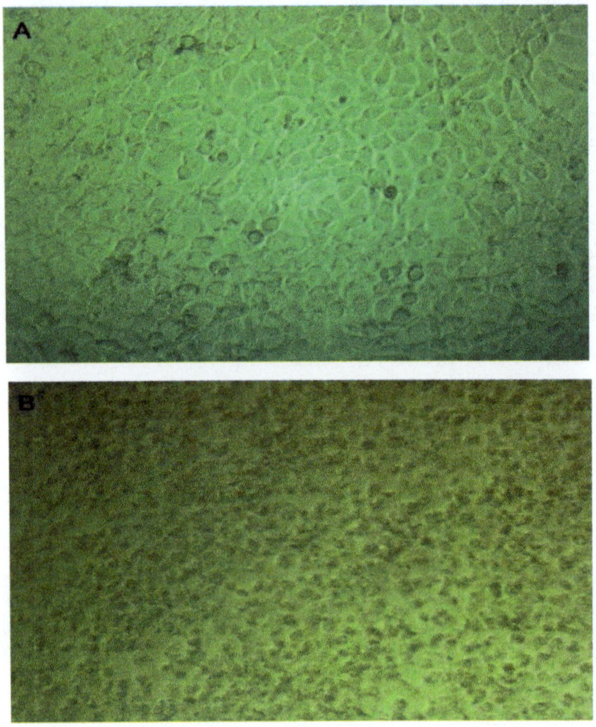

Fig. 3. (A) MCF-7 cancer cells in the control group without treatment with hydroalcoholic extract of *Thymus daenesis* Celak(B) MCF-7 cancer cells after 72 h treatment with hydroalcoholic extract of *Thymus daenesis* Celak at a concentration of 2.5 mg/ml.

Studies have shown that extract of thyme improves the antioxidant potential and thus help preventing from oxidative stress (Rana & Soni, 2008). The findings of some researchers showed that antioxidant compounds such as phenolic compounds can be considered as effective factors on cytotoxic capacity of *A. Campesteris,* phenolic compounds protect cells against reactive oxygen species (ROS) (Angel *et al.,*2009) .

Thymol and carvacrol are important compounds in *Thymus daenesis* Celak to which different biological effects can be attributed. Studies have shown that the thymol and carvacrol function in reducing oxidative stress on the one hand and inhibiting the cyclooxygenase enzymes on the other hand. However, investigations have shown that cyclooxygenase enzymes play a very important role in carcinogenesis mechanism (Keramati *et al.,* 2011).

Cyclooxygenase enzymes can inhibit aromatase enzyme through producing prostaglandins type E2, this enzyme can convert androgen to estrogen (Diaz-Cruz *et al.,* 2005). Since estrogen promotes tumor growth, it is likely that the amounts of estrogen and tumor growth are reduced through inhibiting the enzyme aromatase by inhibiting cyclooxygenase enzymes (Dixon, 2008). So it is likely that phenolic compounds such as thymol and carvacrol of hydroalcoholic extract of *Thymus daenesis* Celak reduce the estrogen level and in turn less tumor growth by inhibiting the aromatase enzyme through inhibiting cyclooxygenase enzymes.

Therapeutic and prophylactic effects of hydroalcoholic extract of Thymus vulgaris on precancerous lesions and carcinoma of the prostate gland cobblestone cells of Wistar albino rats were seen which were related tothymol and carvacrol (Singh & Lucci, 2002).

In a study by Hamta *et al.*(2013) compounds in hydroalcoholic extract of Thymus vulgaris were responsible for inducing apoptosis in cancer cellslines4T1 and anti-cancer and cytotoxic properties of hydroalcoholic extract can be resulted from such compounds as thymol and carvacrol (Hamta & Ghazaghi, 2014). In the present study, cytotoxic effects of hydroalcoholic extract of *Thymus daenesis* Celak can be attributed to phenolic compounds such as thymol and carvacrol, agreeing with results of Hamta *et al.*(2013) study.

Studies show a significant difference at three treatment times (24, 48 and 72h) so that as the time and concentration of hydroalcoholic extract of *Thymus daenesis* Celak is increased, cytotoxicity on MCF-7 cancer cells is also increased. While it doesn't have significant toxicity on natural fibroblast cells. The results of this study are consistent with the findings of Mahdian and co-workers (2015), who studied the effect of hydroalcoholic extract of Brassica *Olerace (Red cabbge)* on inhibiting the growth of breast cancer cells (MCF-7) and normal fibroblast cells (HFF). The results showed that hydroalcoholic extract of *Brassica Olerace (Red cabbge)* cancer inhibited dose-dependent and time-dependent growth of cancer cells, while hydroalcoholic extract of the red cabbage didn't have any toxicity at any time (Mahdian *et al.,* 2015).

The results of this study are also in agreement with the findings of Rezaei and colleagus (2014), who examined cytotoxic effect of hydroalcoholic extract of green fruit and ripe *Cornus mas L*on three cell lines MCF-7 (breast cancer), HepG2 (liver cancer) and CHO (hamster normal cells) by MTT. The results showed that hydroalcoholic extract of *Cornus mas L. fruit* has significant dose-dependent and time-dependent toxicity effect on cancer cells, while it doesn't have any significant toxicity on normal cells (Rezaei *et al.,* 2014).

These results could be a first step in examining and identifying anticancer compounds, however, studies have shown that plant compounds and their derivatives can be considered as part of the standard protocols for cancer treatment and effective weapon to prevent and treat cancer. Due to wide variety of plants, researchers face a long way to research in this field.

4. Conclusion

The results of this study show that hydroalcoholic extract of Thymus *daenesis* Celak has anti-cancer effect which can inhibit the growth of these cells through dose- dependent and time-dependent effect on MCF-7 cancer cells. So that as time spends and in higher doses, growth of cancer cells was more inhibited. Hydroalcoholic extract of *Thymus daenesis* Celak didn't have any significant effect on natural fibroblast cells.

5. References

Abdullaev, F. 2001. Plant-derived agents cancer,*Journal of Pharmacology*. 15(3): 345-354.

Afshari, J., Brook, A., and Moheghi, N. 2011. The cytotoxic effect of *zingiberafficinale* in breast cancer(MCF7) cell line.*Ofogh-e-Danesh*, 17(4): 28-33.

Aggarwal, B.B., Sundaram, C., Malani, N., and Ichikawa, H .2007. Curcumin: the Indian solid gold. *Advances in Experimental Medicine and Biology*, 595: 1-75.

Angel, S., Morana, A., Salvatore, A., Zappia, V., and Galletti, P. 2009. Protective effect of polyphenols from Glycyrrhizaglabra against oxidative stress in Caco-2 cells. *Journal of Medicinal Food*, 12; 1326–1333.

Barazandeh, M., and Bagherzadeh, K. 2007. Investigation on the Chemical Composition of the Essential of *Thymus daenensis* Celak from Four Different Regions of Isfahan Province. *Journal of Medicinal Plant*, 3 (23): 15-19.

Diaz-Cruz, E.S., Shapiro, C.L., and Brueggemeier, R.W.2005. Cyclooxygenase inhibitors suppress aromatase expression and activity in breast cancer cells. *Journal of Clincal Endocrinology & Metabolism*, 90(5): 2563-2570.

Dixon, M.J. Role of ErbB2 in selection for adjuvant tamoxifen or aromatase inhibitors.2008.*Womens Health*, 14(3): 229-231.

Forouzandeh, F., Salimi, S., Naghsh, N., Zamani, N., and Jahani, S.2014.Evaluation of anti-cancer effect of *Peganumharmala* L hydroalcoholic extract on human cervical carcinoma epithelial cell line. *Journal of Shahrekord University of Medical Sciences*, 16(4): 1-8.

Ghasemi Pirbalouti, A., Bahmani, M., and Avijgan, M.2009. Anti-*candida* activity of Iranian medicinal plants. *Electronic Journal of Biology*, 5: 85-88.

Ghasemi Pirbalouti, A., Hashemi, M., and Ghahfarokhi, F.T. 2013. Essential oil and chemical compositions of wild and cultivated *Thymus daenensis* Celak and *Thymus vulgaris* L. *Industrial Crops and Products*, 48: 43-48.

Ghasemi Pirbalouti, A., Malekpoor, F., Enteshari, S., Yousefi, M., Momtaz, H., and Hamedi, B. 2010. Antibacterial activity of some folklore medicinal plants used by Bakhtiari tribal in Southwest. *International Journal of Biology*, 2: 55-63.

Golparvar, A., Ghasemipirbalouti, A., Zinaly, H.,and Hadipanah, A. 2012. Effect OF Harvest Times on Quantity (Morphological) and Quality Characteristics of *Thymus daenensis* Celak. In Isfaha. *Journal of Herbal Drugs*, 2(4): 245-254.

Gordanian, B., Behbahani, M., Carapetian, J., and Fazilati, M. 2014. In vitro evaluation of cytotoxic activity of flower, leaf, stem and root extracts of five *Artemisia* species. *Research in Pharmaceutical Sciences*, 9:91-96.

Hamta, A., and Ghazaghi, S. 2014. The study of *Thymus vulgaris* Cytotoxicity effects on breast cancer cell's line. *Quarterly Journal of Sabzevar University of Medical Sciences,* 21(1):122-130.

Hamta, A., and Parvini, P. 2011. Study of cytotoxic effects of Taxol and Rosemary extracts on cancerous cells derived from DMB Ainduced breast cancer in SD rats. *Journal of Cell & Tissue*, 2: 117-126.

Karimi, A., Ghasemi pirbalouti, A., Malekpoor, F., Yousefi, M,, and Golparvar, A. 2010. Evaluation of Ecotype and Chemotype Diversity of *Thymus Daenensis* Celak on Isfahan and Chaharmahal va Bakhtiari Provinces. *Journal of Herbal Drugs*, 1(3): 1 – 10.

Keramati, k., Sanaie, k., Babakhani, A,. Rakhshan, M., Vaezi, G., and Hareri, A. Effect of *Thymus Vulgaris* hydro- alcoholic extraction on DMBA induced prostate cancer Wistar rat. 2011. *Research in Medicine*, 35(3): 135-140.

Kumaran, A., and Karunakaran, R.J. 2006. Antioxidant and free radical scavenging activity of an aqueous extract of *Coleus aromaticus*. *Food Chemistry*,97: 109-114.

Mahdian, D., Hosseini, A., Mousavi, H., Bihamta, M., and Vahedi, M. 2015. The Evalution of the Effects of Hydro-Alcolic Extract of *Brassica Olerace* (Red cabbge) on Growth inhibition and Apoptosis indution in Breast cancer cell line MCF-7. *Iranian Journal of Obstetrics Gynecology and Infertility*, 18 (151):1-11.

Mosmann, T. 1983. Rapid colorimetric assay for cellular growth and survival: application to proliferation and cytotoxicity assays. *Journal of Immunological Methods*, 1983; 65: 55-63.

O'Hara, M., Kiefer, D., Farrell, K., and Kemper, K. 1998. A review of 12 commonly used medicinal herbs. *Archives of Family Medicine*, 7(7): 523-536.

Osborne, C.K, Hobbs, K., and Trent, J.M. 1987. Biological differences among MCF-7 human breast cancer cell lines from different laboratories.*Breast Cancer Research and Treatment*, 9(12):111-121.

Rana, P., and Soni, G.2008.Antioxidantpotential of thyme extract: alleviation of Nnitrosodiethylamine - in duced oxidative stress.*Human & Experimental Toxicology*. 27(3): 215- 221.

Rezaei, F., Shokrzadeh, M., Majd, A., andNezhadsattari, T. 2014.Cytotoxic Effect of Hydroalcoholic Extract of *Cornus mas* Lfruit on MCF7, HepG2 and CHO cell line by MTTAssay. *Journal of Mazandaran University Medical Sciences*, 24(113):130-138.

Sefidkon, F., and Ahmadi, S.h. 2000. Essential oil of *Saturejakhuzistanica*Jamzad. *Journal of Essential Oil Research*, 12: 427-428.

Shun, Y.M., Wen, Y.H., Yong, C.Y., and Jian, G.S. Two Benzyl Dihydroflavones from Phellinus Igniarius. 2003. *Chinese Chemical Letters*, 14(8): 810-813.

Siegel, R., Ward, E., Brawley, O., and Jemal, A. 2011. Cancer statistics, 2011: the impact of eliminating socioeconomic and racial disparities on premature cancer deaths, *Cancer Journal for Clinicians*. 61(4): 212-236.

Singh, B., andLucci, A. 2002. Role of cycloxygenase-2 in breast cancer,*Journal of Surgical Research*. 108: 173-179.

Analgesic and anti-inflammatory activities of *Zea mays* leaves

Jude E Okokon[1]*, Koofreh Davies[2], Bassey S Antia[3]

[1]*Department of pharmacology and toxicology, Faculty of pharmacy, University of Uyo, Uyo, Nigeria;*
***Email:** *judeefiom@yahoo.com*

[2]*Department of physiology, Faculty of basic medical sciences, University of Uyo, Uyo, Nigeria;*

[3]*Department of chemistry, University of Uyo, Uyo, Nigeria;*

ARTICLE INFO

Topic: *Medicinal Plants*

Key words:
- ✓ *Zea mays*
- ✓ *Anti-inflammatory*
- ✓ *Analgesic*
- ✓ *GC-MS*

ABSTRACT

Background & Aim: *Zea mays* leaf used traditionally in Ibibio ethno medicine in Southern Nigeria to treat malaria and other inflammatory diseases. These anti-inflammatory and analgesic properties were evaluated against experimentally induced inflammation and pains using standard models.
Experimental: The effects of ethanol leaf extract of *Zea mays* (170 -510 mg/kg) on experimentally induced inflammation and pain were studied in rats using Carrageenin, egg albumin and xylene-induced inflammation as well as acetic acid-induced writhing and thermal induced pain models. The GCMS analysis of the most active fraction was carried out.
Results: The extract (170 -520 mg/kg) inhibited inflammation and pains caused by different phlogistic agents used in a dose dependent fashion. The various degrees of inhibitions were statistically significant ($p<0.05$, 0.01, 0.001), though incomparable to that of the standard drugs used (ASA and indomethacin). The GC-MS revealed the present of polyunsaturated fatty acids and phenolic compounds which may be responsible for the observed activities of the extract.
Recommended applications/industries: The present study demonstrates that leaf extract of *Zea mays* might to be useful for the treatment of inflammation and pains.

1. Introduction

Zea mays L. (Family- Poacae) known as maize or corn, is an annual grass plant cultivated for human consumption and rearing of animals. It was introduced to Nigeria in the 16th century (Osagie and Eka, 1998). It is tall with strong erect stalks and a fibrous root system. The plant has long narrow leaves that are spaced alternately on opposite side of the stem and bears ears that are enclosed in modified leaves known as husks (Simmonds, 1979). Besides its nutritive values, maize grains, leaves, cornsilks, stalk, and inflorescence are also used in ethnomedicine for the treatment of several ailments. The corn silk is used as an antidiabetic or diuretic, and decoction of the silk is consumed for the treatment of urinary troubles and gallstones (Foster and Duke, 1990; Gill, 1992; Abo *et al.,* 2008). The ash of the cob is used for the treatment of cough (Gill, 1992) as well as inflammatory diseases. The husks are used in the treatment of pains and arthritis (Owoyele *et al.,* 2010). It is also taken as warm tea for the treatment of malaria in

Ibibio traditional medicine. Biological activities reported on the leaf extract include; anticancer (Balasubramanian and Padma, 2013; Balasubramanian *et al.*, 2014), antioxidant (Balasubramanian and Padma, 2012) and antioxidative stress (Balasubramanian *et al.*, 2015) activities. Anti-inflammatory and analgesic activities have been reported on the husk extract (Owoyele *et al.*, 2010). Eight phenolic compounds (gallic acid, protocatechuic acid, chlorogenic acid, cafeic acid, femlic acid, rutin, resveratrol, and kaempferol) have also been detected in ethanol husk extract of *Zea mays* (Dong *et al.*, 2014). Information on the biological activities of the leaf extract is scarce. We report in this study the anti-inflammatory and analgesic activities of the leaf extract to confirm its uses Ibibio ethno medicine.

2. Materials and Methods

2.1. Plants collection

The plant material *Zea mays* (leaves) were collected in a farmland in Uyo area, Akwa Ibom State, Nigeria in May, 2015. The plant was identified and authenticated by Dr. Margaret Bassey of Department of Botany and Ecological Studies, University of Uyo, Uyo, Nigeria. Hebarium specimen was deposited at Department of Pharmacognosy and Natural Medicine Herbarium.

2.2. Extraction

The plant parts were washed and shade-dried for two weeks. The dried plants' materials were reduced to powder using mortar and pistle. The powdered material was soaked in 50% ethanol. The liquid filtrate was concentrated and evaporated to dryness in vacuo 40°C using rotary evaporator and stored in a refrigerator at -4°C.

2.3. Phytochemical Screening

Phytochemical screening of the crude extract was carried out employing standard procedures and tests (Trease and Evans, 1989, Sofowora, 1993), to reveal the presence of chemical constituents such as alkaloids, flavonoids, tannins, terpenes, saponins, anthraquinones, reducing sugars, cardiac glycosides among others.

2.4. Animals

Albino Swiss mice (20 – 25g) of either sex were obtained from the University of Uyo animal house. They were maintained on standard animal pellets and water *ad libitum*. The animals were divided into 5 groups of 6 mice in each all the models studied. Permission and approval for animal studies were obtained from the College of Health Sciences Animal Ethics committee, University of Uyo.

2.5. Determination of median lethal dose (LD_{50})

The median lethal dose (LD_{50}) of the extract was estimated using albino mice by intraperitoneal (i.p) route using the method of Lorke (1983). This involved intraperitoneal administration of different doses of the extract (1000 -5000 mg/kg) to groups of three mice each. The animals were observed for manifestation of physical signs of toxicity such as writhing, decreased motor activity, decreased body/limb tone, decreased respiration and death. The number of deaths in each group within 24 hours was recorded. The LD_{50} was calculated as geometrical means of the maximum dose producing 0% (a) and the minimum dose producing 100% mortality (b).

$$LD_{50} = \sqrt{ab}$$

2.6. Evaluation of anti-inflammatory activity of the extract

2.6.1. Carrageenin – induced mice hind paw oedema. Adult albino male mice were used after 24 hours fast and deprived of water only during experiment. Inflammation of the hind paw was induced by injection of 0.1 ml of freshly prepared carrageenin suspension in normal saline into the sub planar surface of the hind paw. The linear circumference of the injected paw was measured before and 0.5, 1, 2, 3, 4 and 5 hrs after administration of phlogistic agent. The increase in paw circumference post administration of phlogistic agent was adopted as the parameter for measuring inflammation (Winter *et al.*, 1962; Akah and Nwambie, 1994; Ekpendu *et al.*, 1994, Besra *et al.*, 1996; Nwafor *et al.*, 2010). The difference in paw circumference between the control and 0.5, 1, 2, 3, 4 and 5 hrs after administration of phlogistic agent was used to assess inflammation (Hess and Milonig, 1992). The leaf extract (170, 340 and 510 mg/kg i.p) was administered to various groups of 6 mice each, 1 h before inducing inflammation. Control mice received carrageenin while reference group received ASA (100 mg/kg). The average (mean) oedema was assessed by measuring with vernier calipers. Average inflammation/oedema ($C_t - C_0$) was calculated for each dose (Oriowo, 1982; Akah and Njike, 1990).

2.6.2. Egg-albumin induced inflammation. Inflammation was induced in mice by the injection of egg albumin (0.1ml, 1% in normal saline) into the sub planar tissue of the right hind paw (Akah and Nwambie, 1994; Okokon and Nwafor, 2010). The linear circumference of the injected paw was measured before and 0.5, 1, 2, 3, 4 and 5 hrs after the administration of the phlogistic agent. The leaf extract (170, 340 and 510 mg/kg i.p) and ASA (100 mg/kg orally) were administered to groups (n=6) of 24 h fasted mice 1 h before the induction of inflammation. Control group received 10 ml/kg of distilled water orally. Edema (inflammation) was assessed as the difference in paw circumference between the control and 0.5, 1, 2, 3, 4 and 5 hrs post administration of the phlogistic agent (Hess and Milonig, 1972). The average (mean) edema was assessed by measuring with vernier calipers. Average inflammation/oedema ($C_t - C_0$) was calculated for each dose (Oriowo, 1982; Akah and Njike, 1990).

2.6.3 Xylene – induced ear oedema. Inflammation was induced in mice by topical administration of 2 drops of xylene at the inner surface of the right ear. The xylene was left to act for 15 mins. *Zea mays* leaf extract (170, 340 and 510 mg/kg i.p), dexamethasone (4 mg/kg) and distilled water (0.2 ml/kg) were orally administered to various groups (n=6) of mice 1 h before the induction of inflammation. The animals were sacrificed under light anaesthesia and the left ears cut off. The difference between the ear weights was taken as the oedema induced by the xylene (Tjolsen *et al.*, 1992; Okokon and Nwafor, 2010).

2.7. Evaluation of analgesic potential of the extract

2.7.1. Acetic acid induced writhing in mice. Writhings (abdominal constrictions consisting of the contraction of abdominal muscles together with the stretching of hindlimbs) resulting from intraperitoneal (i.p) injection of 2% acetic acid, was induced according to the procedure described by Santos *et al.* (1994), Correa *et al.* (1996) and Nwafor *et al.* (2010). The animals were divided into 5 groups of 6 mice per group. Group 1 served as negative control and received 10 ml/kg of normal saline, while groups 2, 3 and 4 were pre-treated with 170, 340 and 510 mg/kg doses of *Z. mays* leaf extract intraperitoneally, and group 5 received 100 mg/kg of acetyl salicylic acid. After 30 minutes, 0.2 ml of 2% acetic acid was administered intraperitoneally (i.p). The number of writhing movements was counted for 30 minutes. Antinociception (analgesia) was expressed as the reduction of the number of abdominal constrictions between control animals and mice pretreated with extracts.

2.7.2. Thermally induced pain in mice. The effect of extract on hot plate induced pain was investigated in adult mice. The hot plate was used to measure the response latencies according to the method of Vaz *et al.*, (1996) and Okokon and Nwafor, (2010). In these experiments, the hot plate was maintained at 45±1°C, each animal was placed into a glass beaker of 50 cm diameter on the heated surface, and the time(s) between placement and shaking or licking of the paws or jumping was recorded as the index of response latency. An automatic 30-second cut-off was used to prevent tissue damage. The animals were randomly divided into 5 groups of 6 mice each and fasted for 24 hours but allowed access to water. Group 1 animal served as negative control and received 10 ml/kg of normal saline. Groups 2, 3 and 4 were pre-treated intraperitoneally with 170, 340 and 510 mg/kg doses of *Z. mays* leaf extract respectively, while group 5 animals received 100 mg/kg of acetyl salicylic acid intraperitoneally, 30 minutes prior to the placement on the hot plate.

2.8. Gas chromatography-Mass spectrometry analysis

Quantitative and qualitative data were determined by GC and GC-MS, respectively. The fraction was injected onto a Shimadzu GC-17A system, equipped with an AOC-20i autosampler and a split/ splitless injector. The column used was an DB-5 (Optima-5), 30 m, 0.25 mm i.d., 0.25 μm df, coated with 5 % diphenyl-95 % polydimethylsiloxane, operated with the following oven temperature programme: 50 °C, held for 1 min, rising at 3 °C/min to 250 °C, held for 5 min, rising at 2 °C/min to 280 °C, held for 3 min; injection temperature and volume, 250 °C and 1.0 μl, respectively; injection mode, split; split ratio, 30:1; carrier gas, nitrogen at 30 cm/s linear velocity and inlet pressure 99.8 KPa; detector temperature, 280 °C; hydrogen, flow rate, 50 ml/min; air flow rate, 400 ml/min; make-up (H2/air), flow rate, 50 ml/min; sampling rate, 40 ms. Data were acquired by means of GC solution software (Shimadzu). Agilent 6890N GC was interfaced with a VG Analytical 70-250s double -focusing mass spectrometer. Helium was used as the carrier gas. The MS operating conditions were: ionization voltage 70 eV, ion source 250 0C. The GC was fitted with a 30 m x 0.32 mm fused capillary silica column coated with DB-5. The GC operating parameters were identical with those of GC analysis described above.

2.8.1. Identification of the compounds. The identification of components present in the active fraction of the plants' extract was based on direct comparison of the retention times and mass spectral data with those for standard compounds, and by computer matching with the Wiley and Nist Libraries, as well as by comparison of the fragmentation patterns of the mass spectra with those reported in the literatures (Adams, 2001; Setzer *et al.,* 2007).

2.9. Statistical analysis and data evaluation

Data obtained from this work were analyzed statistically using Students't-test and ANOVA (One-way) followed by a post test (Tukey-Kramer multiple comparison test). Differences between means were considered significant at 1% and 5% level of significance i.e. $P \leq 0.01$and 0.05.

3. Results and discussion

The phytochemical screening of the ethanol leaf extract of *Zea mays* revealed the presence of alkaloids, cardiac glycosides, tannins, saponins, terpenes and flavonoids.

The median lethal dose (LD_{50}) was calculated to be 1732.05 mg/kg. The physical signs of toxicity included excitation, paw licking, increased respiratory rate, decreased motor activity, gasping and coma which was followed by death.

The effect of ethanol extract of *Zea mays* leaf on carragenin-induced oedema is as shown in Table 1. The extract (170 - 510 mg/kg) exerted a significant (P<0.05 – 0.001) anti-inflammatory effect in a dose –dependent manner. The activity of the highest dose was incomparable to that of the standard drug, ASA, 100 mg/kg (Table 1a and 1b).

Administration of leaf extract of *Zea mays* (170 - 510 mg/kg) on egg albumin - induced oedema in mice caused a significant (p<0.05 – 0.001) dose-dependent anti-inflammatory effect against oedema caused by egg albumin. The effect was incomparable to that of standard drug, ASA (100 mg/kg) (Table 2a and 2b).

Anti-inflammatory effect of crude leaf extract of *Zea mays* against xylene-induced ear oedema in mice is shown in Table 3. The extract exerted a dose-dependent anti-inflammatory effects that were significant (P<0.05 - 0.01) but incomparable to that of the standard drug, dexamethasone (4.0 mg/kg).

The administration of *Z. mays* extract (170, 340 and 510 mg/kg) demonstrated a dose-dependent reduction in acetic acid-induced writhing in mice. The reductions were statistically significant (p<0.05 - 0.001) relative to control and the effect of the highest dose(510 mg/kg) at 30 minute was more than that of the standard drug, ASA (Table 4).

The extract (170, 340 and 510 mg/kg) exhibited a dose - dependent effect on thermally-induced pain in mice. This inhibitions were statistically significant (p<0.05) only at the highest dose of the extract (510 mg/kg) relative to the control but incomparable to that of the standard drug, ASA (100mg/kg) (Table 5).

The GC-MS analysis of the ethyl acetate fraction of *Zea mays* leaf revealed the presence of bioactive compounds with major and minor ones as represented in Table 6.

Zea mays leaf is used traditionally for the treatment of various illnesses such as malarial fever, pains and inflammatory conditions. In this study, the ethanol leaf extract was evaluated for analgesic and anti-inflammatory activities using various experimental models.

In the carragenin-induced oedema, the extract (170 - 510 mg/kg) was observed to have exerted a weak effect at the early stage of inflammation (1-2 hr) indicating weak effect probably on histamine, serotonin and kinnins that are involved in the early stage of carragenin-induced oedema (Vane and Booting, 1987). The extract further caused prominent reduction of the later stage of the oedema suggesting its ability to inhibit prostaglandin which is known to mediate the second phase of carragenin induced inflammation (Vane and Booting, 1987).

Table 1a. Effect of *Zea mays* leaf extract on carrageenin- induced oedema in rats.

Treatment/ dose (mg/kg)	Time intervals (h)						
	0	0.5	1	2	3	4	5
Control	2.18 ± 0.04	3.13 ± 0.05	3.13 ± 0.01	3.10 ± 0.06	3.04 ± 0.07	2.97 ± 0.01	2.88 ± 0.06
Extract 170	2.44 ± 0.06	3.72 ± 0.12	3,40 ± 0.07	3.26 ± 0.07	3.36 ± 0.28	3.17 ± 0.20	3.05 ± 0.20
340	2.55 ± 0.06	3.70 ± 0.11	3.55 ± 0.07[a]	3.48 ± 0.14	3.40 ± 0.10	3.18 ± 0.04	3.04 ± 0.13
510	2.45 ± 0.10	3.39 ± 0.10	3.21± 0.03[a]	3.33 ± 0.11	3.08 ± 0.08	2.86 ± 0.09	2.78 ± 0.11
ASA 100	2.21 ± 0.07	2.89±0.04	2.59 ± 0.05[b]	2.75 ± 0.02[a]	2.60 ± 0.02 [a]	2.57 ± 0.08	2.51 ± 0.09

Data are expressed as mean ± SEM. Values were considered significant at $^{a}p<0.05$; $^{b}p< 0.01$ when compared to control. n = 6.

Table 1b. Effect of *Zea mays* leaf extract on carrageenin induced oedema in rats.

Treatment/ Dose (mg/kg)	Average inflammation/oedema (mm)					
	0.5h	1h	2h	3h	4h	5h
Control	0.95 ± 0.01	0.95 ± 0.01	0.92 ± 0.01	0.86 ± 0.01	0.79 ± 0.01	0.70 ± 0.01
Extract 170	1.27± 0.18	0.96 ± 0.13	0.82 ± 0.22	0.92 ± 0.01	0.73 ± 0.25	0.61 ± 0.25
340	1.11± 0.07	0.96 ± 0.07	0.89 ± 0.10	0.81 ± 0.10	0.62 ± 0.01[C]	0..53 ± 0.25 [C]
510	0.90 ± 0.40	0.73 ± 0.03	0.85 ± 0.01	0.60 ± 0.04[C]	0.41 ± 0.07[C]	0.33 ± 0.15[C]
ASA 100	0.68±0.01	0.38 ± 0.01[C]	0.54 ± 0.01[C]	0.39 ± 0.01[C]	0.36 ± 0.01[C]	0.30 ± 0.01[C]

Data are expressed as mean ± SEM. Values were considered significant at $^{c}p < 0.001$ when compared to control. n = 6.

Table 2a. Effect of *Zea mays* leaf extract on egg- albumin induced oedema in mice.

Treatment/ Dose (mg/kg)	Time intervals (h)						
	0	0.5	1	2	3	4	5
Control	2.65 ± 0.07	3.55± 0.25	3.50 ± 0.06	3.45 ± 0.11	3.41 ± 0.07	3.35 ± 0.07	3.25 ± 0.06
Extract 170	2.44 ± 0.37	3.43±0.09	3.09 ± 0.07	3.01 ± 0.07	2.94 ± 0.08	2.87 ± 0.01	2.78 ± 0.04
340	2.38 ± 0.03	3.22±0.12	2.89 ± 0.11[a]	2.82 ± 0.08[c]	2.70 ± 0.06[c]	2.63 ± 0.06 [c]	2.58 ± 0.03 [c]
510	2.31 ± 0.02	3.30 ± 0.09	2.71 ± 0.03[a]	2.72 ± 0.07[c]	2.62 ± 0.06[c]	2.62 ± 0.03[b]	2.51 ± 0.02 [c]
ASA 100	2.61 ± 0.06	2.99 ±0.16[a]	2.89 ± 0.02[a]	2.84 ± 0.02[c]	2.76 ± 0.03[c]	2.64 ± 0.05[b]	2.64 ± 0.05[c]

Data are expressed as mean ± SEM. Values were considered significant at $^{a}p<0.05$; $^{b}p< 0.01$, $^{C}p< 0.001$ when compared to control. n = 6.

Table 2b. Effect of *Zea mays* leaf extract on egg- albumin induced oedema in rats.

Treatment/ Dose (mg/kg)	Average inflammation/oedema (mm)					
	0.5h	1h	2h	3h	4h	5h
Control	0.90 ± 0.01	0.85 ± 0.01	0.80 ± 0.01	0.76 ± 0.01	0.70 ± 0.14	0.60 ± 0.10
Extract 170	0.99± 0.0.9	0.65 ± 0.07	0.55 ± 0.09[c]	0.50 ± 0.11[c]	0.43 ± 0.05 [c]	0.33 ± 0.07 [c]
340	0.83 ±0.10	0.55 ± 0.09[c]	0.50 ± 0.07[c]	0.32 ± 0.06[c]	0.23 ± 0.06 [c]	0.20 ± 0.03 [c]
510	0.99 ±0.08	0.39 ± 0.04[c]	0.41 ± 0.07[c]	0.31 ± 0.05[c]	0.30 ± 0.02[c]	0.20 ± 0.02 [c]
ASA 100	0.38 ±0.01[c]	0.28 ± 0.01[c]	0.23 ± 0.01[c]	0.15 ± 0.01[c]	0.03 ± 0.01[c]	0.03 ± 0.01[c]

Table 3. Effect of *Zea mays* leaf extract on xylene-induced ear oedema in mice.

Treatment/ Dose (mg/kg)	Weight of right ear (g)	Weight of left ear (g)	Increase in ear weight (g)	% Inhibition
Control (normal saline) 0.2ml	0.098 ± 0.01	0.043 ± 0.00	(127.90) 0.055 ± 0.00	-
Extract 170	0.090 ± 0.01	0.043 ± 0.00	(109.30) 0.047 ± 0.00 [NS]	14.54

340	0.080 ± 0.01	0.050 ± 0.01	(60.0)	45.45
			0.030 ± 0.01 [b]	
510	0.056 ± 0.01	0.043 ± 0.01	(30.23)	76.36
			0.013 ± 0.01[c]	
Dexamethasone 4.0	0.043 ± 0.01	0.036 ± 0.01	(19.44)	87.27
			0.007 ± 0.00[c]	

Figures in parenthesis indicate % increase in ear weight. Significant at [a]p < 0.01, [b]p < 0.001 when compared with control. n = 6.

Table 4. Effect of *Zea mays* leaf extract on acetic acid induced writhing in mice.

Treatment/ Dose (mg/kg)	**Time intervals (h)**						
	5	**10**	**15**	**20**	**25**	**30**	**TOTAL**
Control	6.66 ± 0.88	11.66 ± 1.20	24.66 ± 1.85	17.0 ± 0.57	13.00 ± 1.15	11.0 ± 1.00	83.98 ± 6.65
Extract 170	6.33 ± 0.66	5.00 ± 1.15 [a]	18.33 ± 1.45 [a]	14.00 ± 2.00	12.33 ± 0.88	10.66 ± 0.66	66.65 ± 6.80[a]
340	4.00 ± 0.57	4.33 ± 1.85 [b]	13.66 ± 1.33[b]	12.00 ± 1.00[a]	7.33 ± 1.20 [a]	7.66 ± 0.85[a]	48.98 ± 6.80[c]
510	3.00 ± 0.57[a]	4.00 ± 0.57 [b]	7.00 ± 1.00[c]	8.66 ± 0.33[b]	5.33 ± 0.66[b]	6.00 ± 0.57[a]	21.32 ± 3.70[c]
ASA 100	4.00 ± 0.57	6.00 ± 0.57 [a]	8.33 ± 0.88[c]	8.66 ± 0.33[b]	7.66 ± 0.66[a]	4.00 ± 0.57[b]	38.65 ± 3.58[c]

Data are expressed as mean ± SEM. Significant at [a]P < 0.05, [b]P < 0.01, [c]P < 0.001 when compared to control n = 6.

However, ASA (100 mg/kg) a prototype NSAID, a cyclooxygenase inhibitor whose mechanism of action involves inhibition of prostaglandin, produced a considerable inhibition of the paw swelling induced by carragenin injection.

Table 5. Effect of *Zea mays* Leaf extract on hot plate test

Group	**Dose mg/kg**	**Reaction time (sec) (mean ± SEM)**	**% inhibition**
Control	-	4.92 ± 0.23	
Z. mays	170	5.33 ± 0.12	8.33
	340	6.59 ± 0.32	33.94
	510	12.62 ± 0.85 [a]	156.50
ASA	100	29.53 ± 3.48[c]	500.20

Data are expressed as mean ± SEM. Significant at [a]P < 0.05, [b] P < 0.001 when compared to control. n = 6.

The extract also inhibited egg albumin-induced oedema demonstrating that it can inhibit inflammation by blocking the release of histamine and 5-HT, two mediators that are released by egg albumin (Nwafor *et al.*, 2007). However, ASA, a cyclooxygenase inhibitor reduced significantly oedema produced by egg albumin.

The extract exerted a significant (P<0.01) inhibition of xylene -induced ear oedema at higher doses of the extract, suggesting the inhibition of phospholipase A_2 which is involve in the pathophysiology of inflammation due to xylene (Lin *et al.*, 1992). However, dexamethasone, a steroid antiinflammatory agent produced significant reduction in the mean right ear weight of positive control rats indicating an inhibition of PLA_2.

The extract significantly reduced acetic acid-induced writhing and delayed the reaction time of animals (mice) to thermally induced pain. Acetic acid causes inflammatory pain by inducing capillary permeability (Amico-Roxas *et al.*, 1984; Nwafor *et al.*, 2007), and in part through local peritoneal receptors from peritoneal fluid concentration of PGE_2 and $PGF_2\alpha$ (Deraedt *et al.*, 1980; Bentley *et al.*, 1983). The acetic acid-induced abdominal writhing is a visceral pain model in which the processor releases arachidonic acid via cyclooxygenase, and prostaglandin biosynthesis plays a role in the nociceptive mechanism (Franzotti *et al.*, 2002). It is used to distinguish between central and peripheral pain. These results suggest that the extract may be exerting its action partly through the lipoxygenase and/or cyclooxygenase system.

The study also shows that the extract significantly delayed the reaction time of thermally- induced (hot plate) test. This model is selective for centrally acting analgesics and indicates narcotic involvement (Turner, 1995) with opiod receptors.

Phytochemical screening of the leaf extract revealed the presence of alkaloids, cardiac glycosides, tannins, saponins, terpenes and flavonoids and GC-MS analysis of ethyl acetate fraction showed the presence of pharmacological active compounds such as 2,3 dihydro benzofuran and polyunsaturated fatty acids such as 9-

Octadecenoic acid (Z)-, 2- hydroxyethyl ester, Hexadecanoic acid, ethyl ester and Hexadecanoic acid, methyl ester which have been implicated in the anti-inflammatory activity of plants (Ledon *et al*., 2003; Kumar , 2010; Raja *et al*., 2011).

Moreso, anti-inflammatory activities of plants have been linked to antioxidant potentials (Sokeng *et al.,* 2013). The plant extract have been revealed by GCMS to contain phenolic compounds with antioxidant potentials such as p-Hydroxycinnamic acid, ethyl ester and, Phenol, 2,6-dimethoxy-4-(2-propenyl)- (Alamed *et al.,* 2009). Also Triterpene-fatty acid esters and free fatty acids including long chain C16-C20 unsaturated fatty acids have been suggested to be responsible for the anti-inflammatory activity of plants (Li *et al.,* 2004).

Flavonoids are known anti-inflammatory compounds acting through inhibition of the cyclo-oxygenase pathway (Liang *et al.,* 1999). Some flavonoids are reported to block both the cyclooxygenase and lipoxygenase pathways of the arachidonate cascade at relatively high concentrations, while at lower concentrations they only block lipoxygenase pathway (Carlo *et al*., 1999). Some flavonoids exert their antinociception via opioid receptor activation activity (Suh *et al.,* 1996; Rajendran *et al*., 2000; Otuki *et al*., 2005). Flavonoids also exhibit inhibitory effects against phospholipase A2 and phospholipase C (Middleton *et al.,* 2000), and cyclooxygenase and/or lipoxygenase pathways (Robak *et al.,* 1998).

Triterpenes have been implicated in anti-inflammatory activity of plants (Huss *et al.,* 2002; Suh *et al.,* 1998) and reports on their analgesic activities have also been published (Liu, 1995; Krogh *et al.,* 1999; Tapondjou *et al.,* 2003; Maia *et al*., 2006). Ursolic acid is a selective inhibitor of cyclooxygenase-2 (Ringbom *et al*., 1998). Oleanolic acid is known to exert its analgesic action through an opioid mechanism, and possibly, a modulatory influence on vanilliod receptors (Maia *et al.,* 2006).

The anti-inflammatory and analgesic activities demonstrated by the leaf extract in this study may in part be due to its phytochemical constituents which maybe acting through antioxidant action and other mechanisms.

In conclusion, the results of this study demonstrated that *Zea mays* leaf possess anti-inflammatory and analgesic properties. Further investigation is being advocated especially in elucidating cellular mechanisms and establishing structural components of the active ingredients with a view of standardizing them.

4. Conclusion

The present study demonstrates that leaf extract of *Zea mays* might to be useful for the treatment of inflammation and pains.

5. Acknowledgement

Authors are grateful to Messrs Aniefiok Ukpong and Nsikan Malachy of Department of Pharmacology and Toxicology, University of Uyo, Uyo, for their technical assistance.

6. References

Abo, K.A., Fred-Jaiyesimi, A.A., Jaiyesimi, A.E.A. 2008. Ethnobotanical studies of medicinal plants used in the management of diabetes mellitus in South Western Nigeria. *J Ethnopharmacol.,* IS: 67-71.

Adams, R.P. 2001. Identification of Essential oils by Gas Chromatography Quadrupole Mass Spectrometry. Allured Publishing Corporation, Carol Stream, USA

Ahmed, M., Sadhu, S.K., Datta, B.K., Kunu, J.K., Bachar, S.C. 1997. Preliminary studies on the antiinflammatory, analgesic and diuretic activity of stagninol, a sesquiterpene isolated from *Persicaria stagnina*. *Pharmazie.,* 52(6):472-475.

Akah, P.A., Njike, H.A. 1990. Some pharmacological effects of rhizome aqueous extract of *Anchomanes diformis. Fitoterapia.,* 60: 368-370.

Akah, P.A., Nwanbie, A. 1994. Evaluation of Nigerian traditional medicines plants used for rheumatic (inflammatory) disorder. *Journal of Ethnopharmacology.,* 42: 179 – 182.

Alamed, J., Chaiyasit, W., McClements, D.J., Decker, E.A. 2009. Relationships between free radical scavenging and antioxidant activity in foods. *Journal of Agricultural and Food Chemistry.,* 57: 2969-2976.

Amico-Roxas, M., Caruso, A., Trombadore, S., Scifo, R., Scapagnime, U. 1984. Gangliosides antinociceptive effects in rodents. *Archieves of*

International Pharmacodynamics and Therapeutics., 272: 103-117.

Balasubramanian, K., Padma, P.R. 2013. Anticancer activity of *Zea mays* leaf extracts on oxidative stress-induced Hep2 Cells. *J Acupuncture and Meridian Studies.,* 6(3):149-158.

Balasubramanian, K., Padma, P.R. 2012. Screening of Antioxidant Properties of *Zea mays* Leaves at different time periods of growth. *Journal of Pharmacy Research.,* 5(8):4034-4037.

Balasubramanian, K., Vidhya, A., Thiruselvi, M., Sudhadevi, M. and Padma, P.R. 2014. *Zea mays* leaf extracts exhibits anticancer property and enhance the chemotherapeutic action of etoposide in cancer cells. *Indo American Journal of Pharmaceutical Research.,* 4(03): 1530 - 1539.

Balasubramanian, K., Jincy, P.A., Padma, P.R. 2015. Influence of methanolic extract of *Zea mays* leaves against CCL_4 and H_2O_2 induced oxidative stress in *Drosophila melanogaster. Indo American Journal of Pharmaceutical Research.,* 5(01): 566-577.

Bentley, G.A., Newton, S.H., Starr, J. 1983. Studies on the antinociceptive action of agonist drugs and their interaction with opoid mechanisms. *British Journal of Pharmacy.,* 79: 125 - 134.

Besra, S.E., Sharma, R.M., Gomes, A. 1996. Antiinflammatory effect of petroleum ether extract of leaves of *Litchi Chinensis.* Caertn (sapindaceae). *Journal of Ethnopharmacology*., 54:1-6.

Carlo Di, G., Mascolo, N., Izzo, A.A., Capasso, F. 1999. Flavonoids, old and new aspects of a class of natural therapeutic drugs. *Life Science.,* 65: 337–353.

Correa, C.R., Kyle, D.J., Chakravarty, S., Calixto, J.B. 1996. Antinociceptive profile or the pseudopeptide β_2 bradykinin receptors antagonist NPC 18688 in mice. *British Journal of Pharmacology*., 117: 552-556.

Deraedt, R, Jougney, S., Falhout, M. 1980. Release of Prostaglandin E and F in an algogenic reaction and its inhibition. *European Journal of Pharmacy*., 51: 17-24.

Dong, J., Cai, L., Zhu, X., Huang, X., Yin, T., Fang, H., Ding, Z. 2014. Antioxidant Activities and Phenolic Compounds of Cornhusk, Corncob and *Stigma Maydis. J. Braz. Chem. Soc.,* 25(11): 1956-1964.

Ekpendu, T.O., Akah, P.A., Adesomoju, A.A., Okogun, J.I. 1994. Antinflammatory and antimicrobial activities of *Mitracarpus scaber* extracts. *International Journal of Pharmacology*., 32:191-195.

Foster S, Duke JA. 1990. Field Guide 10 Medical Plants: Eastern and Central North America. Houghton MifAin, Boston.

Gill LS. 1992. Ethnomedical Uses of Plants in Nigeria. Uniben Press, Benin, Nigeria, p. 249.

Franzotti EM, Santos CVF, Rodrigues HMSL, Mourao RHV, Andrade MR, Antoniolli AR. 2002. Anti-inflammatory, analgesic activity and acute toxicity of *Sida cordifolia* L. *Journal of Ethnopharmacology.,* 72: 273-278.

Hess SM, Milonig RC. 1972. Inflammation In: Lepow LH, Ward PS. (Eds). Inflammation, Mechanism and control. Academic Press, New-York, USA. pp.1-2.

Huss U, Ringbom T, Perera P, Bohlin L, Vasange M. 2002. Screening of ubiquitous plant constituents for COX-2 inhibition with a scintillation proximity based assay. *Journal Natural Products.,* 65: 1517-1521.

Krogh R, Kroth R, Berti C, Madereira AO, Souza MM, Cechinel-Filho V, Delle-Monache F, Yunes RA. 1999. Isolation and identification of compounds with antinociceptive action from *Ipomoea pes-caprae. Pharmazie.,* 54: 464 – 466.

Kumar PP, Kumaravel S, Lalitha C. 2010. Screening of antioxidant activity, total phenolics and GC-MS study of *Vitex negundo. Afr J Biochem Res., 4* (7): 191-195.

Liang YC, Huang YT, Tsau SH, Lin-Shiau SY, Chen CF, Lin JK. 1999. Suppression of inducible cyclo-oxygenase and inducible nitric acid synthase by apigenia and related flavonoid in mouse macrophages. *Carcinogenesis*., 20: 1945-52.

Ledón N, Casacó A, Rodríguez V, Cruz J, González R, Tolón Z, Cano M, Rojas E.2003. Anti-Inflammatory and Analgesic Effects of a Mixture of Fatty acids isolated and purified from sugar cane wax oil. *Planta Medica.,* 69(4): 367-369

Li, R.W., Leach, D.N., Myers, P., Leach, G.J., Lin, G.D., Brushett, D.J., Waterman, P.G. 2004. Anti-inflammatory activity, cytotoxicity and active compounds of *Tinospora smilacina* Benth. *Phytotherapy Reserch.,* 18: 78-83.

Lin, L.L., Lin, A.Y., Knopt, J.L. 1992. Cytosolic phospholipase A_2 is coupled to hormonally regulated release of arachidonic acid. *Proceeding of National Academy of Science, U. S. A.*, 89: 6147-6157.

Liu, J. 1995. Pharmacology of oleanolic acid and ursolic acid. *Journal of Ethnopharmacology.,* 49: 57- 68.

Lorke, D. 1983. A new approach to practical acute toxicity testing. *Archieves of Toxicology.,* 54:275-286.

Maia, J.L., Lima-Junior, R.C., David, J.P., David, J.M., Santos, F.A., Rao, V.S. 2006. Oleanolic acid, a pentacyclic triterpene attenuates the mustard oil induced colonic nociception in mice. *Biological and Pharmaceutical Bulletin.,* 29: 82–85.

Middleton, E Jr, Kandaswami, C., Theoharides, T.C. 2000. The effects of plant flavonoids on mammalian cells: Implications for inflammation, heart disease, and cancer. *Pharmacological Reviews.,* 52: 673–751.

Nwafor, P.A., Jacks, T.W., Ekanem, A.U. 2007. Analgesic and anti-inflammatory effects of methanolic extract of *Pausinystalia mecroceras* stem bark in rodents. *Journal of Pharmacology.,* 3:86-90.

Nwafor, P.A., Nwajiobi, N., Uko, I.E., Obot, J.S. 2010. Analgesic and anti-inflammatory activities of an ethanol extract of *Smilax krausiana* leaf in mice. *African Journal of Biomedical and Research., 13: 141 -148.*

Osagie, A.U., Eka, O.U.1998. Nutritional quality of plant foods. Post Harvest Research Unit, University of Benin, Benin, Nigeria, pp 34-41.

Okokon, J.E., Nwafor, P.A. 2010. Antiinflammatory, analgesic and antipyretic activities of ethanolic root extract of *Croton zambesicus*. *Pakistan Journal of Pharmaceutical sciences*., 23(4): 383 - 390.

Owoyele, B.V., Negedu, M.N., Olaniran, S.O., Onasanwo, S.A., Oguntoye, S.O., Sanya, J.O., Oyeleke, S.A., Ibidapo, A.J., Soladoyel, A.O. 2010. Analgesic and anti-inflammatory effects of aqueous extract of *Zea mays* husk in male wistar rats. *Journal of Medicinal Food.,* 13 (2):343-347.

Oriowo, M.A. 1982. Anti-inflammatory activity of piperonyl,-4-acrylic isobutyl amide, an extractive from *Zanthoxylum zanthoxyloids. Planta Medica.,* 44: 54 - 56

Otuki, M.F., Ferreira, J., Lima, F.V., Meyre-Silva, C., Malheiros, Â., Muller, L.A., Cani, G.S., Santos, A.R.S., Yunes, R.A., Calixto, J.B. 2005. Antinociceptive properties of mixture of α-amyrin and β-amyrin triterpenes: Evidence for participation of protein kinase C and protein kinase A pathways. *Journal of Pharmacology and Experimental Therapeutics.,* 313: 310–318.

Raja Rajeswari, N., Rama Lakshmi, S., Muthuchelian, K. 2011. GC-MS Analysis of bioactive components from the ethanolic leaf extract of *Canthium dicoccum* (Gaertn.) Teijsm & Binn. *Journal of Chemical and Pharmaceutical Research.,* 3(3):792-798

Rajendran, N.N., Thirugnanasambandam, P., Viswanathan, S., Parvathavarthini, S., Ramaswamy, S. 2000. Antinociceptive pattern of flavone and its mechanism as tested by formalin assay. *Indian Journal of Experimental Biologiocal.,* 38: 182–185.

Ringbom, T., Segura, L., Noreen, Y., Perera, P., Bohlin, L. 1998. Ursolic acid from *Plantago major*, a selective inhibitor of cyclooxygenase-2 catalysed prostaglandin biosynthesis. *Journal of Natural Products.,* 61: 1212–1215.

Robak, J., Shridi, F., Wolbis, M., Krolikowska, M. 1998. Screening of the influence of flavonoids on lipoxygenase and cyclooxygenase activity, as well as on nonenzymic lipid oxidation. *Polish Journal of Pharmacology and Pharmacy.,* 40: 451–458.

Sokeng, S.D., Koubé, J., Dongmo, F., Sonnhaffouo, S., Nkono, B.L.N.Y., Taïwé, G.S., Cherrah, Y., Kamtchouing, P. 2013. Acute and chronic anti-inflammatory effects of the aqueous extract of *Acacia nilotica* (L.) Del. (Fabaceae) pods. *Academia Journal of Medicinal Plants*., 1: 1-5.

Santos, A.R., Cechinel Filho, V., Niero, R., Viana, A.M., Moreno, F.N., Campos, M.M., Yunes, R.A., Calixto, J.B. 1994. Analgesic effects of callus culture from selected species of *Phyllanthus. Journal of Pharmacy and Pharmacology.,* 46 : 755 – 759.

Setzer, W.N., Stokes, S.L., Penton, A.F., Takaku, S., Haber, W.A., Hansell, E., Caffrey, C.R., McKerrow, J.H. 2007. Cruzain Inhibitory activity of leaf essential oils of neotropical lauraceae and essential oil components. *Nat Prod Comm.,* 2(12): 1203–1210.

Simmonds, N.W. 1979. Evolution of Crop Plants. Longman. London. pp. 128-129.

Sofowora, A. 1993.Medicinal Plants and Traditional Medicine in Africa. 2nd edn, Spectrum Book Ltd, Ibadan, Nigeria.

Suh, H.W., Song, D.K., Son, K.H., Wie, M.B., Lee, K.H., Jung, K.Y., Do, J.C., Kim, Y.H. 1996. Antinociceptive mechanisms of dipsacus saponin C administered intracerebroventricularly in the mouse. *General Pharmacology.,* 27: 1167–1172.

Suh, N., Honda, T., Finaly, H.J., Barchowsky, A., Williams, C., Benoit, N.E. 1998. Novel triterpenoids suppress inducible nitric oxide synthase (iNOS) and inducible cyclooxygenase (COX-2) in mouse macrophages. *Cancer Resesearch.,* 58: 717-723.

Trease, G.E., Evans, W. C. 1989. Pharmacognosy, 13th ed. Bailliere Tindal, London.

Tapondjou, L.A., Lontsi, D., Sondengam, B.L., Choi, J., Lee, K.T., Jung, H.J., Park, H.J. 2003. In vivo antinociceptive and antiinflammatory effect of the two triterpenes, ursolic acid and 23-hydroxyursolic acid, from *Cussonia bancoensis. Archives of Pharmacal Research.,* 26: 143–146.

Tjolsen, A., Berge, O.G., Hunskaar, S., Rosland, J.H., Hole, K. 1992. The formalin test: An evaluation of the method. *Pain.,* 51:5-17.

Turner, R.A. 1995. Screening methods in Pharmacology. Vol 1. Academic Press. New York. Pp. 85- 106.

Vane, T., Booting, R. 1987. Inflammation and mechanism of action of anti- inflammatory drugs. *FASSEB J.,* 1:89-96.

Vaz, Z.R., Cechinel, V., Yunes, R.A., Calixto, J.B. 1996. Antinociceptive action of 2-(4-bromobenzoyl)-3-methyl-4-6-dimethoxy bezofuran, a novel xanthoxyline derivative of chemical and thermal models of nociception in mice. *Journal of Pharmacy and Experimental Therapeutics.,* 278: 304 - 312.

Winter, C.A., Risley, E.A., Nuss, G.W. 1962. Carrageenin-induced oedema in hind paw of the rats as an assay of anti-inflammatory drugs. *Proceeding of Society for Experimental Biology Medicine.,* 111:544 -547.

Evaluation of antibacterial activity of methanolic extracts of *Francoeuria Undulata* in two harvest times on several aerobic bacteria causing vaginal infections

Leila Firoozian[1], Leila Amjad[*2], Monir Doudi[3]

[1]*Falavarjan Branch, Islamic Azad University, Isfahan, Iran;*
***Email: Amjad.leila@gmail.com**

[2]*Department of Biology, Falavarjan Branch, Islamic Azad University, Isfahan, Iran;*

[3]*Department of Microbiology, Falavarjan Branch, Islamic Azad University, Isfahan, Iran;*

ARTICLE INFO

Topic: *Medicinal Plants*

Key words:
- ✓ *Francoeuria Undulata*
- ✓ *Antibacterial activity*
- ✓ *Methanol extract*

ABSTRACT

Background & Aim: Vaginal disease has always been a great concern of women. Medicinal plants as natural resources with fewer side effects can effectively treat these infections given the diversity of these infections, resistance to antibiotics and side effects of existing drugs. The present study aimed to compare antimicrobial effects of methanol extract of *Francoeuria Undulata* on growth of several gram-positive and gram-negative bacteria causing vaginal infections.

Experimental: *Francoeuria Undulata* as an indigenous Iranian plant was collected in two harvest times (T_1 and T_2). Methanol extract of aerial parts of the plant was prepared. The effects of various concentrations (62.5, 125, 250 and 500 mg/ml)of methanol extracts were studied onKlebsiella and Enterobacter as gram-negative pathogens. Minimum Inhibitory Concentration (MIC) of bacterial growth and Minimum Bactericidal Concentration (MBC) were determined using macro-dilution method. Data analysis was performed using ANOVA.

Results: The results showed that methanol extracts of aerial parts of *Francoeuria Undulata* inhibit bacterial growth of *Klebsiella pneumoniae* and *Enterobacter aerogenes*. MICs varied from 125mg/ml to 250 mg/ml in the old and new harvest times. Therefore, the smallest diameter of inhibition zone belonged to *Klebsiella pneumoniae* at 62.5mg/ml concentration in the old harvest time and the largestdiameter of inhibitory zone belonged tothe second strains of *Klebsiellapneumoniae* at 500mg/ml concentration in the new harvest time.

Recommended applications/industries: The findings of the study indicated that methanol extracts of *Francoeuria Undulata* at two old and new harvest times had strong antibacterial and inhibitory effects on gram-negative bacteria causing vaginal infections.

1. Introduction

Medicinal plants are divine blessings with an important role in maintaining health and treating various diseases. These herbs are known as valuable resources for treating a variety of diseases for many years (Shanazis, 2007).

Nowadays, bacterial resistance and increased number of different antibiotic-resistant bacterial strains are great concerns of medical science. It is essential to find a suitable herbal alternative to combat pathogens. Valuable biodiversity and natural production of medicinal plants in Iran can lead to production of significant amounts of medicinal plants with proper planning (Rezaei *et al.,* 2008).

Francoeuria Undulata with local name of crisp-leaved fleabane has different species in various regions of Iran. Anticancer and antiviral properties of this plant have been reported in different studies (Algabr, 2012; Amin, 2002).

Barry *et al.* (1970) and Gerging *et al.* (1991) studied antibacterial activity of ethanol extract of this plant on several standard bacterial strains. They showed strong antibacterial activity of this extract on *Escherichia coli* (ATCC 25923), *Staphylococcus aureus* (ATCC25923), *Proteus vulgaris* (ATCC6380) and *Klebsiella pneumoniae* (ATCC 1312) (Ravandeh *et al.,* 2011; Barry *et al.,* 1970).

Female genital infections include a complex of gram-positive cocci (Streptococcus and Staphylococcus) and gram-positive bacilli as normal flora and gram-negative bacilli (Enterobacteriaceae) and gram-variable coccobacilli (*Gardnerellavaginalis*). Genital infections are the most common diseases among womenassociated with high social, emotional and physical consequences (Gerging *et al.,* 1991). Given increased drug resistance to antibacterial and antifungal drugs, it is essential to find herbal compounds with strong antimicrobial properties to treat vaginal infection with fewer side effects and lower costs (Steven, 2010).

Therefore, the study aimed to assess the effects of methanol extracts of aerial parts of *F.undulata* attwo harvest times on several gram-positive and gram-negative aerobic bacteria causing vaginal infections.

2. Materials and Methods

2.1. Extraction of methanolic extract of Francoeuria Undulata

In this study, *Francoeuria Undulata* was collected at two periods from Ardestantown in northeastern Isfahan: a) September 2014 andb) September 2015.

Aerial parts of the plant were dried out at room temperature in the shade. Dried-out samples were powdered using a grinder and kept at 4°C (Nabipour, 2015). Then, powder was soaked in 80% methanol for 72 hours to prepare the extract. For this purpose, 50 grams of the powder was mixed with 500 ml of 80% methanol. The mixture was shaken to mix the powder with the solvent. Then, the flasks containing the mixture were covered with aluminum taps. The flasks were shaken at 150rpm for 72 hours at room temperature. These extracts were filtered with a filter paper and transferred to sterilized plates at ambient temperature until they were dried out. Then, the extracts were condensed with 10%dimethyl sulfoxide (DMSO) solvent. Then, the extracts were prepared at 62.5, 125, 250 and 500 mg/ml concentrations (Cowan, 1999; Skocibusic*et al.,* 2004).

The bacteria were isolated from 100 inpatients and outpatients aged from 20 to 50 who visited the Shahid Beheshti Gynecologic Clinic in Isfahan.

2.2. Antibacterial assay

Blood Agar and EMB (Daruash-Tehran) media were used for primary culture of the isolates. Biochemical and confirmatory tests were used to detect the bacteria (Sokmen *et al.,* 2003; Mardane, 2012).

Bacterial genus and species were detected and confirmed using the above tests (Naghsh, 2013). Antibiogram patterns were determined using antibiotic discs (5μg trimethoprim, 30μg ceftazidime, 30μg cefotaxime, 5μg ciprofloxacin, 10μg gentamicin, 30μg cefalotin, 5μgcefixime, 30μg tetracycline, 10μg streptomycin, 10μg penicillin). Ciprofloxacin was identified as a positive control given antibiotic sensitivity and resistance of each bacterium to various antibiotics and common sensitivity tociprofloxacin.

Isolated bacteria were glycerolizedin a freezer at 20°C. All isolates were revived by standard methods. Fresh cultures of multi-colony bacteria were transferred to Mueller-Hinton broth to prepare bacterial suspension. Turbidity of bacterial suspension was set in accordance with McFarland Standard as1.5×10^{6}cfu/ml. Antimicrobial effects of methanol extracts of aerial parts of *F. undulata*at two harvest times on several gram-positive and gram-negative aerobic bacteria causing vaginal infections were studied using two methods of serial dilutions and well-plate. Various concentrations of the extract were prepared for both old and new harvest times.

In well-plate method, 100 ml of microbial suspension with concentration of 1.5×10^6cfu/ml was evenly spread in Mueller-Hinton agar medium. Then, three wells with 6mm diameter at 2.5cm distance were created in each medium. Then, 100ml of each concentration was transferred to each well. The wells were sealed (bottom of the wells were closed). Negative control was determined as 10% DMSO and 10% Tween80. Positive control was determined as 5µg ciprofloxacin. All media were incubated for 24h at 37°C. Then, bacterial cultures were evaluated in terms of presence or absence of inhibition zone around the wells (Rajabpour *et al.*, 2013). Minimum Inhibitory Concentration (MIC) and Minimum Bactericidal Concentration (MBC) of methanol extracts were determined using tube dilution method (macro-dilution) (Talebi, 2014).

To determine the MICs, 62.5, 125, 250 and 500 mg/ml dilutionsof methanol extracts were prepared. In addition, one ml bacterial suspension with a concentration of 1.5×10^6cfu/ml was added to every dilution. Tubes of positive control (with bacterial medium) negative control (without bacterial medium) were prepared. The tubes were incubated for 24 h at 37°C. After incubation, the tubes were studied in terms of turbidity and growth of inoculated bacteria.

2.3. Statistical analysis

Each test was repeated 3 times. Then, mean and standard deviation were calculated. Data analysis was performed using SPSS20, ANOVA and LSD. The difference between groups was determined at $P<0.001$ significance level.

3. Results and discussion

The results of various concentrations of methanol extracts of the plant in both old and new harvest times using well-plate method are shown in Table 1.

The discs impregnated with 10% DMSO and 10%Tween80were determined as negative controls and 5µg ciprofloxacin disc was determined as positive control. The results showed that methanol extract of either old or new harvest inhibited growth of a large number of *Klebsiella pneumoniae* and *Enterobacter aerogenes*. The inhibitory effect was increased with increasing concentration of methanol extract of the bacteria. Increased inhibition was manifested as increased diameter of inhibitory zone.

The results showed that diameter of the inhibition zone was increased byincreasing concentration of the methanol extract.Increase in both isolates of *Klebsiella pneumoniae* and *Enterobacter aerogenes* represent the presence of Enterobacteriaceae Family. Thisincrease was also observedin both old and new harvest. However, diameter of the inhibitory zone in new extract was smaller than the old extract.

The findings suggested thatthe smallest diameter of inhibition zone belonged to several isolates of *Klebsiella pneumoniae* with 62.5mg/ml concentration of the old extract. There was no significant difference between the old extract and the negative control in terms of inhibition zone. The largest diameter of inhibition zone belonged to several isolates of *K. pneumoniae* with 500mg/ml concentration of the new harvest. There was a significant difference between the new extract and the negative control in terms of inhibition zone. The difference may be attributed tosub-strains, which can be evaluated using molecular identification.

Contents of Table 2 show MICs and MBCs ofthe methanol extracts regarding two types of bacteria. The results showed that125mg/ml concentration of methanol extract of the plant has lethal effects on both bacteria in the new harvest. In addition, 250mg/ml concentration of methanol extract of the plant has lethal effect onboth bacteria in the old harvest.

The results showed significant difference between antibacterial properties of methanol extracts of the plant ($P<0.001$). In other words, antimicrobial effect of the plant decreased in the old harvest compared to the new harvest.

The findings of the study showed that methanol extract of aerial parts of *F. undulata*in the new harvest in 125mg/ml concentration inhibited growth of several aerobic gram-negative bacteria causing vaginal infection. However, methanol extract of aerial parts of the plant in the old harvest at 250mg/ml concentration inhibited growth of aerobic gram-negative bacterial pathogens.

Ethanol extract of the *F.undulata*has the greatest antibacterial effect on gram-negative bacteria (Ravandeh *et al.*, 2011; Barry *et al.*, 1970).

Table 1. Mean ± SD of diameter of inhibition zone of two different genera of aerobic bacteria causing vaginal infections compared to methanol extracts of the plant.

Bacteria		Concentration of the extract (mg/ml)								Control		
		62.5		125		250		500		Positive		Negative
		A	B	A	B	A	B	A	B	A	B	A, B
K.	K1	6	4±0.2	12	10	19.8±0.2	17.7±0.2	26.4±0.3	24±0.3	26	24	6
pneumoniae	K2	9.8±0.2	8	18.3±0.4	15.7	22±0.2	24.2±0.2	30	28±0.2	22	23	6
E. aerogenes	En1	12	10	17.8±0.2	15.5±0.2	21.8±0.2	20	26	26	23	22	6
	En2	12	10±2	18±0.2	14±0.5	22	20±0.2	24.4±0.4	24±0.2	23	22	6

The old and new harvest at 62.5, 125, 250 and 500 mg/ml concentrations
Positive control: Ciprofloxacin
Negative control: 10% DMSOand 10% Tween80.
Diameter of the wells is 6mm diameter.
K1, K2: the first and second strain of *K. pneumoniae*
En1, En2: the first and second strains of *E. aerogenes*
A: new harvest time
B: old harvest time

Table 2. MICs and MBCs of methanol extracts of the plant in the new and old harvest times regarding studied bacteria based on mg/ml

Bacterial species	MIC (mg/ml)		MBC (mg/ml)	
	A	B	A	B
K. pneumoniae (K1, K2)	125	250	62.5	125
E. aerogenes (E1, E2)	125	250	62.5	125

- A: the new harvest
- B: the old harvest

Barry *et al.* (1970) showedstrong antibacterial effect of ethanol extract of aerial parts of Francoeuria on *E. coli*, *Pseudomonas*, *Staphylococcus aureus* and *Proteus* (Ravandeh *et al.*, 2011).

Gerging *et al.* (1991) studied antibacterial effect of *Francoeuria Undulata* and *Francoeuri acripsa* on *Staphylococcus aureus*, *Bacillus subtilis* and *Klebsiella pneumoniae*. They showed that MIC was larger in *Francoeuria Undulate* compared to *Francoeuriacripsa* (Barry *et al.*, 1970).

Mohammadi *et al.* (2010) studied the effect of methanol extracts of *Wilhelm aquila*. They studied gram-positive and gram-negative bacteria due to a specific structure between walls of these two types of bacteria (Khanafari and Hosseini, 2000).

Amjad *et al.* (2010)showed thatmethanol extract of leaves and flowers of *Achillea wilhelmsii* has significant effects on gram-positive bacteria including Staphylococcus. This effect was weaker on gram-negative bacteria. This may be due to presence of lipopolysaccharide cellular wallsof the gram-negative bacteria (Amjad *et al.*, 2010).

Methanolic extract of aerial parts of *F. undulate* inhibits growth of gram-negative bacteria due to specific structure of cellular walls of these of bacteria. These bacteria have an outer membrane, which acts as a solid wall and prevents passage of large and hydrophobic molecules. Since majority of compounds in the extracts are hydrophobic, it can be concluded that methanol extract of the plant inhibits access to gram-negative bacteria as gram-positive bacteria. The extract significantly inhibits growth of gram-negative bacteria, especially the bacteria causing aerobic vaginal and urinary tract infections. The extract can be considered as a natural herbal product (Juven *et al.*, 2009; Mckeegan *et al.*, 2002).

4. Conclusion

The results of the present study indicated that the plants assayed possess antibacterial properties. This explains the use of plants in folk medicine for the treatment of various diseases whose symptoms might involve bacterial infections and underline the importance of the ethnobotanical approach for the selection of plant in the discovery of new bioactive compounds. Further phytochemical research is needed to identifythe active principles responsible for the antibacterial effects of this medicinal plant.

5. References

Algabr, M.N. 2012. Essential oil composition of *Pulicaria jaubertii* from Yemen. *International Journal of Medicinal and Aromatic Plants,* 2(4): 688-690.

Amin, G. 2002. Screening of Iranian plants for antifungal activity. *Daru,* 9(1): 38-48.

Amjad, L., Mohammadi Kamalabadi, M. and Mohammadi Sichani, M. 2010. Antibacterial activity of methanol extracts of flowers and leaves of *Achillea wilhelmsii. Journal of Qom University of Medical Sciences,* 5(3): 50-56.

Barry, A., Garcia, J. and Thrupp, LD. 1970. Interpretation of sensitivity test results. *American Journal of Clinical Pathology,* 53:140-144.

Cowan, M. 1999. Plant products as antimicrobial agent. *Clinic Microbiology Reviews*, 12(14): 564–582.

Gerging, D.N., Larson, T.A. and Hughes, R.A. 1991. Antimicrobial agents. *Chemotherapy,* 35: 1284-1286.

Juven, B.J., kanner, J., Schved, F. and Weisslowicz, H. 2009. Factors that interact with the antibacterial action of Thyme essential oil and its active constituents. *Iranian Journal of Dentist*, 21(3):215-220.

Khanafari, A. and Hosseini, F. 2000. *Scientific microbiology,* Poursina Publication, Vol. I, Second Edition: 140-144.

Mardane, G. 2012. Medical microbiology: detection and clinical follow-up of diseases. *Artistic – Davidson,* 2011: 102-162.

McKeegan, K.S., Borges-Walmsley, M.I. and Walmsley, A.R. 2002. Microbial and viral drug resistance mechanisms. *Trend Microbiology,* 10(110): 8-14.

Mohammadi Sichani, M., Amjad, L. and Mohammadi Kamalabadi, M. 2010. Effects of methanol extract and essential oil of flowers of *Achillea wilhelmsii* on pathogenic bacteria. *Journal of Medical Science,* 13(3): 9-13.

Naghsh, A. 2013. Evaluation of antibacterial activity of essential oils and extracts of flowers of *Artemisia deserti* on several pathogenic bacteria, *Master Thesis, Islamic Azad University, School of Biological Sciences, Flavarjan, pp. 132.*

Rajabpour, M., Arabestani, M., Yousefi Mashouf, R. and Alikhani, M. E. 2013. Determination of MIC at three different antibiotic classes of clinical isolates of *Pseudomonas aeruginosa* from hospitalized patients in Hamedan hospital (2011-2012). *Journal of Medical Microbiology*, 7(3): 18-25.

Ravandeh, M., Valizadeh, J., Noroozifar, M. and Khorasani-Motlagh, M. 2011. Screening of chemical composition of essential oil, mineral elements and antioxidant activity in *Pulicaria undulata* L. Mey from Iran. *Journal of Medicinal Plants Research*, 5(10): 2035-2040.

Rezaei, M. B., Kamkar, G. and Mozaffarian, V. 2008. Studying chemical composition of extract of *Anthemis coelopoda* Boiss. *Research Scientific Journal of Iran Medicinal and Aromatic Plants*, 24: 274-277.

Shahnazi, S. 2007. Evaluation of chemical and antimicrobial properties of the extracts of *Saturejaintermedia* CA. Mey.*Journal of Medicinal Plants*, 1: 85-92.

Skocibusic, M., Bazic, N., Dunnkic, V. and Radonic, A. 2004. Antibacterial activity of *Achillea clavenne* essential oil against respiratory tract patogens. *Fitoteropia*. 75(7-8): 733-736.

Sokmen, A., Vardar-Unlu, G. and Polissiou, M. 2003. Antimicrobial activity of the essential oil and ethanol extract of *Achillea sintenisii* Hub.Mor.(Asteraceae). *Phytotherapy Research*, 17(9): 1005-1010.

Steven Pray, W. 2010. Treating vaginal fungal infection. *Pharmacology*, 35(9): 14-23.

Talebi, F. 2014. Evaluating antibacterial activity of essential oils and extracts of flowers of *Achillea tenuifolia* on several pathogenic bacteria. *Master Thesis, Islamic Azad University, School of Biological Sciences, Flavarjan, pp. 183.*

Effects of some channelling agents on the compaction properties of the mixed stem bark extracts of *Anogeissus leiocarpus* and *Prosopis africana*

Emeje Martins*, **Isimi Christianah, Izuka Amaka, Olayemi Olubunmi**

National Institute for Pharmaceutical Research & Development (NIPRD), Abuja, Nigeria;

Email:** ***martinsemeje@yahoo.com

ARTICLE INFO

Topic: *Medicinal Plants*

Key words:

- ✓ *Micromeritic properties*
- ✓ *Compaction properties*
- ✓ *Tablets*
- ✓ *Anogeissus leiocarpus*
- ✓ *Prosopis africana*

ABSTRACT

Background & Aim: The hot water extract of a mixture of *Anogeissus leiocarpus* and *Prosopis africana* is widely used in the northern part of Nigeria for the treatment and management of asthma. Since investigations of its pharmacological activities already justify its use, and the need for standardization of herbal medicine and develop appropriate dosage forms has continued to grow, the purpose of this study was to evaluate the effects of some common channelling agents (sodium bicarbonate, calcium carbonate and sodium lauryl sulphate) on the compaction properties of the mixed stem bark extracts of *Anogeissus leiocarpus* and *Prosopis africana*.

Experimental: Granules of the mixed extracts (AA1) were produced using the wet granulation method of massing and screening. The micromeritics and flow properties of the extracts as well as the effects of the three common additives were studied, while the compaction properties of the extract formulated alone and in the presence of these additives were interrogated using the Heckel equation.

Results: Our results showed that, all the formulations containing the channelling agents exhibited poor flow. Granules prepared using sodium bicarbonate (NaHCO3) exhibited plastic deformation during consolidation, those formulated using calcium carbonate (CaCO3) showed initial fragmentation before consolidation by plastic deformation and those formulated using sodium lauryl sulphate consolidated essentially by plastic deformation. Inclusion of additives modified the compressibility profiles of the formulations. Tensile strength of the formulations containing NaHCO3 and sodium lauryl sulphate (SLS) were observed to be concentration dependent while those containing CaCO3 showed no appreciable increase in tensile strength with increased pressure. Generally, formulations containing 5% of the additives gave the highest tensile strength, however, those containing CaCO3 were found to be higher than the other two formulations.

Recommended applications/industries: Considering that, none of the channelling agents altered significantly the compaction properties of AA1, they might be useful in developing standardized and robust tablets of *A. leiocarpus* and *P. africana* admixtures for Asthma therapy.

1. Introduction

The World Health Organisation (WHO) reports that 80 % of the world populace use and are dependent on traditional medicine. Traditional medicine is the treatment of ailments with the use of plant (herbal) extracts. Although, herbal medicines are gaining grounds in developing countries because of poor or lack of adequate health facilities, the major problem with the use of herbal extracts is its formulation into suitable dosage forms and also lack of standardization. Oral solid dosage forms are the most acceptable form of dosage form and its wide acceptability has been attributed to its stability, ease of handling and convenience of dosing (Jivrajet *et al*, 2000).

Anogeissus leiocarpus (Family; *Combretaceae*) known as the "chewing stick" tree, is found widely in Sudan, Ethiopia, The Democratic Republic of Congo, Benin, Senegal, Niger and Nigeria (USDA, 2010). Different parts of this plant have been implicated in treatment of various ailments. It has been reported to possess antimicrobial and anthelmintic properties; in combination with other plants has been used to treat diarrhoea and dysentery (Kubmarawa *et al*, 2007). In Ivory Coast, the plant has been used to treat malaria (Okpeton, 2004); and has also been implicated in the treatment of fungal infections such as dermatitis (Batawila, 2005). In Northern Nigeria, it is widely used in the management of respiratory disease such as asthma (Isimi *et al*, 2003) and also in the treatment of cough and tuberculosis (Victor, 2013).

Proposis africana (Family; Fabaceae) also called "iron wood" is widely distributed in Africa. In Nigeria, it is called "*Ayan*" by the Yoruba, "*Okpeghe*" in Idoma, "*Kiriya*" in Hausa and "*Okpei*" in Igbo (Oguntoyinbo *et al.,* 2007). It has been documented to treat dysentery, malaria, toothache, stomach-ache and gonorrhoea. *Prosopis* also has similar actions with *Anogeissus leiocarpus* in treatment of sore throat and bronchitis. Pharmacological investigations (Isimi *et al*, 2003) revealed that the combination of the hot water extract of the stem bark of *Anogeissusleiocarpus* and *Prosopisafricana* (AA1) is effective in the treatment of asthma.

Formulation of phytomedicines into suitable dosage form enhances their stability and acceptability. It is expedient therefore to establish the suitability of various excipients used in these formulations as they can affect the overall efficiency of the phytomedicines. They could act by delivering or modifying drug release at a required site, eliciting disintegration, useful as a means of identification, for aesthetic purposes and to improve overall product stability (Rutesh, 2008). They are essential components of drug products hence, evaluating the effect and performance of these excipients in any product is necessary.

Heckel equation given below is used by researchers to relate the relative density, D, of powder bed during compression to the applied pressure, P. It determines the compaction characteristics and characterizes consolidation behaviour of materials in a tablet formulation.

$$\ln(1-1)/_{D} = KP + A \;\ldots\ldots\ldots\ldots\ldots\ldots \quad (1)$$

The slope of the straight line portion of the curve, K, is the reciprocal of the mean yield pressure, Py of the material. The relative density, D_A, can be calculated from the intercept A, using the equation;

$$DA=1-e^{-A}\ldots\ldots\ldots\ldots\ldots \quad (2)$$

Do is the relative density of a powder at the point when the applied pressure is zero. This connotes the initial phase of powder densification due to particle rearrangement as a consequence of die filling; a high Do value is indicative high densification. DB, is the value indicative of the extent of densification when deformation starts and the phase rearrangement of the particles. It differs from D_A and Do at low pressures.

$$DB = DA - Do \;\ldots\ldots\ldots\ldots\ldots\ldots \quad (3)$$

Materials can be classified into A, B and C based on Heckel plot and compaction behaviour of the material. Type A are characterized with plots that remain linear as applied pressure increases; indicative of plastic deformation. Type B show an initial curved plot followed by a straight line; this implies initial fragmentation of particles followed by plastic deformation. Materials that are type C on the other hand exhibits an initial sharp linear curve which becomes superimposed and flattened as the pressure is increased (York, 1992).

In this study, the compaction properties of extracts of the hot water extract *Anogeissus leiocarpus* and *Prosopisafricana* was evaluated; the types of additive and their effect on this formulation was also evaluated.

2. Materials and Methods

2.1 Plant collection

Anogeissus leiocarpus and *Prosopis africana* stem barks were collected from the National Institute for Pharmaceutical Research (NIPRD) garden.

2.2 Extraction

Stem bark of *Anogeissus leiocarpus* and *Prosopis africana* was collected, washed with distilled water, sun-dried and milled to a coarse (1000 µm) powder. The powders were then mixed in a 1:1 ratio and soaked in distilled water in a ratio 1:10 mass to volume, boiled on an electric heater for 10 minutes and left to soak for 24 hours at room temperature. The liquid extract was filtered through a calico cloth and concentrated to a ratio of 5:1 using a rotary evaporator. The concentrated filtrate was then transferred into a tray and dried in an oven at 60 °C until dry. The dry extract was pulverized using a mortar and pestle and then passed through a 150 µm sieve.

2.3 Granulation

Granules of the extract and channelling agents were prepared by the method of wetting and massing. Sodium bicarbonate, calcium carbonate and sodium lauryl sulphate were employed at concentrations of 5, 10 and 15 % in each formulation while water was used as the granulating fluid. The wet mass was passed through the sieve (1.7 mm), dried in the oven and then kept for further analysis.

2.3.1 Granule properties

2.3.1.1 Particle size evaluation

The particle size of the granules was determined by sieving the granules in the Reitsch test shaker with sieves arranged in decreasing order of aperture. The granules (50 g) were placed on the largest screen, the sieves were shaken for 5mins at amplitude of 1.500 mm/g. Granule weight retained on the sieves and the pan was recorded. The percentage cumulative weight undersize was plotted against sieve aperture.

2.3.1.2 Angle of repose

Forty (40) g of the granules was allowed to flow through a funnel. The height and the radius of the heap were determined and the angle of repose (θ) was computed using the equation below:

$$\theta = \tan^{-1} h/r \ldots \qquad \ldots\ldots 3$$

2.3.1.3 Bulk and tapped density

The bulk and tapped density was conducted using the Stampfvolumeter. The granules (30 g) were poured into the 100 mL graduated cylinder using a glass funnel. The volume occupied by the powder was read off and the bulk density was calculated in gm/ml. The cylinder, which contains the granules, was tapped 100 times and the tapped density was calculated.

2.3.1.4 Carr's index

This was mathematically calculated using the equation below:

$$C\,(\%) = {}^{tapped\ density - bulk\ density}/_{tapped\ density}\ X\,100 \ldots\ldots\ldots 4$$

2.3.1.5 Hausner index

It was calculated using the equation below:

$$H = {}^{tapped\ density}/_{bulk\ density} \ldots\ldots\ldots 5$$

2.4 Compaction properties

Compacts equivalent to 500 mg AA1 were produced by compressing the granules for 60 sec at various compression pressures using a Manesty tableting machine (Shangai, China). Fifty (50) tablets were compressed at each pressure. All readings are average of 3 measurements.

Before each compression, the die (12.5 mm) and flat faced punches were lubricated with 1 % w/v dispersion of magnesium stearate in chloroform. After ejection, the tablets were stored over silica gel in a desiccator for 24 h to allow for elastic recovery and hardening to prevent falsely low yield values and the dimensions of the compact were determined using the micrometer screw gauge (Mitutoyo model IDC1012EB (Mitutuyo corporation, Japan) thickness gauge to the nearest 0.01 mm. The Heckel plots were statistically analysed using the Microsoft Excel computer software. The plots constructed according to the Heckel equation were used to characterize the consolidation behaviour of the formulations.

The tensile strength (*TS*) the tablets were calculated as:

$$TS = {}^{2CS}/_{Dd} \ldots\ldots\ldots 6$$

3. Results and discussion

Figure 1 show more than 50 % of AA1 granules were about 150 µm in size. This implies that the particles of the granules have more cohesive force than gravitational force and are more bounded together.

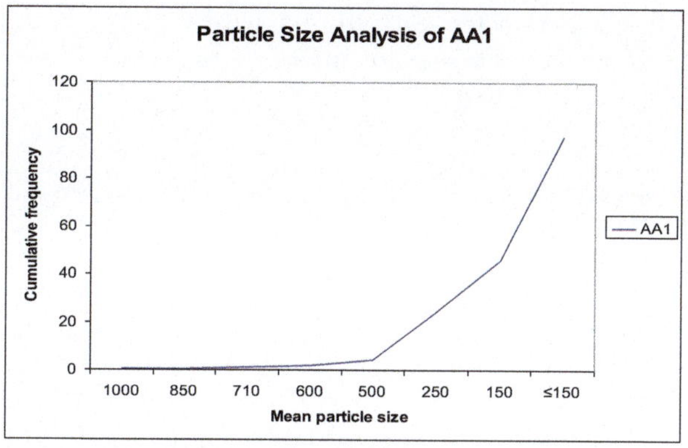

Fig. 1. Particle size analysis of AA1

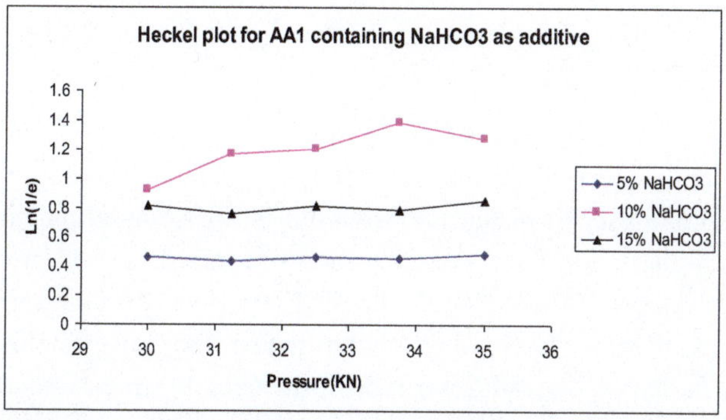

Fig. 2. Heckel plot for AA1 containing $NaHCO_3$ as additive

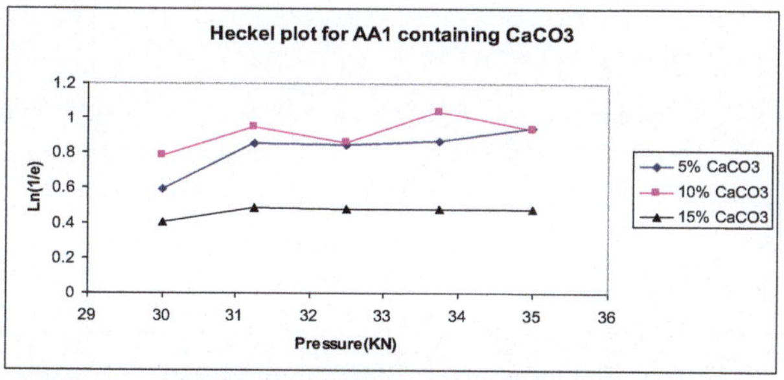

Fig. 3. Heckel plot for AA1 containing $CaCO_3$ as diluent

The flow properties of formulated granules are presented in Table 1. Concentration was observed to have no significant effect on the tapped and bulk density. All the granules were found to have CI > 15 % indicating they are not easily compressible and HI > 1.2 implying the powders are very cohesive. The granules also were found to have poor flow as indicated by angle of repose > 25 %. This is understandable as cohesive materials usually have poor flow.

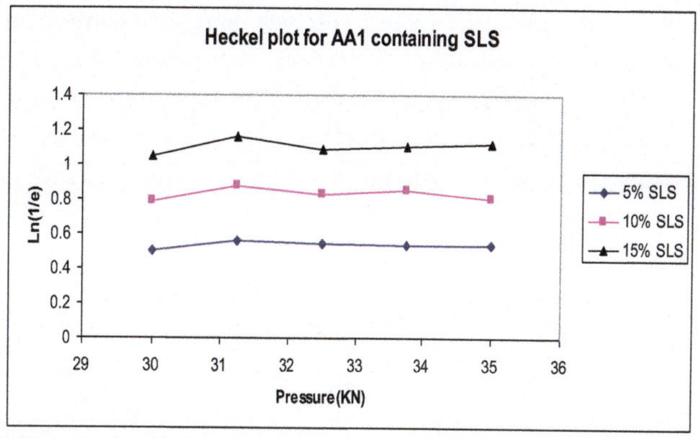

Fig. 4. Heckel plot for AA1 containing SLS as a disintegrant

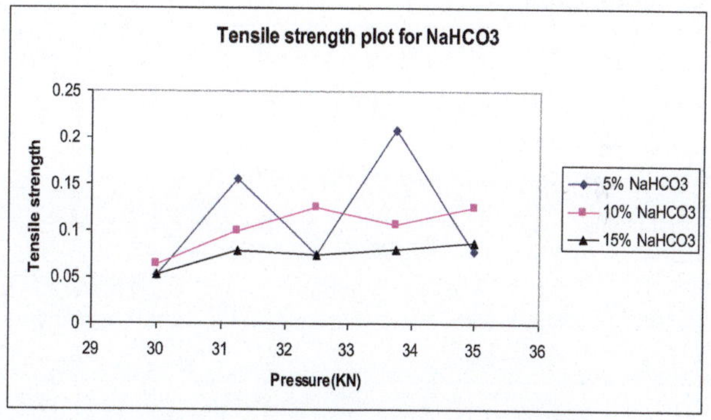

Fig. 5. Compaction plots of AA1 with $NaHCO_3$

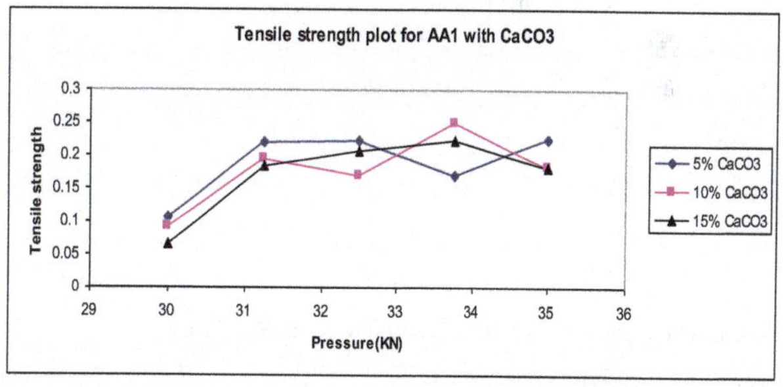

Fig. 6. Compaction plots of AA1 with $CaCO_3$

The Heckel plots presented in Figures 2, 3, 4 show linearity with concentrations employed and at all the pressures, there was no initial curve in the plot thus no initial fragmentation occurred and as such the granules can be said to have deformed plastically.

The Do represents the degree of initial packing in the die as a result of die filling and is said to be related to particle size and of shape of the investigated materials. The type and concentration of additives did not confer any significant effect on the degree of packing as no trend was observed (Table 2). No pattern was observed between particle rearrangement and concentration although DB values for all formulations were generally low; formulations containing SLS had the highest. This suggests that the extent of particle rearrangement in these formulations was low.

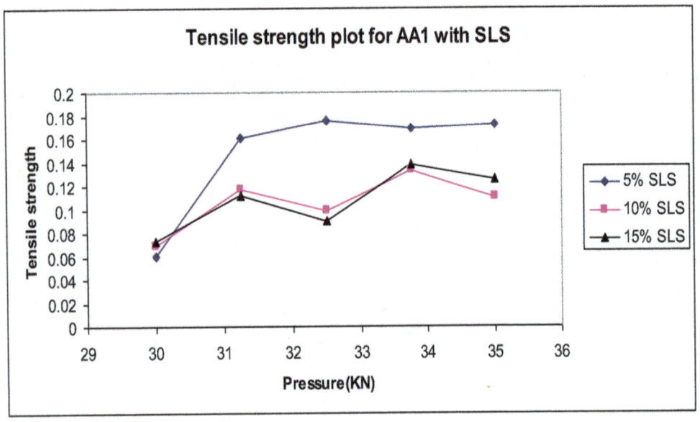

Fig. 7. Compaction plots of AA1 with SLS

Table 1: Powder properties of various batches of AA1

Batch	Bulk density	Tapped density	True density	Angle of repose	Carr's index	Hausner ratio
5 % $NaHCO_3$	0.603 ± 0.003	0.873 ± 0.030	2.637 ±0.240	32.15 ± 2.13	30.47 %	1.438
10 % $NaHCO_3$	0.620 ± 0.010	0.980 ± 0.084	1.440 ±0.050	27.97 ± 0.59	36.73 %	1.581
15 % $NaHCO_3$	0.653 ± 0.007	0.930 ± 0.015	1.762 ± 0.036	30.94 ±1.35	29.78 %	1.424
5 % $CaCO_3$	0.567 ± 0.003	0.920 ± 0.060	1.762 ± 0.083	30.91 ± 2.20	38.37 %	1.623
10 % $CaCO_3$	0.603 ± 0.020	0.987 ± 0.078	1.760 ± 0.090	34.45 ± 2.28	38.91 %	1.637
15 % $CaCO_3$	0.600 ± 0.003	1.010 ± 0.066	2.949 ± 0.071	33.01 ± 1.64	40.30 %	1.675
5 % SLS	0.583 ± 0.008	1.200 ± 0.023	2.615 ± 0.265	28.15 ± 1.60	51.42 %	2.058
10 % SLS	0.567 ± 0.003	0.903 ± 0.013	1.879 ± 0.081	32.40 ± 0.93	37.21 %	1.593
15 % SLS	0.590 ± 0.015	0.950 ± 0.010	1.600 ± 0.060	38.55 ± 0.74	37.89 %	1.610
AA1 only	0.563 ± 0.015	0.800 ± 0.018	1.620 ± 0.040	22.30 ± 0.32	29.63 %	1.421

Da values for all formulations were also found to be low with formulations containing SLS having higher values. There was no significant relationship between the degree of packing and additive concentration although, additive type seemed to influence packing arrangement.

Table 2. Parameters derived from Heckel plots

Batch	Compression parameter	Mean yield pressure	Da	Do	Db
5 % $NaHCO_3$	0.0766	256.41	0.28	0.229	0.051
10 % $NaHCO_3$	0.7751	13.59	-2.31	0.431	-2.741
15 % $NaHCO_3$	0.1141	121.95	0.42	0.371	0.049
5 % $CaCO_3$	0.8826	17.48	-1.82	0.322	-2.142
10 % $CaCO_3$	0.4271	32.15	-0.97	0.342	-1.312
15 % $CaCO_3$	0.2555	847.46	0.08	0.203	-0.123
5 % SLS	0.0942	17.35	0.32	0.223	0.097
10 % SLS	0.0063	-10000	0.57	0.302	0.268
15 % SLS	0.0838	138.87	0.58	0.369	0.211

The mean yield pressure is inversely related to the ability of a material to deform plastically under pressure. The onset of plastic deformation in all formulations at higher additive concentration occurred at higher pressure (Table 2). Values of Py for formulations containing SLS were found to be the lowest, this indicates that additive type influences the pressure at which onset of plastic deformation occurs. Similar findings have been reported in an earlier study where the presence of channelling agents were seen to increase the pressure at which plastic deformation took place (Emeje *et al.*, 2006).

The tensile strength of all compacts was observed to be higher at 5 % (Figure 5, 6, 7) and independent on concentration.

4. Conclusion

Presence of sodium bicarbonate, calcium carbonate and sodium lauryl sulphate did not have any significant effect on the compaction properties of AA1 but tensile strength was influenced by concentration. Therefore, any of these additives may be used to formulate standardized tablets of AA1.

5. References

Batawila, K. 2005. Antifungal activities of five *Combretaceae* used in Togolese traditional medicine. *Fitoterapia*. 76(2): 264-8.

Emeje, M.O., Kunle, O.O. and Ofoefule, S.I. 2006. Compaction characteristics of ethylcellulose in the presence of channelling agents: A technical note AAPS *PharmSciTech*. 7(3): 58.

Isimi, C.Y., Nasipur,i R.N., Ojile, J.B., Ibrahim, Y.K.E. and Emeje, M. 2003. Effects of the diluent type on compressional characteristics of the mixed stem bark extract of *Anogeissus leiocarpus* and *Prosopis africana* tablet formulation. *Acta Pharmaceutica.* 53: 49–56.

Jivraj, I.I, Martini, L.G. and Thomson, C.M. 2000. An overview of the different excipients useful for the direct compression of tablets. *Pharmaceutical Science Technology*. 2: 58-63.

Kubmarawa, D., Ajoku, G.A., Enwerem, N.M. and Okorie, D.A. 2007.Preliminary phytochemical and antimicrobial screening of 50 medicinal plants from Nigeria. *African Journal of Biotechnology*. 6:1690–6.

Okpekon, T. 2004. Antiparasitic activities of medicinal plants used in Ivory Coast. *Journal of Ethnopharmacology*. 90(1): 91-7.

Oguntoyinbo, F.A., Sanni, A.I., Franz, C.M., Wilhelm, H. and Holzapfel, W.H. 2007. *In vitro* fermentation studies for selection and evaluation of Bacillus strains as starter cultures for the production of okpehe, a traditional African fermented condiment. *International Journal of Food Microbiology*. 113: 208–18.

Rutesh, H.H. 2008. Overview of Pharmaceutical excipients used in tablets and capsules, Division of Pharmaceutical Sciences, Lon Island University. 1-3.

USDA, 2010. GRIN - Germplasm Resources Information Network. National Germplasm Resources Laboratory, Beltsville, Maryland

Victor, Y.A. 2013. *In-Vitro* Assessment of Antioxidant and Antimicrobial Activities of Methanol Extracts of Six Wound Healing Medicinal Plants. *Journal of Natural Sciences Research*. 3(1): 74-82.

Effect of using different levels of Dill seeds on performance, some blood biochemical and intestinal microbial population in Ross 308 broiler chicks

Yaser Rahimian[1,2]*, Farshid Kheiri[1], Mohammad Alavi[3], Mehran Aboozar[4]

[1] *Department of Animal Science, Shahrekord Branch, Islamic Azad University, Shahrekord, Iran;*
***Email: yas.rahimiyan.yr@gmail.com**

[2] *Extension Agent, Agriculture Organization of Jihad, Chaharmahal and Bakhtiari Province, Shahrekord, Iran;*

[3] *Department of Herbal Plant Science, Shahrekord Branch, Islamic Azad University, Shahrekord, Iran;*

[4] *Department of Animal Science, Abhar Branch, Islamic Azad University, Abhar, Iran;*

ARTICLE INFO

Topic: *Medicinal Plants*

Key words:

- ✓ *Broiler chicks*
- ✓ *Dill seeds*
- ✓ *Performance*
- ✓ *Blood biochemical*
- ✓ *Intestinal microbial population.*

ABSTRACT

Background & Aim: Dill "*Anethum graveolens*" is an annual medical plantin the celery family "*Apiaceae*". It is the sole species of the genus "*Anethum*".The health advantages of dill seed include its ability to increasedigestive health, as well as providingrelief from insomnia, hiccups, diarrhea, dysentery, menstrual disorders, respiratory disorders, and cancer. This experiment aimed to determine the effects of using different levels of Dill seeds on performance, some blood biochemical parameters and intestinal microbial population in Ross 308 broiler chicks.
Experimental: 300 one-day-old male broiler chickswere divided into the four treatments with six replicates and 15 birds each as randomized design. The treatments contained basal diet with no Dill seeds kept as control, and200,400 and 600 gof Dill seedsper each ton of diets respectively. The live bodyweightsgain, feed intake and feed conversion ratio of birdswere calculated weekly. At the end of the experimentfour male birdsform each replicates were slaughtered and dressing percentage were calculated. In addition, some carcass traits and chick's visceral partwere weighed separately as percentage of carcass and some organs weight.
Results: Data indicated that using Dill seeds increased feed intake (FI) in treatmentscompared to control.Alsobody weight (BW) (g/d) and Pre-slaughter weight (g) were higher in groups that werefed by dill seedscompared to the control. Additionally, therewere significant differences ($p<0.05$) for feed conversation ratio (FCR) among treatments.
Recommended applications/industries: In conclusion, increasing levels of Dill seeds improved performance and some blood biochemical parametersof broilers chicks.

1. Introduction

Recently, considerable research has been done to explore some alternative to antibiotics as growth promoters (Jamroz, 1989; Cyberhorse, 1999). Herbal plants or its products including plant extracts, essences or the components of the essential oils hold promise as alternatives to antibiotics (Burger and Wachter, 1998). Many studies have been conducted to determine the efficacy of herbal on broilers performance. Because of the importance of poultries as an economic and nutritious form of animal protein and the fast growing traitsof this animal, researchers have devoted studies to the use of some herbal in avian (Jamroz *et al.*, 2003). A series of medicinal and spicy herbs were used as additives, given as powder into the fodder, singular or mixed, either as aqueous, oily extracts or as essential oil (Rezaian, 2006).

Dill is called (*Anethum graveolens*) belongs to *Apiaceae* family and the only type of *Anethum* which is cultivated in some part of Iran. Its essence includes limonene and carron, which make more than90 percent of this essence.Based on the properties of Dill which prohibits raising up the level of cholesterol (Zheng *et al.,* 1992 and Bahramikia *et al.,* 2009), anti-cancerous (Panda, 2008), anti-diabetes (Al-Ismail *et al.*, 2004), and antioxidant (Satyanarayana *et al.*, 2008), the objective of this study was to evaluate the effect of using different levels of Dill (*Anethumgraveolens*) seeds on performance and some blood biochemical in Ross 308 broiler chicks.

2. Materials and Methods

The experiment was done at the Broiler farm of Islamic Azad University, Shahrekord, Iran.

2.1. Birds and the diets

A total of 300 one-day-old maleRoss 308 broiler chicks with an average weight of 39.50±50 g were divided intofourtreatments and also were subdivided intothe six replicates with 15 birds in each. Dill seeds werepurchased from a local market in Shahrekord, Iran and were grounded to obtain a fine and uniform powder. Additionally, soybean meal and corn grains were analyzed in the lab todetermine of dry matter, crude protein, calcium, phosphorus and its crude fiber withAssociation of Official Analytical Chemists (AOAC, 2000) method.The basal diet was balanced based on corn and soybean meal as recommended by National Research Council (NRC, 1994) as shown in (table 1). The treatments were separated as basal diet with no drill seeds kept as control and 200, 400 and 600 g per ton, respectively. During this experiment, diets and fresh water were provided *adlibitum*. The live body weight gains, feed intake andfeed conversion ratio of birds were calculated weekly.

2.2. Investigation of the carcass characteristics

At the end of experimental period, four male broiler chicks form each replicates (initially 96 chicks)were slaughtered and then dressing and some visceral organ percentage were calculated. The internal organs were removed after slaughter.

2.3. Microbial population determination

To determine the microbial count, about7 cm from the length of the ileum was sampled to investigate the microbial population. Also 1 g of ileum content was usedto make 10-fold dilution using buffered peptone water and0.1 mL of the appropriate ileum dilution was spread on Lactobacillus MRS1 Agar-Hi Media Laboratories to detectlactic acid bacteria and Violet Red Bile Agar) todetect *E. coli* and *Klebsiella* form. The plates were stored and incubated at 37.5 $^{\circ C}$ for 48 h. After counting the number ofcolonies in each plate, the number so obtained was multiplied by inverse of the dilution and the result was stated asthe number of colony forming unit (cfu) in 1 g of the sample described by (Kheiri *et al.,* 2015).

2.4. Statically analyzing

To determine the effect of dill powder on blood parameters, performance and carcass traits data were analyzed statistically by one way-ANOVA with SAS 9.1 (2001) software. Additionally Duncan's (1995) multiple range test was used to detect the differences ($P<0.05$) among different group means.

3. Results and discussion

Results of using Dill seeds effects on performance of broilers were shown in Table 1. Results revealed that the use of different levels of Dill seeds had increased feed intake (FI) significantly ($p<0.05$) Result showed that body weight BW (kg) difference was more significant when the birds were fed by Dill seeds. Additionally, feed conversion ratio (FCR) was lesser in Dill seeds group and there were significant differences compared to the control ($p<0.05$). The usage of Dill seeds had significant influences on FI, BW, FCR and carcass yield. According to Richter (2010) Dill could completely improve digestive process and the digestibility of foods.

Table 1. Composition (%) of the experimental diets for broiler chicks

Ingredients %	0-14 (days)	14-21 (days)	21-42 (days)
Corn grain	54.8	59.4	65
Soybean meal	39.6	35.5	30
Soybean Oil	1.45	1.50	1.70
Di Calcium Phosphate	1.70	1.45	1.30
Oyster shells	1.05	0.95	0.86
Methionine - D-L	0.310	0.250	0.230
Lysine -L	0.22	0.10	0.10
Edible Salt	0.3	0.3	0.25
Vitamin Premix*	0.25	0.25	0.25
Mineral Premix*	0.25	0.25	0.25
Theronine -L	0.09	0.04	0.04
Calculated nutrient content			
ME(Kcal per Kg)	2850	2900	2940
CP (%)	21.8	20.4	18.4
Ca(%)	0.91	0.82	0.74
Available Phosphorus (%)	0.46	0.41	0.37
Lysine (%)	0.180	0.120	0.130
Methionine+Cystine (%)	0.92	0.84	0.75

*Supplied per each kilogram of broiler feed: 7.500 IU of vitamin A, 2000IU vitamin D3, 30 mg vitamin E, 1.5 µg vitamin B12, 2mg B6, 5 mg Vitamin K, 5 mg vitamin B2, 1 mg vitamin B1, 40 mg nicotinic acide, 160µg vitamin Biothine, 12 mg Calcium pantothenate, 1mg Folic acid, 20 mg Fe, 71 mg Mn, 100µg Se, 37mg Zn, 6 mg Cu, 1.14 mg I, 400 µg Cu.

The beneficial effects of medical plantor active substances in poultry nutrition may include the stimulation of appetite and the improvement of endogenous digestive enzyme secretion, antibacterial, and antioxidant activities (Kheiri *et al.,* 2015). Bahadori *et al.* (2013) showed that the use different levels of dill powder had no significant effect on feed intake in earlier growth period ($p>0.05$). The feed intake ofbirds in Dill groups was higher than control and other treatments at grower and whole of the rearing period significantly ($p<0.05$). In Rafiei-Tari *et al.* (2016) study, feed intake was also influenced by dietary treatment of herbal plant as birds that received diet containing Dill seeds showed a significantly ($P<0.05$) lower feed intake over the course of their experiment.

Table 2. The effect of using Dill seeds on broilers chicks performance

Treatments	FI(g/d)	BW(g/d)	FCR	Pre-slaughter weight (g)	Carcass(%)
Control	98.2^{b}	48.0^{b*}	1.96^{b}	2360.6^{a}	70.1
200 g per ton Dill seeds	99.8^{b}	49.1^{ab}	1.94^{ab}	2355.2^{ab}	70.5
400 g per ton Dill seeds	100.2^{a}	49.4^{ab}	1.92^{ab}	2342.7^{ab}	70.8
600 g per ton Dill seeds	101.6^{a}	50.4^{a}	1.90^{ab}	2295.5^{b}	71.11
SEM	2.52	1.41	0.093	82.44	1.75

*Means in each column followed by the same letters are not significantly different($P<0.05$).

Table 3. The effect of using Dill seeds on some visceral organs percentage

Treatments	Intestine (%)	Liver (%)	Gizzard (%)	Abdominal Fat (%)
Control	5.56^{ab}	2.29	1.79^{a}	3.41^{a}
200 g per ton Dill seeds	5.05^{b}	2.40	1.64^{ab}	2.69^{b}
400 g per ton Dill seeds	5.10^{b}	2.16	1.53^{ab}	2.21^{c}
600 g per ton Dill seeds	5.07^{b}	2.04	1.55^{ab}	1.94^{d}
SEM	0.31	0.21	0.096	0.42

*Means in each column followed by the same letters are not significantly different ($P<0.05$).

Bahadori *et al.* (2013) noted that thigh weight percentage was significantly higher in experimental groups than control group ($p<0.05$), and they had lower weight of breast than control group ($p<0.05$). They also demonstrated that the use of the highlevel of Dill powder in broiler diet hadlower percent of inner fat significantly ($p<0.05$) than control group. Rafiei-Tari *et al.* (2016) demonstrated that carcass weight andcarcass components were not positively influenced by the dietary treatments with Dill seeds.

Table 4. The effect of using Dill seeds on some blood biochemical.

Treatments	Triglyceride (mg/dl)	Cholesterol (mg/dl)	HDL (mg/dl)	LDL (mg/dl)
Control	72.50[a]	134.10[a]	68.11[c]	62.10[a]
200 g per ton Dill seeds	69.00[b]	132.50[b]	70.10[b]	58.34[b]
400 g per ton Dill seeds	66.01[b]	130.20[b]	70.11[a]	55.11[b]
600 g per ton Dill seeds	62.00[c]	128.11[c]	72.02[a]	54.20[c]
SEM	1.01	1.11	0.98	1.11

*Means in each column followed by the same letters are not significantly different ($P<0.05$).

Table 5. The effect of using Dill seeds on (*Escherichia Coli and Klebsiella*) bacteria (cfu.g).

Treatments	Dilution 1	Dilution 2	Dilution 3
Control	2.45[a]	1.86[a]	1.10
200 g per ton Dill seeds	2.16[a]	1.74[ab]	0.99
400 g per ton Dill seeds	1.94[ab]	1.36[ab]	0.96
600 g per ton Dill seeds	1.75[ab]	1.29[ab]	0.88
SEM	036	0.46	0.26

*Means in each column followed by the same letters are not significantly different ($P<0.05$).

Data from table 4 showed that serum triglyceride, cholesterol and low density lipoprotein decreased and HDL increased significantly ($p<0.05$).

Scientific research on the effect of Dill seeds on serum biochemical in poultry is limited. Bahadori *et al.* (2013) suggested that there were not significant effects of Dill seeds on cholesterol and serum blood high-density lipoprotein levels in broilers. It has been argued that dill has dose-dependent cholesterol-lowering effects (Zhang *et al.*, 2007). They also showed that birds fed by Dill seeds showed significantly ($P<0.05$) lower very low-density lipoprotein and triglyceride serum compared to control group. Yazdanparast and Alavi (2008) reported that the dill extract could reduce broilers cholesterol and triglyceride properties.

In the present study, the intestinal microbial population of gram-negative (*Escherichia Coli and Klebsiella*) bacteria decreased significantly in treated groups ($P<0.05$).

Ghaedi *et al.* (2014) who observed that inclusion of black pepperin the diet lowered microbial colony in the illeal content of broiler chickens. Faghani *et al.* (2014) demonstrated that the reduction in microbial load of broiler chickens intestinal could bedue to the antibacterial effect of some herbals on intestinal microbiota. Our findings about intestinal microbiota are in agreement with Faghani *et al.* (2014) and Ghaedi *et al.* (2014).

4. Conclusion

Briefly, we could demonstrate that the using of Dill seeds as medical plantand its advantages on broilers chicks' performance.These beneficial actsmay be due to the biological functionsof this medical plantto improve performanceor may be due toits role as appetite stimulant, carminative, digestibility enhancer, antioxidant and antimicrobial properties. Additionally, further studies are needed for more discussion and explanations.

5. Acknowledgements

We are thankful to the Agricultural and Veterinary Staff of Islamic Azad University, Shahrekord Branch, for the cooperation and assistance in order to run this test. In addition, the authors sincerely acknowledge the sincere assistance provided by Professor Abdollah Ghasemi Pirbalouti.

6. References

AOAC. 2000. Official methods of analysis, Association of official analytical chemists. AOAC Press, Gaithersburg, USA.

Al-Ismail, K.M. and Aburjai, T. 2004. Antioxidant activity of water and alcohol extracts of chamomile flowers, anise seeds and dill seeds. *Journal of Science Food and Agriculture*. 84: 173-178.

Bahramikia, S. and Yazdanparast, R. 2009. Efficacy of different fractions of Anethum graveolens leaves on serum lipoproteins and serum and liver oxidative status in experimentally induced hyper cholesterolaemic rat models. Journal of Chinese Medicine. 37: 685-699.

Duncan, D.B. 1955. Multiple range test and F-test. *Biometrics*, 11:1- 42.

Bahadori, M.M., Irani, M., Ansari Pirsaraei, Z., Koochaksaraie, R. R. 2013. The Effects of dill powder in diet on some blood metabolites, carcass characteristics and broiler performance. *Global Veterinaria*., 10, 500-504

Burger A., Wachter, H. 1998. Hunnius, pharmaceutical dictionary.8th Edition. Walter de Gruyter, Berlin.

Cyberhorse. 1999. International animal health products. The Australian Company ACN 003 185 699, Australia. h*ttp://www.cyberhorse.net.au/an/protexin.htm*.

Faghani, M., Rafiee, A., Namjoo, A.R., Rahimian, Y. 2014. Performance, cholesterol profile and intestinal microbial population in broilers fed turmeric extract. *Research opinion in animal and veterinary sciences*.,4(9): 500-503

Ghaedi, H., Nasr, J., Kheiri, F., Rahimian, Y., Miri, Y. 2014. The effect of virginiamycine and black pepper (Piper nigrum L.) extract on performance ofbroiler chicks. *Research Opinion in Animal and Veterinary Science*., 4: 91-95.

Jamroz, D., Orda, J., Kamel, C., Williczkiewicz, A., Wertelecki, T., Skorupin'Ska, J. 2003. The influence of phytogenic extract on performance, nutrients digestibility, carcass characteristic and gut microbial Status in broiler Chickens. *Journal of Animal Feed Science*., 12(3), 583-596.

Jamroz, A.M. 1989. Antimicrobial activities of essential oils: A Pharmacognostical Study. Dissertation, Rijksuniversiteitte Leiden.

Kheiri, F., Rahimian,Y., Nasr, J. 2015. Application of sumac and dried whey in female broiler feed. *Archive Animal Breeding*. 58, 205–210.

NRC, National Research Council. 1994. Nutrient requirements of poultry.9th Rev. Ed., Washington, DC. National Academy Press.

Panda, S. 2008. The effect of Anethum graveolens L. (Dill) on corticosteroid induced diabetes mellitus: involvement of thyroid hormones, *Phytotherapy Researches*., 22(12): 1695-1697.

Rafiei-Tari.A, Karimi, K., Hosseini, S.A. Meimandipour, A. 2016.Growth performance, carcass characteristics and serum biochemical of Japanese quails fed with oat bran (Avena sativa) and Dill Seed (Anethumgraveolens). *Iranian Journal of Applied Animal Science*., 6(2), 423-428.

Rezaian, M. 2006. Modification of fixation process in avian histologic sections, *Journal of Histotechnol*, 29, 123–127.

Richter C. 2010. Celebrating dill, herb of the year 2010. Available at: http://www.richters.com/show.cgi

SAS Institute, SAS/STAT user's guide for personal computer. 2001. Release 6.12 SAS Institute, Inc., Cary, N.C., USA.

Satyanarayana, S., K. Sushruta, G.S. Sarma N. Srinivas and R.G.V.N. Subba. 2004. Antioxidant activity of the aqueous extracts of spicy food additives evaluation and comparison with ascorbic acid in *in vitro* systems. *Journal of Herbal Pharmacotherapy*.4: 1-10.

Yazdanparast, R., Alavi, M. 2001. Anti hyperlipidaemic and anti hypercholesterolaemic effects of Anethum graveolens leaves after the removal of furocoumarins, Cytobios, 105: 85-91.

Zhang Y., Zhang H., Hua S., Ma L., Chen C., Liu X., Jiang L.,Yang Y., Zhang P., Yu D., Guo Y., Xue H., Tan X., Liu J. 2007. Identification of two herbal compounds with potential cholesterol-lowering activity. *Biochemistry and Pharmacolgy*.74, 940-947.

Regulation of Intestinal GLP-1 and GLUT2 genes underlie hypoglycemia in Desplatsia subericarpa (Bocq)-Fed Wistar Rats

Omotuyi Idowu Olaposi[1]*, Ovuakporie-Uvo Oghale[2], Idu MacDonald[2]

[1]*Center for Bio-computing and Drug Development, Adekunle Ajasin University Akungba Ondo State, Nigeria;*

***Email:** olaposi.omotuyi@aaua.edu.ng

[2]*Department of Plant Biology and Biotechnology, University of Benin, Benin City, P.M.B. 1154. Edo State, Nigeria;*

ARTICLE INFO

***Topic:** Medicinal Plants*

Key words:
- ✓ *Glucagon-like peptide-1*
- ✓ *Glucose transporter 2*
- ✓ *Kidney injury molecule-1*
- ✓ *Interleukin-1-β*
- ✓ *Diabetes*
- ✓ *Desplatsia subericarpa*

ABSTRACT

Background & Aim: Indigenous people of West Africa use the whole-leaf of *Desplatsia subericarpa* (Bocq) in anti-diabetic soup delicacy. This study was designed to validate the anti-diabetic claims and delineating possible mechanisms.

Experimental: RT-PCR method was used to investigate regulation of intestinal glucose transporter 2 (GLUT2) and glucagon-like peptide-1 (GLP-1), and pancreatic insulin, L-type voltage-gated calcium channel genes. Insulin exocytosis was also monitored using ELISA method. The kidney sample was investigated for biomarkers of injury (kidney injury molecule-1 (KIM-1) and interleukin-1-β (IL-1β)).

Results: GLP-1 up-regulation, GLUT2 down-regulation and increased insulin exocytosis but not increased insulin gene expression was observed in animals after a 3-day culinary exposure to *D. Subericarpa* leaves. This mechanism may explain hypoglycemia in streptozotocin-induced diabetes in animals in this study. KIM-1 and IL-1-β genes were marked up regulated in normal animals exposed (14-day) to *D. Subericarpa*.

Recommended applications/industries: *D. Subericarpa* whole leaf contains phytochemicals principles with anti-diabetic potency but may be nephrotoxic. Therefore, for clinical use, selective fractionation of active components from the toxic components is desirable.

1. Introduction

Desplatsia subericarpa is an understory dense tree growing up to 10 meters tall. The bole is about 4-10 cm in diameter. The glabrous papery leavesare alternate and simple with stipules.Drupe is 6-10cm long and 5-7.5 cm wide (Burkill, 2000; Keay, 1958). *D.Subericarpa* has been identified following an ethnopharmacological survey of neglected plants with food and therapeutic uses in Southern Nigeria. Folklorically, the fresh leaves of *D. subericarpa* are eaten as vegetables while the dried leavesaremade into a decoction useful in managing diabetic conditions yet without scientific data to validate this claim and explain its mode of action, safety in humans.

Glucagon-like peptide 1 (GLP-1) is a potent incretinhormone produced in the L-cells of thedistal ileum and colon. In the L-cells, tissue-specific post-translational processing of the proglucagon gene generates GLP-1(Ezcurr *et al.,* 2013; Velasquez *et al.*, 2010), which acts onβ cells GLP-1 receptor, and mediates its glucose responsiveness by promoting insulin exocytosis in GLUT2 (the normally expressed high K_m glucose transporter of β cells)-dependent manner (Chen *et al.,* 1990). Indeed, GLP-1/GLP-1R signaling and GLUT2, mediate glucose-stimulated insulin secretion, and their blockage impair glucose sensing with resulting hyperglycemia (MacDonald *et al.*, 2002).

TGR5 is a bile acid activated G-protein coupled receptor, which plays key regulatory roles in energy expenditure and diet-induced obesity through intestinal (GLP-1) mechanisms (McKillop *et al.,* 2016; Pols *et al.,* 2010; Wacker *et al.,* 2014). Pharmacological targeting of TGR5 has been identified as a promising incretin-based strategy for managing type 2 diabetes and metabolic disorders such as non-alcoholic fatty liver disease. Therefore, in this study,TGR5/glucagon-like peptide-1 (GLP-1)/insulin pathway[11] along the intestino-hepato-pancreatic axis was investigated in *Desplatsia subericarpa* Bocq.-fed Wistar Rats. Furthermore, we investigated blood glucose regulation in streptozotocin-induced diabetic rats fed *Dsubericarpa* Bocq-based diet, and finally evaluate nephrotoxicity following sub-chronic exposure. Our results support intestinal GLP-1 up-Regulation and GLUT2 down-regulation in *Desplatsia subericarpa* Bocq.-fed Wistar Rats which may play significant role in its antidiabetic claims.

2. Materials and Methods

2.1 Plant materials

Desplatsia subericarpa Bocq. leaves were collected in January 2016 from Ugbogiobo village located in Ovia North Local Government Area of Edo State, Nigeria. Leaves were dried in a cool dry place for two weeks and oven died for 30 minutes at 40° C to ensure leaves were crispy. Dried leaves were pulverized using a mechanical mill, sieved and used as feed formulation as described below. A voucher specimen was deposited in the University of Benin Herbarium (UBHm0284).

2.2 Animal studies

6-week-old male inbred Wistar Rats were used with strict compliance with the NIH Guide for the Care and Use of Laboratory Animals. All the protocols were also reviewed and approved by Laboratory Animal Ethical Committee of AdekunleAjasin University, Akungba-Akoko. The Animals (now referred to as subjects) were maintained on a standard rat chow and water *ad libitum* for 5 days prior to grouping and experimentation.

2.3 D. subericarpa-regulated anti-diabetic transcriptional program along intestinal-pancreatic-hepatic axis

Subjects were housed three (3) per cage under a 12-h light/dark condition. Subject randomization and grouping for this study has been presented (fig.1) for clarity. 6-hr prior to sacrifice, food and water were withheld; anesthesia was induced in the subjects using chloroform. The Intestine, pancreas, liver and blood samples (cardiac puncture) were collected for further analysis.

2.4 Diabetes study

Diabetes was induced by intraperitoneal injection of single dose of freshly prepared solution of streptozotocin (in 0.1 M sodium citrate buffer, pH 4.5), 45 mg/kg) to overnight fasted subjects. Three days after administration, hyperglycemic subjects were grouped into diabetic control (100% feed/honey) and diabetic treatment groups (10% *D. subericarpa* leaf powder/90% rat chow mixed in honey), basal group was also fed like diabetic control but without streptozotocin treatment. Blood samples were taken three (3) times over of 9 feeding days for non-fasting blood glucose determination using the glucose oxidase method (Barham & Trinder, 1972).

2.5 Blood insulin quantification

Blood samples taken via cardiac puncture were stored in heparinized tubes, centrifuged at 3500 rpm for 15 minutes to separate the plasma for insulin quantification using insulin ELISA kits (EZRMI-13K) according to the manufacturer's instructions.

2.6 Total RNA isolation, Reverse transcription and PCR amplification

RNA samples were extracted from tissues (n=3) using acid guanidiniumthiocyanate-phenol-chloroform extraction method. Genomic DNA contaminant was digested using DNase I (Fermentas, Ontario, Canada) treatment. The reaction mixture contains 2 μL of DNase I, 5 μL of reaction buffer and 23 μL RNA sample. The mixture was incubated at 37°C for 30 minutes. DNase I inactivation was achieved by adding 5 μL EDTA (25 mM) followed by 65°C incubation for 10 minutes[13]. RNA yield and purity were then spectrophotometrically determined. Prior to cDNA conversion, all RNA samples were diluted to 100 ng concentration using nuclease free water. MMLV Reverse Transcriptase 1st-Strand cDNA Synthesis Kit (NEB) was used for RNA-to-cDNA conversion according to the manufacturer's instruction. PCR amplification for the determination of genes whose primers (SnapGene software) are listed below was done using the following protocol: PCR amplification was performed in a total of 25 μl volume reaction mixture containing 2 μlcDNA (40 ng), 2 μl primer (100 pmol) 12.5 μl ReadyMix Taq PCR master mix (Sigma Aldrich) and 8.5 μl nuclease-free water. Initial denaturation at 95 °C for 5 minutes was followed by 20 cycles of amplification (denaturation at 95 °C for 30 seconds, annealing at 55 °C for 30 seconds and extension at 72 °C for 60 seconds) and ending with final extension at 72 °C for 10 minutes.

2.5 Primers

GLUT2F-5'-GACCTGGATTGAGACAACAACTCCG-3'
GLUT2R-5'-TATTATTACCTCTTGAGGTGCATTGATCACACC-3'
GLP-1-F-5'-TCCCAAAGGAGCTCCACCTG-3'
GLP-1-R-5'-TTCTCCTCCGTGTCTTGAGGG-3'
FAS-F-5'-AGAGACGGCAGCAGCG-3'
FAS-R-5'-GATCCTTCAGCTTTCCAGACCG-3'
G6PDD-F-5'-AAAGCACACGCCCTCTTGC-3'
G6PDD-R-5'-CTTGGTGGAAGGCATCACCC-3'
INSULIN-F-5'-AACCCTAAGTGACCAGCTACAATCA-3'
INSULIN-R-5'-AAACCACGTTCCCCACACAC-3'
LT-VDCC-F-5'-CTAGGCAAGCTCTCTACCAC-3'
LT-VDCC-R-5'-AGTAACCAGGTTGGTTCATG-3'
IL1□-F-5'-GGCTCATCTGGGATCCTCTCC-3'
IL1□-R-5'-GACACTGCCTTCCTGAAGCTC-3'
KIM-1-F-5'-GGTGCCTGTGAGTAAATAGATCA-3'
KIM-1-R-5'-TAAACTTCAACTACCTTAAACACAATAAGATG-3'
□-Actin-F-5'-GTCGAGTCCGCGTCCAC-3'
□-Actin-R-5'-AAACATGATCTGGGTCATCTTTTCACG-3'

2.6. Image processing and statistical analysis

In-gel amplicon bands (n=3) were captured using iPhone-5s camera (Noir), image post-processing was done on Keynote platform and band quantification was done using Image-J software. Data presented here expressed as Mean ± Standard Error of Mean (SEM). Statistical analyses were performed using t-test ($P < 0.05$ vs. basal control) using Graph Pad Prism version. 7 (GraphPad Software, Inc. La Jolla, CA, USA) software.

3. Results and discussion

3.1 Intestinal GLP1 up-regulation and GLUT2 down-regulation following culinary administration of D. subericarpa

Our understanding of ethnopharmacological uses of D. *subericarpa* leaves is infantile at this stage and to our knowledge; this study provides the first systematic study at unraveling its antidiabetic activity. First, our choice of administering the whole-leaf in culinary exposure was informed by the consensus that the leaf is traditionally made into vegetable decoction for managing diabetic complications. To mimic this, normal rat chow and the dried leaf powder were mixed together in 90:10 and 70:30 ratios respectively. To aid consumption in animals, 100mL of pure honey was used to formulate the diet. The feed (Fig. 1) was administered *ad libitum* for 48 hr period. RT-PCR gel electrophoresis of RNA samples isolated from the intestinal crypt of the animals following feeding period showed up-regulated GLP-1 expression and down-regulated GLUT2 genes. GLUT2 is the major route for glucose absorption across the brush-border membrane (Kellett & Helliwell, 2000) and its inhibition has been identified as a antidiabetic mechanism in some plants extracts(Nistor Baldea *et al.,* 2010). Uncharacterized components of D. *subericarpa* leaves interfere with the expression of GLUT2, which appears more robust hypoglycemic mechanism than inhibition or blockage of mobilization to the brush-border.

We propose a plausible mechanism underlying GLUT2 gene downregulation as interference with sterol response element-binding protein (SREBP)-1c, which is known to facilitate glucose-stimulated GLUT2 gene expression (Im *et al.,* 2005). Note that direct inhibition of (SREBP)-1c has been chosen rather than inhibition membrane-bound transcription factor site-1 protease (S1P)(Brown & Goldstein, 1999), which catalyzes its post-translational maturation because direct inhibition of S1P would have resulted in hepatic downregulation of fatty acid synthase and glucose-6-phosphate dehydrogenase whose regulation are controlled by (SREBP)-1a(Inoue *et al.*, 2005). Our result show increased expression of hepatic fatty acid synthase and glucose-6-phosphate dehydrogenase (Fig. 3), providing clear evidence against S1P inhibition.

Next, GLP-1 expression pattern was investigated. GLP-1 is an enteroendocrine L-cells hormone produced following accumulating nutrients such as glucose within the gastrointestinal tract. Indeed, repression of GLUT2 should cause glucose accumulation within the gastrointestinal space resulting in increased GLP-1 expression and release, which in turn stimulates insulin and inhibits glucagon release with concomitant hypoglycemic effects (Ezcurra *et al.,* 2013; Velasquez *et al.,* 2010). Additionally, GLP-1 upregulation may proceed though TGR5 activation as naturally occurring TGR5 agonists have been previously shown to modulate GLP-1 biosynthesis and secretion(Jafri et al., 2016).*D. subericarpa* may contain TGR5 phytochemical agonists; some of these scaffolds have been characterized in plants such as *Olea europraea* (Sato *et al.,* 2007).

3.2 Pancreatic Insulin release not gene expression is regulated by culinary administration of D. Subericarpa

The desired goal in treatment of type-2 diabetes is to improve cell health (Marchetti *et al.*, 2009), increase insulin release, and tissue absorption of blood glucose via GLUT4, which is rapidly translocated to the membrane of target tissue downstream insulin/Insulin-receptor signaling pathway (Leto & Saltiel, 2012). We tested whether D. *subericarpa* leaves also alter insulin and L-type voltage gated channel transcription in the pancreas (Fig. 2D). While our data showed that none of these genes is significantly upregulated in the test groups (*vs.* control ($p < 0.05$), Fig. *2D, ii&iii*), blood insulin release is however dose-dependently increased in the treatment groups (Fig. 2D, *iv*). Increased blood insulin levels following *D. subericarpa* may have resulted from increased GLP-1 expression as stimulation of insulin secretion from pancreatic β-cells via glucagon-like peptide 1 receptor (GLP-1R)/GLP-1 (or other agonists) is well documented (Meloni *et al.,* 2013) Paradoxically, blunted GLUT2 expression may result in low blood glucose, which should act synergistically with GLP-1 to activate insulin release pathway in pancreatic β-cells (MacDonald *et al.,* 2002), clearly insulin release mediated by *D. subericarpa* may involve GLP-1 but glucose-independent manner. Interestingly, TGR5 agonists are the scaffolds, which mediate secretion of GLP-1 in the absence of glucose(Lan *et al.,* 2012), whether GLP-1 is sufficient for insulin release in the absence of glucose is yet to be determined.

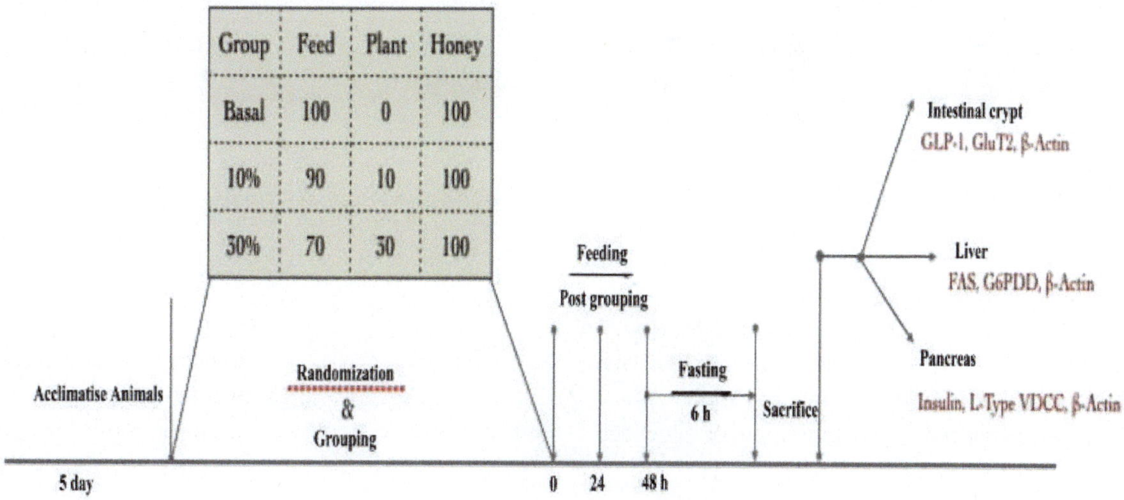

Fig. 1. Experimental Design (normal rats)

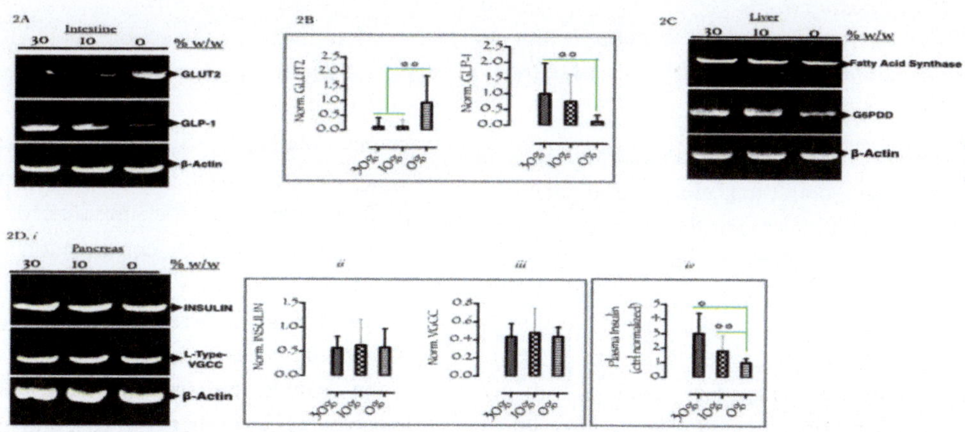

Fig. 2. Querying anti-diabetic mechanism(s) of *D. subericarpa* leaves using gene expression studies.

(A) Representative gel image showing intestinal mRNA levels of GLUT2, GLP-1and □□actin.

(B) Column depiction of □□actin-normalized GLUT2 and GLP-1 levels in the intestine from band density estimate of n=3 independent samples.

(C) Representative gel image showing liver mRNA levels of fatty acids synthase (FAS), glucose-6 phosphate dehydrogenase (G6PDD) and □□actin.

(D) (*i*) Representative gel image of pancreatic expression of insulin, L-type voltage-gated calcium channel (LT-VGCC) and □□actin. Column representation of band density following quantification and normalization of insulin (*ii*) and LT-VGCC (*iii*). Column represents plasma insulin profile of experimental animals and control.

(All experiments were sampled in triplicate (n=3), ** (*p< 0.05vs. control*), * (*p< 0.01 vs. control*)

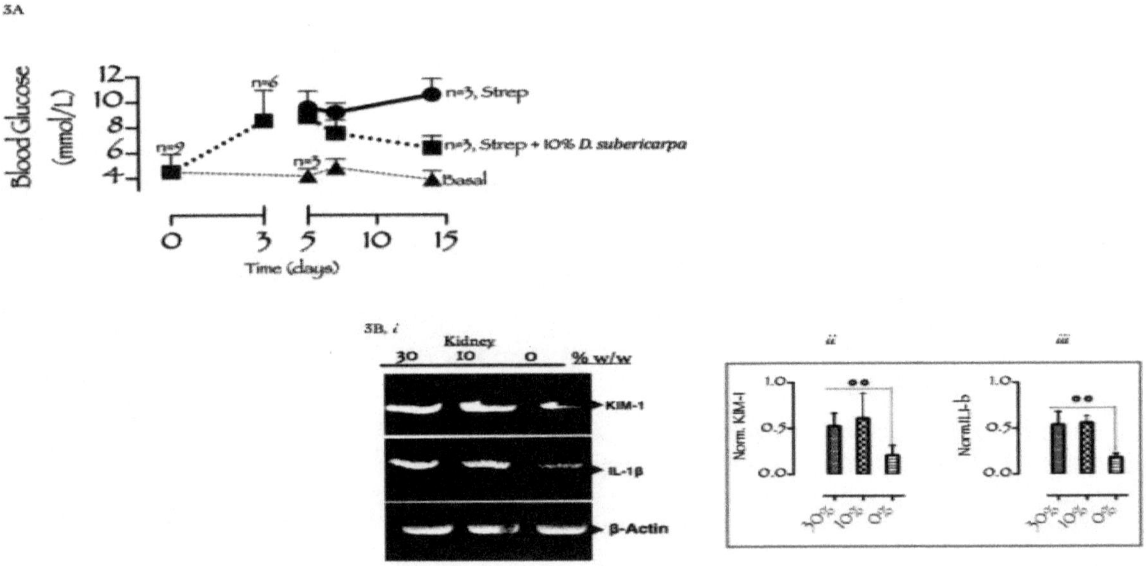

Fig. 3. *D. subericarpa* leaves exhibit anti-diabetic potency and toxicity in experimental animals (A). Line graph showing blood glucose profile with time in streptozotocin-induced hyperglycemia (treated and untreated) and basal control groups. (B, *i*) Gel image representation of mRNA levels of kidney toxicity biomarkers (Kidney injury molecule-1 (KIM-1) and interleukin-1 (IL-1)-□, column representation of band density following quantification and normalization of KIM-1 (*ii*) and IL1-□□ (*iii*) following □□actin normalization. (All experiments were sampled in triplicate (n=3), ** (*$p < 0.05$ vs. control*))

3.3 *D. Subericarpa reverses hyperglycemia in experimental animals but exhibit sub-chronic nephrotoxicity*

To test the usability of *D. subericarpa* leaves in experimental diabetic condition, nine (9) animals were subjected to similar initial feeding conditions (normal rat chow with honey base), six (6) of the animals were induced with diabetes using streptozotocin (single dose, 45 mg/kg, *i.p.)*; day-3 post streptozotocin treatment, hyperglycemia was observed in all the treatment groups. Three (3) of the diabetic animals were chosen for treatment (10% *D. subericarpa*) for 9 days. Blood samples were drawn periodically (once every 3 days) from the tail of the animals for blood glucose determination. Indeed, *D. subericarpa* leaves in the diet of diabetic rats partially reversed hyperglycemia associated with streptozotocin treatment (Fig. 3A). This result clearly supports the folkloric use of *D. subericarpa* leaves in diabetic condition. Since diabetes is treated chronically, it should be interesting to know how the kidney functions in a 14-day treatment period.

Here, kidney injury molecule 1 (KIM-1)(Andreucci *et al.*, 2016) and interleukin 1 □ expression(Faubel *et al.,* 2007) patterns were investigated as biomarkers for kidney damage. Surprisingly, both genes were upregulated in both test subjects (Fig. 3B,*i-iii*). This finding may not be absolutely peculiar to *D. subericarpa* leaves as consumption of mixed Chinese herbs have resulted in renal tubular acidosis with hypokalaemic paralysis, rhabdomyolysis and subsequent acute renal failure (Lee *et al.,* 1999).

In conclusion, we have demonstrated that *D. subericarpa* leaves have potent anti-diabetic principles acting via GLUT2 gene downregulation and GLP-1 upregulation mechanisms. We have also shown its applicability in animal model of diabetes. Its application in humans may be limited in whole-leaf form as renal IL-1□ and kidney injury molecule 1 (KIM-1) expression were significantly increased in animals administered *D. subericarpa* leaves. Thus, reciprocal regulation of GLP-1 and GLUT2 genes by *D. subericarpa* leaves provides preliminary indication that the leaves contain TGR5 agonists, since TGR5 activation is upstream GLP-1 gene upregulation. Taking a cue from previous studies, we hypothesize that the unidentified compounds may likely be of sterol class especially the triterpenes, which has demonstrated potent TGR5 agonism *in vitro* and *in vivo*(Schaap *et al.,* 2014); GLUT2 downregulation in SREBP-dependent manner also lends credence to our speculation as sterols likewise regulate the activity of SREBP(Nohturfft *et al.,* 1999).It may be instructive to suggest immediate isolation and characterization of SREBP-1c inhibiting/TGR5 activating principle, which may be different from the nephrotoxic components for anti-diabetes drug development.

4. Conclusion

This study was designed to validate the anti-diabetic claims and delineating possible mechanisms by following the gene expression pattern of intestinal glucose transporter 2 (GLUT2), glucagon-like peptide-1 (GLP-1), pancreatic insulin, L-type voltage-gated calcium channel genes. Similarly, The kidney sample was investigated for biomarkers of injury (kidney injury molecule-1 (KIM-1), interleukin-1-β (IL-1β)).

Upregulated GLP-1, increased insulin exocytosis but not increased insulin gene expression coupled with GLUT2 down-regulation following culinary exposure to *D. Subericarpa* leaves solidly support its anti-diabetic claims. The anti-diabetic pharmacology may be blunted by nephrotoxicity as KIM-1 and IL-1-β genes were marked up regulated in normal animals exposed (14-day) to *D. Subericarpa*. We therefore report that the whole leaf indeed *D. Subericarpa* contains phytochemical principles with potent anti-diabetic potency but may be nephrotoxic; for future clinical use, selective fractionation of active components from the toxic components is desirable.

5. Acknowledgements

The technical assistance of Dr. Elekofehinti of Federal University of Technology Akure, Nigeria is acknowledged. The authors also acknowledged the First Bank of Nigeria for providing Solar-power supply facility to Center for Bio-Computing and Drug Development where the study was conducted.

6. References

Andreucci, M., Faga, T., Riccio, E., Sabbatini, M., Pisani, A., & Michael, A. 2016. The potential use of biomarkers in predicting contrast-induced acute kidney injury. *Int J Nephrol Renovasc Dis, 9*, 205-221.

Barham, D., & Trinder, P. 1972. An improved colour reagent for the determination of blood glucose by the oxidase system. *Analyst, 97*(151), 142-145.

Brown, M. S., & Goldstein, J. L. 1999. A proteolytic pathway that controls the cholesterol content of membranes, cells, and blood. *Proc Natl Acad Sci U S A, 96*(20), 11041-11048.

Burkill, H. M. 2000. *The useful plants of West Africa.* (2 ed. Vol. 5). United Kingdom: families S-Z, Addenda. Royal Botanic Gardens, Kew, Richmond,.

Chen, L., Alam, T., Johnson, J. H., Hughes, S., Newgard, C. B., & Unger, R. H. (1990. Regulation of beta-cell glucose transporter gene expression. *Proc Natl Acad Sci U S A, 87*(11), 4088-4092.

Ezcurra, M., Reimann, F., Gribble, F. M., & Emery, E. 2013. Molecular mechanisms of incretin hormone secretion. *Curr Opin Pharmacol, 13*(6), 922-927.

Faubel, S., Lewis, E. C., Reznikov, L., Ljubanovic, D., Hoke, T. S., Somerset, H., . . . Edelstein, C. L. 2007. Cisplatin-induced acute renal failure is associated with an increase in the cytokines interleukin (IL)-1beta, IL-18, IL-6, and neutrophil infiltration in the kidney. *J Pharmacol Exp Ther, 322*(1), 8-15.

Im, S. S., Kang, S. Y., Kim, S. Y., Kim, H. I., Kim, J. W., Kim, K. S., & Ahn, Y. H. 2005. Glucose-stimulated upregulation of GLUT2 gene is mediated by sterol response element-binding protein-1c in the hepatocytes. *Diabetes, 54*(6), 1684-1691.

Inoue, N., Shimano, H., Nakakuki, M., Matsuzaka, T., Nakagawa, Y., Yamamoto, T., . . . Yamada, N. 2005. Lipid synthetic transcription factor SREBP-1a activates p21WAF1/CIP1, a universal cyclin-dependent kinase inhibitor. *Mol Cell Biol, 25*(20), 8938-8947.

Jafri, L., Saleem, S., Calderwood, D., Gillespie, A., Mirza, B., & Green, B. D. 2016. Naturally-occurring TGR5 agonists modulating glucagon-like peptide-1 biosynthesis and secretion. *Peptides, 78*, 51-58.

Keay, R. W. J. 1958. *Flora of West Africa* (2 ed. Vol. 1, part 2). London, United Kingdom: Crown Agents for OverseaGovernment and Administrations.

Kellett, G. L., & Helliwell, P. A. 2000. The diffusive component of intestinal glucose absorption is mediated by the glucose-induced recruitment of GLUT2 to the brush-border membrane. *Biochem J, 350 Pt 1*, 155-162.

Lan, H., Lin, H. V., Wang, C. F., Wright, M. J., Xu, S., Kang, L., . . . Kowalski, T. J. 2012. Agonists at GPR119 mediate secretion of GLP-1 from mouse enteroendocrine cells through glucose-independent pathways. *Br J Pharmacol, 165*(8), 2799-2807.

Lee, C. T., Wu, M. S., Lu, K., & Hsu, K. T. 1999. Renal tubular acidosis, hypokalemic paralysis, rhabdomyolysis, and acute renal failure--a rare presentation of Chinese herbal nephropathy. *Ren Fail, 21*(2), 227-230.

Leto, D., & Saltiel, A. R. 2012. Regulation of glucose transport by insulin: traffic control of GLUT4. *Nat Rev Mol Cell Biol, 13*(6), 383-396.

MacDonald, P. E., El-Kholy, W., Riedel, M. J., Salapatek, A. M., Light, P. E., & Wheeler, M. B. 2002. The multiple actions of GLP-1 on the process of glucose-stimulated insulin secretion. *Diabetes, 51 Suppl 3*, S434-442.

Marchetti, P., Lupi, R., Del Guerra, S., Bugliani, M., D'Aleo, V., Occhipinti, M., . . . Masini, M. 2009. Goals of treatment for type 2 diabetes: beta-cell preservation for glycemic control. *Diabetes Care, 32 Suppl 2*, S178-183.

McKillop, A. M., Moran, B. M., Abdel-Wahab, Y. H., Gormley, N. M., & Flatt, P. R. 2016. Metabolic effects of orally administered small-molecule agonists of GPR55 and GPR119 in multiple low-dose streptozotocin-induced diabetic and incretin-receptor-knockout mice. *Diabetologia*. 59(12):2674-85.

Meloni, A. R., DeYoung, M. B., Lowe, C., & Parkes, D. G. 2013. GLP-1 receptor activated insulin secretion from pancreatic beta-cells: mechanism and glucose dependence. *Diabetes Obes Metab, 15*(1), 15-27.

Nistor Baldea, L. A., Martineau, L. C., Benhaddou-Andaloussi, A., Arnason, J. T., Levy, E., & Haddad, P. S. 2010. Inhibition of intestinal glucose absorption by anti-diabetic medicinal plants derived from the James Bay Cree traditional pharmacopeia. *J Ethnopharmacol, 132*(2), 473-482.

Nohturfft, A., DeBose-Boyd, R. A., Scheek, S., Goldstein, J. L., & Brown, M. S. 1999. Sterols regulate cycling of SREBP cleavage-activating protein (SCAP) between endoplasmic reticulum and Golgi. *Proc Natl Acad Sci U S A, 96*(20), 11235-11240.

Pols, T. W., Auwerx, J., & Schoonjans, K. 2010. Targeting the TGR5-GLP-1 pathway to combat type 2 diabetes and non-alcoholic fatty liver disease. *Gastroenterol Clin Biol, 34*(4-5), 270-273.

Sato, H., Genet, C., Strehle, A., Thomas, C., Lobstein, A., Wagner, A., . . . Saladin, R. 2007. Anti-hyperglycemic activity of a TGR5 agonist isolated from Olea europaea. *Biochem Biophys Res Commun, 362*(4), 793-798.

Schaap, F. G., Trauner, M., & Jansen, P. L. 2014. Bile acid receptors as targets for drug development. *Nat Rev Gastroenterol Hepatol, 11*(1), 55-67.

Velasquez, D. A., Beiroa, D., Vazquez, M. J., Romero, A., Lopez, M., Dieguez, C., & Nogueiras, R. 2010. Central GLP-1 actions on energy metabolism. *Vitam Horm, 84*, 303-317.

Wacker, D. A., Wang, Y., Broekema, M., Rossi, K., O'Connor, S., Hong, Z., . . . Robl, J. A. 2014. Discovery of 5-chloro-4-((1-(5-chloropyrimidin-2-yl)piperidin-4-yl)oxy)-1-(2-fluoro-4-(methyls ulfonyl)phenyl)pyridin-2(1H)-one (BMS-903452), an antidiabetic clinical candidate targeting GPR119. *J Med Chem, 57*(18), 7499-7508.

Chemical composition and anti-inflamatory, anti-nociceptive and antipyretic activity of rhizome essential oil of *Globba sessiliflora* Sims. collected from Garhwal region of Uttarakhand

Kumar Ravendra[1*], Prakash Om[1], Pant Anil K[1], Kumar Mahesh[2], Isidorov Valary A[3], Szczepaniak Lech[3]

[1]*Department of Chemistry, College of Basic Sciences and Humanities, G.B. Pant University of Agriculture & Technology, Pantnagar, U.S. Nagar, Uttarakhand, India;*
*Email: ravichemistry.kumar@gmail.com

[2]*Department of Vet. Epidemiology and Preventive Medicine, College of Veterinary & Animal Sciences. G.B. Pant University of Agriculture & Technology, Pantnagar, U.S. Nagar, Uttarakhand, India;*

[3]*Institute of Chemistry, Białystok University, Division of Environmental Chemistry, UL. Hurtowa 1,15-399, Białystok, Poland;*

ARTICLE INFO

Topic: *Medicinal Plants*

Key words:
- ✓ *Globba sessiliflora* Sims
- ✓ *Essential oil*
- ✓ *Zingiberaceae*
- ✓ *β-eudesmol,*
- ✓ *Anti-inflamatory*
- ✓ *Anti-nociceptive*
- ✓ *Antipyretic activity*

ABSTRACT

Background & Aim: Family Zingiberaceae is worldwide in distribution. Plants of the zingiberaceae family are used in traditional herbal folk medicine besides their uses in spices, cosmetic, ornamental, food preservatives etc. In Uttarakhand the herbs grow from sub-tropical to temperate region. *Globba sessiliflora* Sims rhizomes were collected at maturity stage in November from Garhwal region of Uttarakhand, India. In present communication the medicinal use of various zingiberaceous herb provoked us to study the chemical diversity and pharmacological activity determination of this important traditional herb.

Experimental: The essential oil was extracted using hydrodistillation method and analyzed by GC-MS. Anti-inflamatory, anti-nociceptive and antipyretic activities of essential oil were experimently determined using mice model.

Results: The major compounds identified were β-eudesmol (27.6%), (*E*)-β-caryophyllene (24.3%), α-humulene (3.0%), (6*E*)-nerolidol (4.1%), caryophyllene oxide (9.7%), γ-eudesmol (6.4%) and τ-muurolol (8.3%) besides other minor constituents. Essential oil of *G. sessiliflora* rhizome showed good anti-inflamatory, anti-nociceptive and antipyretic activities at the dose level of 100 mg/kg body weight. The oral administration of the essential oil exhibited no toxicity at 400, 600 and 800 mg/kg b.wt. concentration. Ibuprofen, indomthacin and paracetamol were used as standard drugs for comparison.

Recommended applications/industries: *G. sessiliflora* essential oil can be used as herbal remedy for its nontoxicity anti-inflamatory, anti-nociceptive and antipyretic activities

1. Introduction

The complex biological response by harmful factors like pathogens, irritants and damaged cells results in inflammation. The common symptoms are redness of skin, edema, stiffness, pain and difficulty in of joint function which may be acute or chronic. Inflammation could result in a chronic stage which may indicate a factor of pathogenesis. A self defence mechanism may cause inflammation in primary phase which can be treated with chemotherapic agents to treat and eliminate symptoms and disease (Shailasree *et al.*, 2012).

The nociceptive pathway is described in three-neuron chain which transmits nociceptive information to the cerebral cortex from the periphery (Besson and Chaouch, 1987; Almeida *et al.,* 2004). The dorsal root ganglion has the first order neurons in their hair cell bodies. From here, two axons are projected to the peripheral tissues and the dorsal horn of the spinal cord. From the spinal cord, the second order neurons originate and ascend to the thalamus or the regions of the brainstem. From the thalamus, the third order neurons are ascended to the cerebrocortex (Besson and Chaouch, 1987; Abelson, 2005).

The secondary impact of infection is tissue damage, inflammation, graft rejection, malignancy or other diseased states which results in fever or pyrexia (Chattopadhyay *et al.*, 2005). The body's natural defense system generates in an environment for non survival of the infectious agent or damaged tissues. The enhanced formation of pro-inflammatory mediator's (cytokines like interleukin 1β, α, β and tumor necrosis factor-α) is normally caused by the infected or damaged tissues. The proinflammatory factors results the increase the synthesis of prostaglandin E2 (PGE2) near preoptic hypothalamus area and triggers the hypothalamus area to increase the body temperature (Saper and Breder, 1994).

The clinical treatment of inflammatory diseases is dependent on drugs which belong either to the non-steroidal or steroidal chemical therapeutic agents. The early steps in the biosynthetic pathway of prostaglandins by inhibition of COX enzymes are affected by the nonsteroidal anti-inflammatory drugs (NSAIDs) such as aspirin, indomethacin and ibuprofen and reduce the untoward consequences of inflammation (Albert *et al.,* 2002). However NSAIDs cause side effects like gastric injury and ulceration, renal damage and bronchospasm due to their non-selective inhibition of both isoforms of the COX enzymes (Tapiero *et al.,* 2002). The controversy of the use of steroidal drugs as anti-inflammatory agents is because of their multiple side effects (Vanden Worm *et al.,* 2001). Therefore, a demand has arisen for the search of newer anti-inflammatory drugs of natural origin with potential activity and with minor side effects as substitutes for chemical therapeutic agents. Some Indian medicinal plants and their active principles which have anti-inflammatory activity are documented by Chatterjee and Pal (1984).

The available analgesic drugs in the market are often associated with several adverse effects and are either too potent or too weak. Opiods are known to cause side effects which includes; sedation, respiratory depression, potential for addiction and tolerance whereas NSAIDS are known to cause gastric irritation that may lead to gastric bleeding. There is need for new analgesic compounds (Mattison *et al.,* 1998). Plants of medicinal value in ethnopharmacology are an important source of natural products with potential therapeutic effects (Blumenthal, 2000; Bisset, 2001). Study of plant species that are used in traditional herbal medicine as pain killers, therefore, form a logical search strategy for new analgesic drugs (Farnsworth, 1989; Mattison *et al.,* 1998).

High selectivity of irreversible inhibition of COX-2 expression by antipyretic drugs is the cause of reduction of increase body temperature by possible inhibition of biosynthesis of PGE2. The natural COX-2 inhibitors have lower selectivity with less side effects and less toxic to hepatic cells, glomeruli, cortex of brain and heart muscles. To combat the pro-inflammatory mediators, a number of plant extracts have been screened those inhibit leukotriene and prostaglandins synthesis modulating cyclooxygenase pathway by inhibition of COX-1 and COX-2 enzymes (Oj *et al*., 2007, Alberto *et al.,* 2009).

The members of family Zingiberaceae are currently of interest to phytochemist and pharmacologist all the world-over and work on their chemistry and pharmacology has been intensified recently. The research in family Zingiberaceae has evolked much attention after patent issue on haldi (*Curcuma longa* L.). Several species of ginger like *Zingiber officinale* Rosc. *Z. capitatum* Roxb and *Z. roseum* Rosc are known to grow in Kumaun and Garhwal region of Uttaranchal (Strachey, 1979). Numbers of plants from this family are used in traditional system of medicine (Hussain *et al.,* 1992). Plants of this family have been attributed to have anti-inflammatory, antiulcer, antioxidant and antimicrobial properties (Jaganath *et al.,* 2000).

Globba (Zingiberaceae-Zingiberales) consists of 100 species of small perennial herbs from East Asia and Malaysia. Flowers of *Globba* are strinking orange, yellow, purple or white, contrasting with the often green inflorescence bracts (Endress, 1994; Takano and Okada, 2003). *Globba* L. genus is represented by 17 species in India mainly distributed in the Himalaya, South India and Andman-Nicobar Islands (Karthikeyan *et al.,* 1989). In Uttarakhand the genus is represented by three species *G. orixensis* Roxb, *G. racemosa* Smith and *G. sessiliflora* Sims (Uniyal *et al.,* 2007). *G. sessiliflora* is erect, pemrennial herbs, with a creeping short rhizome which emits fleshy roots (Babu 1977).

We have earlier studied the mono and sesquiterpene composition of the rhizomes and aerial parts of *G. sessiliflora* Sims at flowering stage. β-caryophyllene, α-cadinol, selin-11-en-4α-ol, caryophyllene oxide, γ-eudesmol and myrcene were the major constituents in the rhizome volatile oil. The oil from aerial part revealed the presence of myrcene, β-caryophyllene, selin-11-en-4α-ol, β-longipinene, manool, germacrene D and β-eudesmol as major constituents. The oils showed significant myorelaxant effect on isolated duodenum smooth muscles of Wistar rats. The antioxidant activity of the oils were evaluated using reducing power assay, 2,2-diphenyl-1-picrylhydrazyl (DPPH) assay and the chelating effect on Fe^{2+}. Both rhizome and aerial part oils exhibited good to moderate antioxidant and myorelaxant activity in a dose-dependent manner (Kumar *et al.,* 2012).

In present study we worked on the chemical composition of essential oil of mature rhizomes of *G. sessiliflora* after litter fall collected from Garhwal region of Uttarakhand and anti-inflammatory, antinociceptive and antipyretic activity of rhizome essential oil of *G. sessiliflora.*

2. Materials and Methods

2.1. Plant material

G. sessiliflora rhizomes were collected in November, from the Dehradun- Mussoorie highway, Garhwal region of Uttarakhand, India. The identification and authentication of the plant was made by Dr. D. S. Rawat, Assistant Professor and plant taxonomist, Department of Biological Sciences, G.B. Pant University of Agriculture and Technology, Pantnagar. The voucher specimen has been deposited in the Department of Biological Sciences, GBPUAT, Pantnagar for future reference.

2.2. Isolation of essential oil

Essential oil from rhizomes was isolated by hydrodistillation in a Clevenger-type apparatus for 8 hours. The oil was extracted with CH_2Cl_2 and dried over anhydrous Na_2SO_4. The solvent was removed under vacuum and the oil was stored at 4°C for further analysis.

2.3. GC-MS analysis of essential oil

10% solution of essential oil was prepared in CH_2Cl_2 and filtered to obtain clear solution. GC-MS analysis of oleoresin solution (0.2 μl) was performed using Autosystem XL (Perkin-Elmer, USA) fitted with Elite-5MS fused silica column (30 m × 0.25 mm; 0.25μm film thickness), with split-splitless injector. Helium flow rate through the column was 1 ml/min in constant flow mode. The initial column temperature was 40°C rising 325°C at a rate 3°C/min. The MS detector temperature was 280°C. The constituents were detected in the full scan mode from *m/z* 41 to 620.

A hexane solution of C_8-C_{28} *n*-alkanes was previously separated under the above conditions, and their retention times were determined. Linear temperature programmed retention indices (LTPRI) were calculated from the results of the separation of the oleoresin and *n*-alkanes according to eq.:

$$LTPRI = 100(t_x - t_n)/ (t_{n+1} - t_n) + 100n,$$

Where t_x, t_n and t_{n+1} are the retention times of component *x*, and *n*-alkanes with the number of carbon atoms in the molecule *n* and *n*+1, respectively. After integration the fraction of each component in the total ion current (TIC) was calculated.a

Components of essential oil were identified with the help of NIST II, mass spectra library. Identification was considered reliable if the calculated values of LTPRI confirmed the results of library search at mass spectra library ($LTPRI^{Exp} - LTPRI^{Lit} \leq 10$ index units) (Adams, 2007).

2.4. Analysis of anti-inflammatory, antinociceptive and antipyretic activity of Essential oil

The investigations of different biological activities of the essential oil were carried out on Swiss strain albino mice weighing 18-23 g and purchased from the Indian Veterinary Research Institute(IVRI), Izatnagar, Bareilly, India. The mice were divided into different experimental groups. Each group consisted of six mice. All the groups were maintained under standard laboratory conditions of food and water. Prior to conduct the experiment, all the mice in each group were weighed individually to calculate the dose of drugs for each group. The animals were maintained in laboratory environment for two weeks to get them acclimatized. All experiments were conducted between 900, 1700 hours. All the animals were sustained under observation for one week, after the completion of experiments to observe acute or sub acute toxicity, if any [Experiments protocols were approved by the institutional animal ethics committee, CPCSEA, New Delhi (Ref: IAEC/Chem/CBSH/118)].

2.5. Animal model for anti-inflammatory, antinociceptive and antipyretic activities

Total four different groups of mice with six in each group were taken for conducting various pharmacological activities. The experiments were conducted using two different doses (50 mg/kg and 100 mg/kg b. wt.). These concentrations were selected as per IC_{50} calculations. 50 and 100 mg of oleoresins were separately triturated by the addition of small amount of Tween-20 and saline water was poured to make the final volume of 10 ml. Paracetamol, Ibuprofen and indomethacin were used as positive and saline water as negative control respectively. The essential oil, standard drug and saline water were given at the dose rate of 0.1 mL/10 gm weight of the experimental animals.

2.6. Anti-inflammatory assay

2.6.1. Acute Anti-inflammatory assay

Anti-inflammatory activity was determined by carrageenan induced hind paw edema method (Winter *et al.,* 1962). Acute inflammation was produced by subplantar injection of 0.1 mL of 1% suspension of carrageenan. The measurement of paw volume was made by plethysmometer (UGO Basile, Italy) at intervals of 1, 3 and 24 h after the injection of carrageenan. Standard anti-inflammatory drug, ibuprofen suspension was used orally at a dose of 40 mg/kg b.wt. The anti-inflammatory effect was measured as the reduction of volume displacement by hind foot in comparison to control.

2.6.2. Sub-acute Anti-inflammatory assay

The formaldehyde induced arthritis method was used to determine the subacute activity of the rhizome essential oil (Selye, 1949). 0.1 ml formaldehyde (1%) solution was injected in the right hind paw of the mice on first day for the experiment. Doses of the oleoresins (50 and 100 mg/kg b. wt.) were administered orally daily in the morning till the end of the experiment study period for 10 days. Whereas control group received only saline water. Ibuprofen at a dose of 10 mg/ kg b.wt. was orally given used as standard anti-inflammatory drug. Paw volume of all the mice were measured plethysmometrically in the evening hours for 10 days till the end of the experiment.

2.7. Antinociceptive assay

2.7.1. Writhing effect

The pain sensation in experimental mice was created by administering Glacial acetic acid intraperitoneally. Initially 0.2 mL of essential oil, standard drug (Ibuprofen – 40 mg/kg body wt) and control (saline water) were administered orally to each group of mice. Glacial acetic acid (1% at dose of 0.1 mL/10 g body weight) was administered intraperitoneally after 40 min to each mice. The numbers of writhing per minute were counted for every mice. The inhibition of writhing and percentage of pain protection in mice was calculated as per following formula:

$$\% \text{ writhing} = (T/C) \times 100$$

$$\% \text{ inhibition} = \frac{C-T \times 100}{C}$$

Where:

T = treatments (group II-III); C= control saline group (I)

2.7.2. Hot plate method

The standard hot-plate test was used to determine the analgesic response latencies (Langerman *et al.,* 1995). The mice were placed into Perspex cylinder on the heated surface of the hot-plate (maintained at 55.0 ± 0.5 ^{0}C). The time (sec) to discomfort reaction (licking paws or jumping) was recorded to record response latency. The measurements were recorded initially and after 30, 60, 120, and 150 min of oral administration of the essential oil at the dose rate of 50 and 100 mg/kg b.wt. For positive control, standard drug indomethacin (5 mg/kg b. wt.) was used. Saline water (0.2 mL) given orally as a negative control. A latency period of 20 sec. was marketed as complete analgesia and the measurements were stopped if it exceeded the latency period to avoid injury.

2.8. Antipyretic assay

To measure the antipyretic activity, pyrexia was induced using yeast as per the method given by Rao *et al.* (1997) generally being practiced. To record the basal body temperature a thermometer was inserted in to the rectum after restraining the mice. All the experimental groups were given a subcutaneous injection of 10 ml/kg b.wt. of 20% suspension of Brewer's yeast *(Sacchromyces cerevisiae)* except in control group. The mice were allowed to remain quiet in the cage for 18 hour, to rise in their body temperature. At nineteenth hour, again the rectal temperature was recorded. Immediately, 0.1 ml/10 gm body wt. of the oleoresins in the calculated doses of 50 mg/kg and 100 mg/kg b. wt. and paracetamol (33 mg/kg b. wt.) were given orally. Control group received 0.2 ml normal saline water only. The rectal temperature was recorded at hourly intervals in all the groups up to 3 hours. The percentage reduction in rectal temperature was calculated by considering the total fall in temperature to normal level as 100%.

% Reduction = $\{(B\text{-}Cn/B\text{-}A) \times 100\}$

Where:

A=normal temp B= Pyrexia temp C= temp at hourly interval

2.9. Assessment of toxicity

The acute toxicity was performed according to OECD guidelines (423, OECD/OCDE, 2001). The Lethality of essential oil of *G. sessiliflora* was checked by oral administration of essential oil at 400, 600 and 800 mg/kg b.wt. Behavioral changes were recorded for 24 hr. The numbers of casualties were recorded after upto 48 hr.

2.10. Statistical analysis

Data were expressed as mean±S.E. Results were analyzed using programme 43 (software) one way ANOVA and $p<0.05$ was considered to be statically significant.

3. Results and discussion

3.1. Essential oil composition

The rhizomes were collected in the month of October-November after litter fall and the essential oil analysed by GC and GC-MS representing 98.1% of the oil. Table 1 shows the chemical composition of the oil studied. The oil was very rich in oxygenated sesquiterpenes (65.8%), major component of the oil was β-eudesmol (27.6%). The other major oxygenated sesquiterpenes components in oil were caryophyllene oxide (9.7%), τ-muurolol (8.3%), γ-eudesmol (6.4%), (6*E*)-nerolidol (4.1%), (*E*)-sequisabinene hydrate (2.4%), 1-*epi*-cubenol (2.6%) and β-bisabolenol (2.2%). Other oxygenated sesquiterpenoids were found to be less than 1%. Sesquiterpene hydrocarbons contribute to 29.2% of the oil. Among sesquiterpene hydrocarbons, (*E*)-β-caryophyllene (24.3%) was found in highest amount. Other hydrocarbons identified were α-humulene (3.0%), (*E*)-β-elemene (0.4%), β-selinene (1.0%) and α-selinene (0.5%). (*E*)- α- bergamotene, (*E, E*)- α- farnesene and γ-cadinene were found in trace amounts. The oil had low amount of oxygenated monoterpenoids (1,8-cineole, linalool, borneol, 4-terpineol, α-terpineol, bornyl acetate), contributing to 1.4% of the oil. Monoterpene hydrocarbons (sabinine, β-pinene, p-cymene, limonene) were found in trace amount in the oil.

It is interesting to note that the essential oil of mature rhizome of *G. sessiliflora* collected from garhwal region has different chemical makeup, collected from kumaon region (Kumar *et al.,* 2012). In the essential oil collected from both the regions have sabinene, p-cymene, linalool, α-terpineol, β-caryophyllene, α-humulene, caryophyllene oxide and 1-*epi*-cubenol present in their essential oils. however γ-eudesmol (6.4%) and β-eudesmol (27.6%) were present in essential oil collected from Garhwal region were as γ-eudesmol (3.0%) and β-eudesmol (4.1%) in the essential oil collected from kumaun region. The eesential oil of *Globba sessiliflora* from Kumaun region has the presence of selin-11-en-4α-ol (12%), Manool (1.0%) and Sandaracopimara-8(14)-diene (1.5%) which were not present in the oil collected from Garhwal region.

Table 1. Chemical Composition of rhizome essential oil of *G. sessiliflora* Sims.

S. N.	Compound	t_R, min	$LTPRI^{exp}$	$LTPR^{Lit}$ (Adams,1995)	% contribution
1	sabinine	8.26	970	976	t
2	β-pinene	8.44	975	978	t
3	*p*-cymene	10.19	1021	1020	t
4	limonene	10.38	1028	1031	t
5	1,8-cineole	10.49	1033	1034	0.3
6	linalool	13.32	1098	1098	0.3
7	borneol	16.41	1168	1165	t
8	4-terpineol	16.81	1177	1177	t
9	α-terpineol	17.46	1192	1189	0.3
10	bornyl acetate	21.37	1281	1288	0.5
11	(*E*)-β-elemene	25.87	1386	1391	0.4
12	(*E*)-α-bergamotene	26.47	1400	-	t
13	(*E*)- β-caryophyllene	27.08	1415	1418	24.3
14	α-humulene	28.53	1451	1453	3.0
15	β-selinene	29.88	1484	1484	1.0
16	α-selinene	30.08	1488	-	0.5
17	(*E,E*)-α-farnesene	30.17	1491	1494	t
18	γ-cadinene	30.62	1502	1508	t
19	(6*E*)-nerolidol	32.79	1558	1561	4.1
20	caryophyllene oxide	33.48	1576	1575	9.7
21	(*E*)-sesquisabinene hydrate	33.63	1580	1584	2.4
22	humulene epoxide II	34.53	1603	1603	0.6
23	1-*epi*-cubenol	35.32	1625	1627	2.6
24	γ-eudesmol	35.40	1625	1633	6.4
25	(*E*)-Sesquilavandulol	35.57	1631	1633	0.6
26	β-eudesmol	36.23	1648	1639	**27.6**
27	τ-muurolol	36.35	1652	1647	8.3
28	6-hydroxy-caryophyllene	36.81	1665	1670	0.3
29	aromadendrene oxide	36.90	1667	1669	0.4
30	(6*R*,7*R*)-bisabolone	39.37	1735	1736	t
31	(*E,Z*)-farnesol	39.62	1742	1742	t
32	β-bisabolenol	41.31	1790	1786	2.2
33	occidol acetate	47.24	1971	1970	0.6
34	isokaurene	47.45	1978	1988	1.0
35	coranorin-*E*	51.57	2112	-	0.7
	Total				**98.1**
	Monoterpene hydrocarbons				0.0
	Oxygenated monoterpenes				1.4
	Sesquiterpene hydrocarbons				29.2
	Oxygenated Sesquiterpenes				65.8
	Diterpenes				1.7

t= trace <0.1%

Table 2: Acute anti-inflammatory activity of rhizome essential oil of *G. sessiliflora* (Mean±SE, n=6)

Group	Treatments	Dose (mg/kg) b.wt.	Change in paw thickness		% Inhibition
			0 hr	4 hr	
I	Control	0.2 mL	2.18±0.02	2.17±0.04	00.48
II	Ibuprofen	40	2.97±0.05	1.78±0.04[a]	40.06
III	GSREO	50	2.67±0.23	2.21±0.15[b]	17.22
IV	GSREO	100	2.86±0.12	1.90±0.42[a]	33.56

[a]= significant (p<0.05) as compared to control

[b]= significant (p<0.05) as compared to drug (Ibuprofen), GSREO: *G. sessiliflora* rhizome essential oil

Table 3. Effect of rhizomes essential oil of *G. sessiliflora* on formaldehede induced sub acute inflammation (Mean±SE, n=6)

Groups	Dose (mg/kg) b.wt.	Volume of inflammation(cm³)										
		Day 0	Day 1	Day 2	Day 3	Day 4	Day 5	Day 6	Day 7	Day 8	Day 9	Day 10
Control (I)	0.2 mL	2.14 ± 0.06	2.20 ± 0.10	2.16 ± 0.13	2.25 ± 0.12	2.15 ± 0.07	2.18 ± 0.08	2.16 ± 0.15	2.29 ± 0.11	2.16 ± 0.12	2.19 ± 0.11	2.23 ± 0.13
Ibuprofen (II)	10	2.18 ± 0.08	2.35 ± 0.09[a]	2.28 ± 0.12	2.34 ± 0.03	2.31 ± 0.08[a]	2.31 ± 0.11[a]	2.29 ± 0.10	2.28 ± 0.10	2.26 ± 0.09	2.17 ± 0.O5	2.16 ± 0.06
GSREO (III)	50	2.09 ± 0.08	2.31 ± 0.10	2.38 ± 0.13[a]	2.35 ± 0.04	2.34 ± 2.26[a]	2.28 ± 0.07[a]	2.29 ± 0.06	2.26 ± 0.04	2.24 ± 0.13	2.11 ± 0.11	2.14 ± 0.09
GSREO (IV)	100	2.10 ± 0.06	2.39 ± 0.06[a]	2.31 ± 0.03[a]	2.32 ± 0.05	2.26 ± 0.02[a]	2.25 ± 0.03	2.17 ± 0.11[b]	2.12 ± 0.05[a,b]	2.11 ± 0.06	2.10 ± 0.06	2.10 ± 0.06

[a] = significant (p<0.05) as compared to control, [b] = significant (p<0.05) as compared to Ibuprofen GSERO: *G. sessiliflora* Rhizome Essential Oil

Table 4. Antinociceptive activity of rhizome essential oil of *G.sessiliflora* (Writhing effect) (Mean±SE, n=6)

Groups	Treatments	Dose (mg/kg. b.wt.)	No of Writhings	% Writhings	% Inhibition
I	Control	0.2 mL	217.00±1.26	100.0	-
II	Ibuprofen	40	123.5±3.44	56.91	43.08
III	GSREO	50	143.83±0.75	66.28	33.71[a]
IV	GSREO	100	129.16±0.75	59.52	40.47[a]

a = significant (p<0.05) as compared to control, b = significant (p<0.05) as compared to Ibuprofen

GSREO: *G. sessiliflora* Rhizome Essential Oil.

Table 5. Antinociceptive activity of rhizomes essential oil of *G. sessiliflora* (Hot Plate Method) (Mean±SE, N=6)

Groups	Dose (mg/kg) b.wt.	Hot plate reaction time (min)				
		0	30	60	120	150
I(Control)	0.02 mL	3.01±0.00	3.11±0.01	2.95±0.01	2.84±0.02	3.03±0.02
II(Indometha)	5	3.27±0.03	3.83±0.03[a]	4.93±0.04[a]	4.07±0.09[a]	3.84±0.03[a]
III(GSREO)	50	2.93±0.04	3.35±0.41[a,b]	3.12±0.03[a,b]	2.61±0.30[a,b]	2.66±0.01[a,b]
IV(GSREO)	100	3.37±0.19	3.37±0.04[a,b]	3.41±0.03[a,b]	3.14±0.03[a,b]	2.87±0.12[a,b]

[a]= significant ($p<0.05$) as compared to saline water, b = significant ($p<0.05$) as compared to Indomethacin
GSREO: *G. sessiliflora* Rhizome Essential Oil.

Table 6. Effect of rhizome essential oil of G. sessiliflora on yeast induced pyrexia in mice (Mean±SE, N=6

Groups	Treatment	Dose (mg/kg) b.wt	Body temp. (^{0}C)		Temp after administration of drug (^{0}C)		
			Before injection of Brewer yeast	After injection of Brewer yeast	1 hr	2 hr	3 hr
I	Control	0.2 mL	37.55±0.02	38.87±0.03	38.87±0.03 (2.36±1.07)	38.89±0.03 (3.77±5.46)	38.81±0.03 (6.05±3.70)
II	Paracetamol	33	37.53±0.06	38.82±0.04	37.63±0.04[a,b] (92.86±3.28)	37.54±0.02[a,b] (99.47±5.49)	37.49±0.01[a,b] (103.60±5.20)
III	GSREO	50	37.64±0.03	38.85±38.91	38.26±0.06[a,b] (50.66±10.04)	38.13±0.03[a,b] (52.23±22.96)	37.84±0.07[a,b] (83.40±8.09)
IV	GSREO	100	37.54±0.03	38.86±0.01	37.65±0.03[a] (91.90±3.28)	37.44±0.04[a,b] (108.08±3.78)	37.34±0.03[a,b] (115.05±2.89)

Percentage reduction in temperature is given within parenthesis, [a] = significant ($p<0.05$) as compared to control, [b] = significant ($p<0.05$) as compared to drug, GSREO: *G. sessiliflora* rhizome essential oil

However the oil of collected from Garhwal region shows the presence of two diterpines isokaurene (1.0%) and coranorin- E (0.7%). Nootkatone was not detected at maturity stage collected from Garhwal region. Rhizome and aerial part essential oils contain nootkatone which was less than 3% of the oil in earlier stage collection from Kumaun region. The variation in the makeup of essential oils may be because of climatic variations in the two different regions of Uttrakhand.

3.2. Anti-inflammatory Assay

3.2.1. Acute Anti-inflammatory Assay

The paw volume of carrageenan induced paw edema was remained unchanged in saline treated control. In comparison to the control, the essential oil showed some anti-inflammatory activity. Maximum inhibition (40.06%) was recorded in Ibuprofen treated group and it was almost parallel to essential oil at the dose level 100 mg/kg b. wt. (Table 2).

3.2.2. Sub-acute Anti-inflammatory Assay

In ibuprofen treated mice, significant decrease in the paw volume was noticed from day 3 and value came to normal by day 10. Essential oil (50 mg/kg b.wt.) showed decreased in the sub-acute inflammation from day 1 and 100 mg/kg b. wt. dose of essential oil showed a decrease in the sub-acute inflammation from day 4 and reverted to normal by day 10 (Table 3).

Carrageenan induces acute inflammation method is used for the detection of anti-inflammatory activity in the drugs (Di Rosa and Willoughby, 1971). It has been reported that the edema is developed to carrageenan injection is a biphasic event. In first phase histamine and serotonin are released while in phase two (3-5 hours) is said to be synergised by prostaglandins. The edema is maintained between first and second phase due to kinin. It has also been reported that the second phase edema is sensitive to clinically effective steroids and non steroids anti-inflammatory agents. A variety of clinically ineffective agents can reduce initial phase (Vinegar *et al.,* 1969).

Essential oil of *Globba sessiliflora* used in this study, showed anti inflammatory activity probably due to the inhibition of the cyclo-oxygenage pathway. It has been reported earlier that the essential oil show anti-inflammatory activity due to its interference with the production of prostaglandins (Smith and Willis, 1971; Seibert et al., 1994; Miguel, 2010). In the carrageenan induced paw edema, essential oil showed activity at higher dose level.

For studying sub acute anti-inflammatory activity, arthritis was induced by formaldehyde injection on the first day and the test samples were administered orally every day for 10 days. During present investigation, oleoresins exhibited significant anti-artritis effect. Essential oil had anti-inflammatory effect corresponding to standard drug ibuprofen.

3.3. Antinociceptive assay

3.3.1. Writhing Effect

Essential oil showed significant analgesic activity with 34.79% inhibition at 50 mg/kg and 43.24% inhibition at the dose level of 100 mg/kg b. wt. As compared to standard drug ibuprofen (43.08 %, inhibition) (Table 4).

3.3.2. Hot Plate Method

Perusal of **table 5** reveals that the discomfort reaction time in indomethacin treated mice was maximum at 60 minute while essential oil exhibited a dose dependent manner increase in the paw licking and jumping time.

The abdominal constitution response induced by glacial acetic acid is a sensitive procedure to establish peripherally acting analgesics. This response is thought to involve local peritoneal receptors. Essential oil, significantly attenuated the acetic acid induced squirm.

In this work, we also measured the central nociceptive reactivity to thermal stimuli in mice using the hot plate test. In central analgesic activity, essential oil revealed efficacy against thermal stimulus.

3.4. Antipyretic Assay

Globba sessiliflora essential oil produced significant antipyretic effect in a dose dependent manner. Negative control mice did not show any reduction in the body temperature on oral administration of saline. The maximum inhibition was obscured at 3 hr (Table 6).

An appreciable antipyretic effect was noticed by essential oil at dose level of 100 mg/kg b. wt. which was comparable to paracetamol. Previous studies already suggested that intensification of lipid per oxidation at increase body temperature is indicated by pyrexia and is associated by increase in oxidative stress. The use of antioxidants retards the process of lipid per oxidation (Brzezinska-Slebodziniska, 2001).

We have earlier reported that essential oil of *G. sessiliflora* exhibits antioxidant activity (Kumar *et al.*, 2012).

3.4. Toxicity

On oral administration of 400, 600, 800 mg/kg.b.wt. of *G. sessiliflora* essential oil, no behavioural or physiological change was observed for 24 hr and on subsequent day. None of the treated mice died. All reflexes (pedal and corneal) and rectal temperature as well heart, respiration rates were within normal physiological limits in the extract treated mice.

4. Conclusion

From the experimental results it can be concluded that the herb can be a good natural source of β-eudesmol, (*E*)-β-caryophyllene, α-humulene (6 *E*)-nerolidol, caryophyllene oxide, γ-eudesmol and τ-muurolol etc. The herb exhibited moderate to good pharmacological activity hence the results will be helpful to generate data base on this plant so that it can be exploited scientifically and judiciously for traditional system of medicine besides its academic importance.

5. References

Abelson, K., 2005. Acetylcholine in spinal pain modulation: An *in vivo* study in the rat. Digital Comprehensive Summaries of Upsulla Dissertations from the faculty of Medicine. 19. 55pp. Uppsula. ISBN 91-554-6178-6.

Adams, R.P., 1995. Identification of essential oil components by gas chromatography, mass Spectrometry. Allured Publishing Corporation, Carol Stream, Illinois, USA.

Albert, D., Z¨undorf, I., Dingermann, T., M¨uller, W. E., Steinhilber, D., Werz, O., 2002. Hyperforin is a dual inhibitor of cyclooxygenase-1 and 5-lipoxygenase. *Biochemical Pharmacology.* 64,1767–1775.

Alberto, M.R., Zampini, I.C., Isla, M.I.,2009. Inhibition of cyclooxygenase activity by standardized hydroalcoholic extracts of four Asteraceae species from the Argentine Puna. Braz J Med Biol Res. 42(9),787-90.

Almeida, T. I., Roizenblatl, S. and Tufik, S., 2004. Afferent pain pathways: a neuroanatomical review. *Brain Research,* 1000,40-56.

Babu, C.R., 1977. Herbaceous flora of Dehradun. CSIR, New Delhi, pp 502.

Besson, J. M., Chaouch, A., 1987. Peripheral and spinal mechanisms of Nociception. *Physiology Reviews*, 67,67-186.

Brzezinska-Slebodzinska, E., 2001. Fever induced oxidative stress. The effect on thyroid status and the 5'-mono deiodinase activity, protective role of selenium vitamin. Journal of Physiology and Pharmacology. 52,275-284.

Chattopadhyay, D., Arunachalam, G., Ghosh, L., 2005. Antipyretic activity of Alstonia macrophylla Wall ex A. DC: an ethnomedicine of Andaman Islands. J Pharm Phar Sci.8 (3), 558-64.

Chatterjee, G. K., Pal., S. P., 1984. Search for anti-inflammatory agents from Indian Medicinal Plants-A review. *Indian Drugs.* 21, 413.

Di Rosa, M., Willoughby, D.A., 1971. Screens for anti-inflammatory drugs. Journal of Pharmacy and Pharmacology. 23,297-298.

Endress, P.K., 1994. Diversity and evolutionary biology of tropical flowers. Cambridge University Press, Cambridge.

Farnsworth, N. R. 1989. Screening plants for new medicines. In Wilson E.O. Editor, Biodiversity, Part II, National Academy Press, Washington, pp 83-97.

Hussain, A., Virmani, O.P., Popli, S.P., Misra, L.N., Gupta, M.M., 1992. Dictionary of Indian medicinal plants. Director, Central Institute of Medicinal and Aromatic Plants, Lucknow. 161-162.

Jaganath, I.B., Ng, L.T. 2000. Herbs: The green Pharmacy of Malaysia. Vinpress Sdn. Bhd. Malaysia Agriculture and Research and Development Institute. 95-99.

Karthikeyan, S., Jain, S.K., Nayar, M.P., Sanjappa, M., 1989. Floral Indicae Enumeratio: Monocotyledonae. Botanical survey of India, Calcutta, pp 293-294.

Kumar, R., Prakash, Om., Pant, A.K., Isidorov, Valery A., Mathela., C.S. 2012. Chemical composition, antioxidant and myorelaxant activity of essential oils of Globba sessiliflora Sims. 24(4),385-391.

Langerman, L., Zakowski, M.I., Piskoun, B., Grant, G.J., 1995. Hot plate versus tail-flick: Evaluation of acute tolerance to continuous morphine infusion in rat model. Journal of Pharmacological and Toxicological Methods. 34,23-27.

Mattison, N., Trimple, A. G., Larsen, I., 1998. New drug development in the United States, 1963 through 1994. *Clinical Pharmacology Therapeutics Journal.* 43, 290-301.

Maria G. M., 2010. Antioxidant and Anti-Inflammatory Activities of Essential Oils: A Short Review. Molecules. 15, 9252-9287.

OJ, Oh., H. Y. Min, Lee, S.K.,2007. Inhibition of inducible prostaglandin E2 production and cyclooxygenase-2 expression by curdione from Curcuma zedoaria. Arch Pharm Res. 30(10),1236-9.574.

423, OECD/OCDE, 2001. Acute oral toxicity-Acute toxic class method. Guideline for the testing of chemicals, guidance document on acute toxic class method.

Rao, R.R., Babu, R.M., Rao, M.R.V., Babu, M.G.V. 1997. Studies on antipyretic, analgesic and hypoglycaemic activities of root of *Gynandropsis gynandra* Linn. Indian Drugs. 34,12:690- 694.

Seibert, K., Zhang, Y., Leahy, K., Hauser, S., Masferrer, J., Perkins, W., 1994. Pharmacological and biochemical demonstration of the role of cyclooxygenase 2 in inflammation and pain. Proceedings of the National Academy of Sciences. 91,12013-12017.

Smith, J.B., Willis, A.L., 1971. Aspirin selectivity inhibition prostaglandin production in human platelets. Nature New Biology. 231,235-239.

Strachey, L., 1979. Catalogue of plants of Kumaun and of adjacent portion of Garhwal and Tibbet. Revised by Duthie JE pp 269, 1918, Reprint in 1974 periodicals publication Dehradun

Shailasree, S., Ruma, K., Kini, K.R., Niranjana, S.R., Prakash, H.S., 2012. Potential anti-inflammatory bioactives from medicinal plants of Western Ghats, India. Phcog Commn. 2,2-12.

Saper, C.B., Breder, C.D., 1994. The neurologic basis of fever. N Engl J Med, 330(26), 1880-1886.

Takano, A., Okada, H., 2003. Taxanomy of Globba (Zingiberaceae) in Sumatra, Indonesia. Syst Bot 28,524-546

Tapiero, H., Ba, G. N., Couvreur, P., Tew, K. D., 2002. Polyunsaturated fatty acids (PUFA) and eicosanoids in human health and pathologies. *Biomedicineand Pharmacotherapy.* 56,215–222.

Uniyal, B.P., Sharma, J.R., Chouddhery, U., Singh, D.K., 2007. Flowering plants of Uttarakhand (a checklist). Bishen Singh, Mahendra Pal Singh, Dehradun, pp 235.

Vanden Worm, E., Beukelman, C. J., Vanden Berg, A. J. J., Kores, B. H., Labadie, R. P., Van Dijk, H. 2001. Effects of methoxylation of apocynin and analogson the inhibition of reactive oxygen species production by stimulated human neutrophils. *European Journal of Pharmacology*. 433,225–230.

Vinegar, R., Schreiber, W., Hugo, R., 1969., Biphasic development of carrageenan edema in rates. Journal of Pharmacology and Experimental Therapeutics. 166,1:96-103.

Winter, C.A., Risley, E.A., Nuss, G.W., 1962. Carrageenan-induced edema in hind paws of the rats as an assay for antiinflammatory drugs. Proceedings of the Society for Experimental Biology and Medicine. 111,544-547.

Comparative study of the effect of Eucalyptus extract on *Candida albicans* and human pathogenic bacteria

Zahra Dehbashi[1], Forough Forghani[1], Seyed Kazem Sabbagh[2*], Saeideh Saeidi[3]

[1]*Department of Obstetrics' & Gynecology, Faculty of Medicine, Zabol University of Medical Science, Zabol, Iran;*

[2]*Department of Biology, Faculty of Science, Yazd University, Yazd, Iran;*
***Email: sksabbagh@yazd.ac.ir**

[3]*Laboratory expert of Microbiology, Institute of Plant Biotechnology, University of Zabol, Zabol, Iran;*

ARTICLE INFO

Topic: *Medicinal Plants*

Key words:
- ✓ *Anti-fungal activity*
- ✓ *Anti-microbial activity*
- ✓ *Minimum inhibitory concentration*
- ✓ *E. globules*
- ✓ *Candida albicans*

ABSTRACT

Background & Aim: During recent decades, infections disease resulting from opportunistic fungi such as *Candida albicans* and resistance increasing of human pathogenic bacteria to current antibiotics has led to many problems for treating of these diseases. The aims of the present study was to investigate anti-fungi and anti-bacterial effects of Eucalyptus extract on *Candida albicans* species isolated from clinical samples and some standard human pathogenic bacteria.
Experimental: Eucalyptus extract was provided using rotary apparatus and maceration method. Thirty isolates of *Candida albicans* were isolated from referred patients to gynecologist and then were purified and identified by valid keys. Finally, 30 isolated were used to growth inhibitory activity assay. Minimum bactericidal concentration (MBC) and minimum inhibitory concentration (MIC) of eucalyptus extract against 5 standard bacteria inculding: *Staphylococcus aureu, Shigella dysenteriae, Listeria monocytogenes, Vibrio cholera* and *Bacillus cereus* were evaluated using micro broth dilution method.
Results: Our results indicated that in compare to bacterial strains, fungus isolates showed more sensitivity to eucalyptus extract. The highest and lowest MIC of extract was recorded at 12.5 and 3.1 ppm for *S. aureus* and *B. cereus,* respectively. As *MIC,* the maximum MBC (20ppm) and minimum MBC (5ppm) of extract was recorded fro *S. aureus* and *B. cereus* respectively. Minimum inhibitory concentration of extract to fungal growth inhibitory was 50 ppm, whereas the maximum inhibiting concentration was 150 ppm.
Recommended applications/industries: The positive and interesting results suggest the essential oil of *E. globulus* could be exploited antibiotic for the treatment of candidiasous disease caused by C*andida albicans* fungi, and some human pathogenic bacteria studied in this work.

1. Introduction

Although, fungal infections compared to bacterial and virus infections, was not much prevalent in the past, but they have been responsible for considerable increase of diseases during recent decades (Baker *et al.,* 2012). Risk factors such as long and wide use of antibiotics, croton drugs, immuno suppressants medicament and basic disorders such as diabetes, AIDS and malignancies caused by fungal diseases, especially increased more than in the past (Goswami *et al.,* 2000; Merenstein *et al.,* 2013). Vaginal yeast infections known as candidiasis, is a disease caused by growth of more yeast around genital aerea of women (Consolaro *et al.,* 2004; Giraldo *et al.,* 2000). This is an important disease during the years in women who are sexually acitve, and it is increasingly spreading (Hay and Ashbee, 2010). *Candida albicans* species is the main causal agent that generates candida virginities disease with growth in two biological forms: yeast and mycelia forms in medium culture (De Vos *et al.,* 2005). This dimorphic fungus growth mainly in the human body as digestive and genital systems, and culture of, and also is present on vaginal secretion of 10-25% of women without symptoms disease (Cates *et al.,* 1990; Mathema *et al.,* 2001). The sexual contact is not usually the main cause of fungus spread in candidiasis or yeast infection. Antibiotics, birth control pills, steroid consuming and also tight clothing, severe obesity and warm weather, cause increase numbers of yeast.

One of the most widespread methods of candidiasis controlling is the use of fungicides such as fluconazole, ketoconazole, itraconazole (Amber *et al.,* 2010; Schuster *et al.,* 2008). Resistant of *C. albicans'* isolates to normal treatment by topical medications such as miconazole and fluconazol antifungal cream has been reported (Hoehamer *et al.,* 2010; Moosa *et al.,* 2004). Bactreia are another pathogenic factor in human. Currently, human pathgenic bacteria are controlled using chemical drugs including different antibiotics. Regarding to broad-spectrum and fast-acting of antibiotics, they are the first choice of patients (Biyela *et al.,* 2004; Levy, 1998; Neo, 2011). Continous and immethodical consumption of chemical drugs cause resistance to these combinations which result in weakened or neutralized effect of drugs and finally leads to raising the drug doze and tendency to apply new and more powerful formulae. Another disadvantage of using these drugs is their side effects which lead to emergence of diseases more dangerous than the primary ones (Pinto *et al.,* 2009). During recent years, medical plants are being used as an appropriate alternative for chemical drugs without their negative side effects. Eucalyptus plant (*Eucalyptus globules*, *Myrtaceae*) is a flowering tree and shrub which have been adapted to hot and humid climate of Iran and is frequently used as medical plants to cure for the common cold. Antifungal and antibacterial effects of eucalyptus extract in human (Cermelli *et al.,* 2008; Hammer *et al.,* 1999; Saeeidi *et al.,* 2014) and plant diseases (Ghorbani *et al.,* 2014; Wilson *et al.,* 1997) have been assessed, and it has been shown that in most cases in exprimental condition, eucalyptus has had good inhibiting effects on the growth of tested fungi and bacterial. Extract of Eucalyptuse has anti-inflammatory, antiseptic, antibacterial and expectorating properties and has resulted to inhibit inflammation of nasal mucosa, pharyngeal mucosa, otitis, sinuses inflammation and vaginitis (Noumi *et al.,* 2011). Analysis of chemical compound of eucalyptus extract content has shown that these compounds contain cineol, cytrol (Maciel *et al.,* 2010), piperitone, α-Phellandrene and trepene (Gilles *et al.,* 2010) . Because of biological and pharmacological properties of essential oil of Eukalyptus species and its applications as anesthetic, anodyne, antiseptic, astringent, deodorant, diaphoretic, in the international pharmacopeia and marke we were firstly interested, to investigate antifungal effects of eucalyptus extract on *C. albicans* isolates obtained from clinical samples and secondly to compare this with anticacterial effects of this extract against some human pathogenic standard bacteria.

2. Materials and Methods

2.1. Sample preparation

The plant used in this study was purchased from commercial source and based on morphological and botanical descriptions were identified as Eucalyptus *globules* by an expert botanist. The leaves of plant were dried in the shadow under the appropriate conditions, were grinded in a grinder and homogenized to a fine powder and then were maintain at room temperature for further studies.

2.2. Plant extraction

Plant extraction, was carried out using maceration method. For this propose, 10 gr dried powder of the eucalyptus leaf was put in 0.5 lit Erlenmeyer flask containing 100 ml ethanol (96%) and water. The flask content was mixed using a shaker in the room temperature with the speed of 130 rpm for 24 h, and then was filtered from Whatman No. 2. The solvent was separated and concentrated from the extract using a rotary evaporator (Heidolph, Germany), and was dried after being passed from a microbial filter with 0.45 micro meter pores in 60 °C temperature for two days (Saeedi et al., 2012). The obtained extract was wieghted and solved in DSMO solvent and was kept in refrigrator in 4°C until being used in anti-microbial tests. To determine the Maximum Inhibiting Concentration (MIC) of the extracts, was done using dilution method

2.3. Fungal isolates

Fungi isolates were isolated from patients' vaginas referred to the medical center using a sterile swab, by a gynecologist and then were quickly transferred to a sterile falcon tube containing sterile water for further culture and purification. Two solid culture medium including: Sabouraud Dextrose Agar and Sabouraud Dextrose Broth (Merck, Germany) were used for fungal culture and purification. One drop of fungi suspension was spread in a line across over the solid SDA medium in plates. All plates were transferred to an incubator at 37°C and then were examined after 24 hrs incubation. Growth individual colonies were cultured again on the solid medium and fresh colonies were used for purification and identification. Each purified colony was identified according to the standard keys based on morphological critari. Isolates were kept for further studies in -20°C (Otang et al., 2012). To prepare a suspension of fungal spores, a piece of *C. albicans* cultured on Sabouraud Dextrose Agar medium were transferred to liquid physiologic serum and kept in 37°C. After fungi growth in liquid medium, the concentration of fungal suspension was measured using a spectrophotometer (Unico, USA) in 530 µm wavelength. Based on the obtained light absorption, a suspension with a concentration of 10^6 cells/mL was adjusted.

2.4. Bacterial strains

Standard bacteria strains including: *Staphylococcus aureus* ATCC1189, *Shigella dysenteriae,* ATCC1188, *Listeria monocytogenes* ATCC1298, *Vibrio cholera* ATCC1611, *Bacillus cereus* ATCC1015 were used to determine inhibiting effects of eucalyptus extract. After preliminary preparations, a colony of bacteria was cultured in 10 ml Tryptic Soy Broth (TSB, Merck, Germany) medium and was incubated in 37 °C for 18 hrs; then, 100 ml of the fresh grown suspension of each bacterium was transferred to the solid TSB medium and was incubated in 37 °C for 18 hours.

2.5. Preparing McFarland microbial suspension

To prepare a microbial suspension, one day before experiment, a piece of stock culture (solid medium) was transferred to nutrient agar medium (Merck, Germany). After growth of bacterial cells on the surface of culture medium, the surface was washed using a normal salt solution and concentrated microbial suspension was obtained. A drop of bacterial suspension was poured in leaded sterile tubes containing normal saline and its turbidity was measured using a spectrophotometer in 530 µm wavelength and was diluted with normal saline and then the turbidity of a bacterial suspension was equal to the turbidity of 0.5 McFarland suspension. The final concentration of the bacterial suspension was adjusted to 1.5×10^8 CFU.

2.6. The Minimum Inhibitory Concentration (MIC) Method

The minimum inhibitory concentration (MIC), is the lowest concentration of an antibiotic or plant extract that can inhibits the growth of a particular organism as bacteria or fungi. The MIC of eucalyptus extract was determined using broth micro-dilution method. For this proposes, one drop of each bacterial suspension (1.5×10^8 CFU) was added to well of micro-titer plate containing Muller liquid Hinton nutrient medium (MHB). A serial dilution (ppm) of plant extract was done for each bacterial strain. Micro-titer plates were incubated at 37°C and the MIC was recorded after 24 h.

2.7. The Minimum Bacterial Concentration (MBC)

The lowest concentration of plant extract which is able to reduce the viability of the initial bacterial inoculums by ≥99.9% is called MBC. The MBC is complementary to the MIC. MBC was determined by sub-culturing the test dilutions on to a fresh solid medium and incubated further for 18- 24 h. The highest dilution that yielded no bacterial/fungal growth on solid medium was taken as MBC.

2.8. Statistical analysis

The mean values of studied parameters were taken from the measurements of three replicates and the "Standard Error" of the means was calculated. One-way ANOVA was applied to determine the significance of the results between different treatments and then Duncan multiple range tests ($p < 0.05$) were performed. All the statistical analyses were done using the Statistical Package for Social Sciences (SPSS) for Windows (version 18.0).

3. Results and discussion

The result of this study showed that various concentrations of eucalyptus extract can inhibit the growth rate of *Candida albicans* isolates in excremental condition. Increase of plant extract concentration resulted to high growth inhibitory effect on solid medium. Minimum inhibitory concentration was 50 ppm, whereas the maximum inhibiting concentration was 150 ppm (Fig. 1).

The results of investigating the effect of eucalyptus extract on bacteria indicated that eucalyptus extract was able to inhibit growth of all tested bacteria. The maximum inhibiting concentration (MIC) and maximum bacterial concentration (MBC) (MBC) was recorded for *staphylococcus aureus* strain and the minimum inhibitory concentration (MIC) minimum bacterial concentration (MBC) was recorded for *Bacillus cereus* strain, and (Fig. 1).

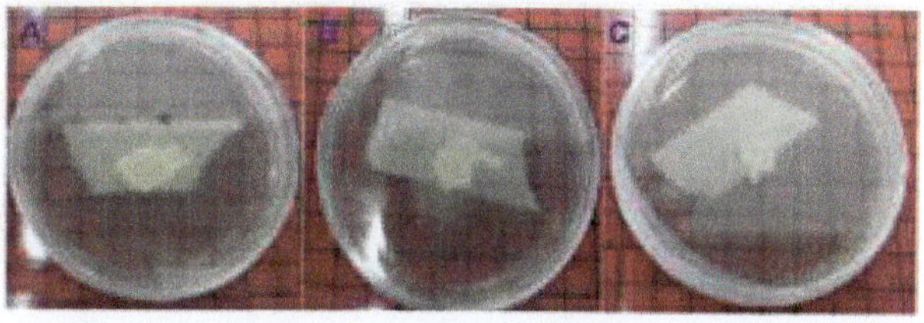

Fig. 1. the control sample of candida albicans in the medium without extract (A): isolate of candida albicans in 100 ppm concentration of eucalyptus essence, (B): isolate of candida albicans in 150 ppm of eucalyptus extract (C).

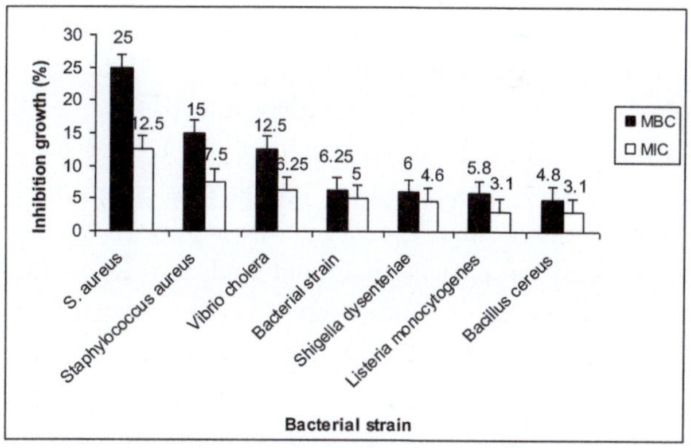

Table 1. The results of minimum inhibiting concentration and minimum bacterial concentration of eucalyptus extract against human pathogenic bacteria.

The growth inhibition effect assay showed that the sensitivity of 30 tested isolates varied from 50-150 ppm of eucalyptus extract. The mean of inhibitory effect of eucalyptus extract was calculated to be 120 ppm.

Although aggressive and systemic fungal diseases are hardly prevalent (2% of the patients), the mortality rate resulting from these infections have been reported to be 26-56 percent. Regarding to, resistance of fungi including different species of Candida to current fungicides, many scientists have been interested to develop new treatment with the least side effects on humans to disease control (Patterson *et al.,* 1996). In recent years, many human pathogenic fungi have been resisted to antibiotics. So, many laboratories have attempted to find alternative drugs. Currently, medicinal plants are one the most appropriate alternative controlling factors. The provenance of medicinal plants using is traditional medicine that has resulted from experimental activities. So, based on these experiments, use of medicinal plants has open up new perspective in order to apply them in pharmaceutical industries for treatment of infectious disease

The present study, investigated the inhibitory effect of eucalyptus extract on *Candida albicans* isolates, as well as its comparative effect on inhibitory of some human pathogenic bacteria. The study of inhibitory effect of two essential oil of eucalyptus and lavender plant on the growth of clinical strains of *Candida albicans* isolated from animals infected by mucosal and cutaneous infections and comparing them with *C. albicans* resistant and sensitive to Itraconazole fungicide showed that the highest effect of Eucalyptus essential oil was at concentrations of 32 and 64 pm while, the highest effect for lavender essential oil was at concentrations of 8-16 ppm. Based on the obtained results of the present study and compared to effective concentrations, of plant extract, these values are lower than the ones for our data. This fact could be resulted from higher permeable nature of essential oil than extract.

Application of eucalyptus extract for male rats having diabetes led to reducing diabetes symptoms and indictors such as hyperglycemia and polyphagia as well as considerably reducing *Candida albicans* in the liquid around kidney and liver (Bokaeian et al., 2010). Uses of medical plants as synthetic medicines and determining their inhibitory effect has been investigated in various plants. The effect of plant extract of *Myrtus communis* as topical ointment application to inhibit the growth of *C. albicans* and comparing its effect with clotrimazole ointment shows that like clotrimazole, *M. communis* extract reduced itching in vaginal area of women having candidacies and this effect is similar to the effect of antibiotics (Genani *et al.,* 2011). Antibacterial effect of essential oil related to 26 species of eucalyptus species on six strains of gram-positive bacteria showed that all species were able to inhibit the growth of bacteria in concentrations of 15-250 ppm under experimental condition, but none of them had any effects on gram-negative bacteria (Takahashi, 1966). In the present study, all gram-positive bacteria showed sensitivity to eucalyptus extract. Seed oil of eucalyptus has fungicide effect on *Fusarium oxysporum* species wich produce canceous toxin in human (Kottearachchi *et al.,* 2012). These results confirm effectiveness of eucalyptus extract in inhibiting the growth of fungi. The results of our research showed that with increase of the extract, the inhibitory effect against fungi and bacteria was increased. The reason for this increase might be the change in effective material of plants due to alterations in plant culture condition and climate and this may consequently affect microorganisms differently. The inhibitory effect of essential oil of Eucalyptus plant on gram-positive bacteria S*taphylococcus aureus* and gram-negative bacteria E*scherichia coli* has been proved (Bachir and Benali, 2012). The result of Saeidi et al's study showed that Eucalyptus extract has considerable MIC in 5 mg/ml against S*taphylococcus aureus* , and the highest amount of MBC is observed in 10 mg/ml concentration (Saeeidi *et al.,* 2014). The minimum inhibitory concentrations of eucalyptus extract against:S. *aureus, B. cereus, E. faecalis, Alicyclobacillus acidoterrestri* and *Propionibacterium acne* were recorded as 3.9, 3.9, 7.8, 31, and 7.8 mg/ml, respectively (Takahashi *et al.,* 2004) which is in accordance with the results of the present study. Findings of another study showed that inhibition zone diameters of ethanolic extract of eucalyptus at concentrations of 5, 7.5, 10 and 20 μl/ml was observed 1.4, 1.9, and 3.2 mm against *staphylococcus aureus* and 1.3, 1.5, 2, and 2.4 mm inhibitory zone against E*scherichia coli* (Ghalem and Mohamed, 2008).

4. Conclusion

It should be noted that during recent years, several reports about resistance of a series of *C. albicans* species-to chemical fungicide have been released. Based on the obtained data in this study, the results indicate that the extract of eucalyptus plays an important role in inhibiting the growth of *C. albicans* isolates and tested bacteria, and thus it can be used as an appropriate alternative for chemical anti-fungal medicine. Performing complementary tests with standard fungal isolates and various species of eucalyptus plants can be effective in introducing proper medicine in pharmaceutical industry.

5. References

Amber, K., Aijaz, A., Immaculata, X., Luqman, K., and Nikhat, M., 2010. Anticandidal effect of Ocimum sanctum essential oil and its synergy with fluconazole and ketoconazole. *Phytomedicine*. 17 (12): 921-925.

Bachir, R.G., and Benali, M., 2012. Antibacterial activity of the essential oils from the leaves of *Eucalyptus globulus* against Escherichia coli and *Staphylococcus aureus*. *Asian Pacific Journal of Tropical Biomedicine*. 2 (9): 739-742.

Baker, R.D., Angulo, O., Barroso-Tobila, C., Carbonell, L.M., Cespedes, R., Chick, E.W., Clark, B.M., Duque, O., Edington, G.M., and Fetter, B.F., 2012, The pathologic anatomy of mycoses: human infection with fungi, actinomycetes and algae, Springer Science & Business Media.

Biyela, P., Lin, J., and Bezuidenhout, C., 2004. The role of aquatic ecosystems as reservoirs of antibiotic resistant bacteria and antibiotic resistance genes. *Water Science & Technology*. 50 (1): 45-50.

Bokaeian, M., Nakhaee, A., Moodi, B., and Khazaei, H.A., 2010. Eucalyptus globulus (eucalyptus) treatment of candidiasis in normal and diabetic rats. *Iranian Biomedical Journal*. 14 (3): 121-129

Cates, W., Rolfs, R.T., and ARAL, S.O., 1990. Sexually transmitted diseases, pelvic inflammatory disease, and infertility: an epidemiologic update. *Epidemiologic Reviews*. 12 (1): 199-220.

Cermelli, C., Fabio, A., Fabio, G., and Quaglio, P., 2008. Effect of eucalyptus essential oil on respiratory bacteria and viruses. *Current Microbiology*. 56 (1): 89-92.

Consolaro, M.L., Albertoni, T.A., Yoshida, C.S., Mazucheli, J., Peralta, R.M., and Svidzinski, T.E., 2004. Correlation of Candida species and symptoms among patients with vulvovaginal candidiasis in Maringá, Paraná, Brazil. *Review Iberoam Micology* 21(4): 202-205.

De Vos, M., Cuenca-Estrella, M., Boekhout, T., Theelen, B., Matthijs, N., Bauters, T., Nailis, H., Dhont, M., Rodriguez-Tudela, J., and Nelis, H., 2005. Vulvovaginal candidiasis in a Flemish patient population. *Clinical Microbiology and Infection*. 11(12): 1005-1011.

Genani, F., Akbari, S., Delfan, B., Tolabi, T., Ebrahim zadeh, and Motamedi, M., 2011. Coamparsion study of effect of Myrtus communis vaginal -cream and clotrmazol on treatment of vaginal candisiosis *Yafteh*. 13(1): 35-43.

Ghalem, B.R., and Mohamed, B., 2008. Antibacterial activity of leaf essential oils of Eucalyptusglobulusand Eucalyptus camaldulensis. *African Journal of Pharmacy and Pharmacology*. 2(10): 211-215.

Ghorbani, F., Panjehkeh, N., Nasrollanejad, S., Salari, M., and Sabagh, S., 2014. Inhibitory effect of essential oils of Eucalyptus sp. and Zataria multiflora on fungal growth of Macrophomina phaseolina. *Archives of Phytopathology and Plant Protection*. 47(19): 2410-2413.

Gilles, M., Zhao, J., An, M., and Agboola, S., 2010. Chemical composition and antimicrobial properties of essential oils of three Australian Eucalyptus species. *Food Chemistry*. 119(2): 731-737.

Giraldo, P., von Nowaskonski, A., Gomes, F.A., Linhares, I., Neves, N.A., and Witkin, S.S., 2000. Vaginal colonization by Candida in asymptomatic women with and without a history of recurrent vulvovaginal candidiasis. *Obstetrics & Gynecology*. 95(3): 413-416.

Goswami, R., Dadhwal, V., Tejaswi, S., Datta, K., Paul, A., Haricharan, R., Banerjee, U., and Kochupillai, N., 2000. Species-specific prevalence of vaginal candidiasis among patients with diabetes mellitus and its relation to their glycaemic status. *Journal of Infection*. 41(2): 162-166.

Hammer, K.A., Carson, C., and Riley, T., 1999. Antimicrobial activity of essential oils and other plant extracts. *Journal of Applied Microbiology*. 86(5): 985-990.

Hay, R., and Ashbee, H., 2010. Mycology. *Rook's Textbook of Dermatology, Eighth Edition*.1-93.

Hoehamer, C.F., Cummings, E.D., Hilliard, G.M., and Rogers, P.D., 2010. Changes in the proteome of Candida albicans in response to azole, polyene, and echinocandin antifungal agents. *Antimicrobial Agents and Chemotherapy*. 54: 1655-1664.

Kottearachchi, N.S., Sammani, A., Kelaniyangoda, D.B., and Samarasekara, R., 2012. Anti-fungal activity of essentialoils of Ceylon Eucalyptus species for the control of Fusarium solaniandSclerotiumrolfsii. *Phytopathology and Plant Protection*. 45(3): 2026-2035.

Levy, S.B., 1998. The challenge of antibiotic resistance. *Scientific American*. 278: 32-39.

Maciel, M., Morais, S., Bevilaqua, C., Silva, R., Barros, R., Sousa, R., Sousa, L., Brito, E., and Souza-Neto, M., 2010. Chemical composition of Eucalyptus spp. essential oils and their insecticidal effects on Lutzomyia longipalpis. *Veterinary Parasitology*. 167(1): 1-7.

Mathema, B., Cross, E., Dun, E., Park, S., Bedell, J., Slade, B., Williams, M., Riley, L., Chaturvedi, V., and Perlin, D.S., 2001. Prevalence of vaginal colonization by drug-resistant Candida species in college-age women with previous exposure to over-the-counter azole antifungals. *Clinical Infectious Diseases*. 33(5): e23-e27.

Merenstein, D., Hu, H., Wang, C., Hamilton, P., Blackmon, M., Chen, H., Calderone, R., and Li, D., 2013. Colonization by Candida species of the oral and vaginal mucosa in HIV-infected and noninfected women. *AIDS Research and Human Retroviruses*. 29(1): 30-34.

Moosa, M.-Y.S., Sobel, J.D., Elhalis, H., Du, W., and Akins, R.A., 2004. Fungicidal Activity of Fluconazole against Candida albicans in a Synthetic Vagina-Simulative Medium. *Antimicrobial Agents and Chemotherapy*. 48(1): 161-167.

Neo, H., 2011. Worlds of food: Place, power, and provenance in the food chain. *Asian Journal of Social Science*. 39(3): 409-410.

Noumi, E., Snoussi, M., Hajlaoui, H., Trabelsi, N., Ksouri, R., Valentin, E., and Bakhrouf, A., 2011. Chemical composition, antioxidant and antifungal potential of Melaleuca alternifolia (tea tree) and Eucalyptus globulus essential oils against oral Candida species. *Journal of Medicinal Plants Research*. 5(17): 4147-4156.

Otang, W.M., Grierson, D.S., and Ndip, R., 2012. Ethnobotanical survey of medicinal plants used in the management of opportunistic fungal infections in HIV/AIDS patients in the Amathole District of the Eastern Cape Province, South Africa. *Journal of Medicinal Plnat Research. 6 (11): 2071*. 2080.

Patterson, T.F., Revankar, S.G., Kirkpatrick, W.R., Dib, O., Fothergill, A.W., Redding, S.W., Sutton, D.A., and Rinaldi, M.G., 1996. Simple method for detecting fluconazole-resistant yeasts with chromogenic agar. *Journal of Clinical Microbiology*. 34(7): 1794-1797.

Pinto, R.J., Marques, P.A., Neto, C.P., Trindade, T., Daina, S., and Sadocco, P., 2009. Antibacterial activity of nanocomposites of silver and bacterial or vegetable cellulosic fibers. *Acta Biomaterialia*. 5(6): 2279-2289.

Saeedi, S., SABBAGH, S., and SABORI, R.E., 2012. A Study of antibacterial activity of plant extract and essential oil of Myrtus communis against resistant strains of *Staphyloccocus aureus* bacteria to selective antibiotics. Rostamineh. 4(1): 21-32.

Saeeidi, S., Sabbagh, S.K., and Bazi, S., 2014. Antibacterila Effect of Eucalyptus globules Againts Resistance Staphyloccocus aureus. 5(4): 50-58.

Schuster, M.G., Edwards, J.E., Sobel, J.D., Darouiche, R.O., Karchmer, A.W., Hadley, S., Slotman, G., Panzer, H., Biswas, P., and Rex, J.H., 2008. Empirical fluconazole versus placebo for intensive care unit patients: a randomized trial. *Annals of Internal Medicine*. 149(2): 83-90.

Takahashi, E., 1966. Effect of silicon on resistance of rice to radiation. *Jpn J Soil Sci Plant Nutr*. 37: 183-188.

Takahashi, T., Kokubo, R., and Sakaino, M., 2004. Antimicrobial activities of eucalyptus leaf extracts and flavonoids from Eucalyptus maculata. *Letters in Applied Microbiology*. 39(1): 60-64.

Wilson, C., Solar, J., El Ghaouth, A., and Wisniewski, M., 1997. Rapid evaluation of plant extracts and essential oils for antifungal activity against Botrytis cinerea. *Plant Disease*. 81(2): 204-210.

The comparison of antibacterial effect of *Schrophularia striata Boiss.* and *Stachys schtschegleevii Sosn.* extracts on pathogens isolated from urinary tract infections

Somayeh Azami[1*] , Bijan Fahimi[1], Mehdi Bagheri[2], Shabnam Mohsenzadeh[3]

[1]*Department of Laboratory Sciences, Faculty of Medical Sciences, Shahrood Branch, Islamic Azad University, Shahrood, Iran;* [*]**Email:** *azamis@iau-shahrood.ac.ir*

[2]*Research Committee, Semnan University of Medical Sciences, Semnan, Iran;*

[3]*International Jolfa Branch, Islamic Azad University, Jolfa, Iran;*

ARTICLE INFO

Topic: *Medicinal Plants*

Key words:

- ✓ *Antibacterial activity*
- ✓ *MIC*
- ✓ *MBC*
- ✓ *Schrophularia striata*
- ✓ *Stachys schtschegleevii*

ABSTRACT

Background & Aim: The present study was aimed to evaluate and compare the antibacterial activity of *Schrophularia striata Boiss.* and*Stachys schtschegleevii Sosn.* Extracts against seven clinical isolates. The test isolates were *Streptococcus agalactiae, Enterococcus faecalis, Staphylococcus saprophyticus, E. coli, Klebsiella pneumoniae, Proteus mirabilis and Enterobacter dissolvens. E. coli* (ATCC 25922) and *S.aureus* (ATCC 29213) were used as quality control strains.

Experimental: Clinical isolates were identified using standard microbiological methods.The methanol extracts from the aerial parts of these plants were assessed using agar well diffusion and broth microdilution methods. Considering the wide application of ciprofloxacin in treatment of Urinary Tract Infections (UTIs), susceptibility test was performed towards antibiotic.

Results & Discussion: The methanol extracts of *Schrophularia striata* and *Stachys schtschegleevii* exhibit both high bacteriostatic and bactericidal activities. The Minimum Inhibitory and Bactericidal Concentration (MIC and MBC) values of *Schrophularia striata* extract ranged between 0.39-12.5 mg/ml and 0.78-25 mg/ml, respectively. The extract of *Stachys schtschegleevii* was effective in MIC and MBC ranges of 1.56-12.5 mg/ml and 3.12-50 mg/ml, respectively. On comparing the efficiency of the two extracts, *Stachys schtschegleevii* extract exhibited the highest activity against gram-negative bacteria, whereas, the extract of *Schrophularia striata* inhibited the growth of *Streptococcus agalactiae* and *Staphylococcus* spp.

Industrial and practical recommendations: On considering antibacterial activity of both the extracts, these herbal extracts may treat urinary tract infections caused by some of the test isolates.

1. Introduction

The genus Scrophularia (Schrophulariaceae) comprises about 200 species of flowering plants, commonly known as 'figwort (GRIN, 2011) which are widely distributed in the world, especially in the Mediterranean area (Amiri *et al.*, 2011). In traditional medicines, some species of the genus have been found to possess antibacterial, antifungal (Fernandez *et al.*, 1996; Ahmad *et al.*, 2012a; Tasdemir *et al.*, 2008), antitumor (Tasdemir *et al.*, 2008; Garcia *et al.*, 1998), anti-inflammatory (Diaz *et al.*, 2004), diuretic and cardiac stimulant activities (Ahmad *et al.*, 2012b), and have been used in the treatment of gastrointestinal disorders (Loi *et al.*, 2005). Scrophularia genus contains biologically active compounds, e.g., irridoids, irridoids glycosides (Miyase and Mimatsu, 1999; Boros and Stermitz, 1990; Stevenson *et al.*, 2002), phenylpropanoids and terpenoids (Monsef-Esfahani *et al.*, 2010).

Another medicinal plant considered in this study, *Stachys schtschegleevii Sosn.* (Lamiaceae), is one of the 34 Iranian Stachys species (Rechinger, 1982; Mozaffarian, 1996). This plant (traditionally named poulk), has been used in infectious, rheumatic, inflammatory and respiratory diseases (Rezazadeh *et al.*, 2005). The antibacterial property of the essential oil and methanol extract obtained from the leaves of *Stachys schtschegleevii* has been assessed (Sonboli *et al.*, 2005; Abichandani *et al.*, 2010). Phytochemical studies on this plant revealed the presence of phenolic compounds (Nazemiyeh *et al.*, 2006), and terpenoids (Sonboli *et al.*, 2005; Norouzi-Arasi *et al.*, 2004).

In respect of high resistance of nosocomial isolates responsible for urinary tract infections (UTIs) to antibiotics, introducing of the new antimicrobial agents is critical in treatment of such infections. UTI is one of the most common infectious diseases worldwide. Moreover, UTIs account for 35- 45% of the nosocomial infections (Kamat *et al.*, 2009). *Escherichia coli* is the most frequent pathogen in acute infections (Beyene and Tsegaye, 2011; Amin *et al.*, 2011). In this study we evaluated and compared the antibacterial activity of methanol extracts of *Scrophularia striata* and *Stachys schtschegleevii* against some of bacterial uropathogens.

2. Materials and Methods

2.1. Plant materials

Schrophularia striata Boiss. and *Stachys schtschegleevii Sosn.* were collected from Shahvar mountain and the Abr Forest (Shahrood, Semnan province, Iran) in April 2014. Voucher specimens (No. 582 and 673) were deposited at the Herbarium of the Research Center for Agriculture and Natural Resources (Shahrood).

2.2. Preparation of the extracts

The aerial parts of these plants washed, dried and powdered (40g). Methanol extracts (200 ml) were concentrated in rotary evaporator (Heidolph, Germany) at 45 ℃ for 30 min. The dried extracts were stored at refrigerator. Extracts were resuspended in dimethyl sulphoxide (DMSO), (Merck, Germany) to achieve the stock concentration 250 mg/ml. The stock solutions were sterilized using 0.22 μm filters.

2.3. Bacterial isolates

Seven bacterial uropathogens including *Streptococcus agalactiae, Enterococcus faecalis, Staphylococcus saprophyticus, E. coli, Klebsiella pneumoniae, Proteus mirabilis, Enterobacter dissolvens* and standard strains *E. coli* (ATCC 25922) and *Staphylococcus aureus* (ATCC 29213) were used to assess the antibacterial activity of both the plant extracts. Pathogens were isolated from midstream urine samples of hospitalized patients in Imam Hossein hospital of Shahrood. Urine samples were cultured on 5% blood agar, MacConkey, and Eosin-Methylene blue (EMB) agar (Merck, Germany) using calibrated loops for semi-quantitative method (Beyene and Tsegaye, 2011) and incubated for 24 h at 37℃. Samples with colony count $\geq 10^5$ CFU/ml were considered positive. The isolates were identified using standard microbiological methods (Cheesbrough, 2002).

2.4. Antibacterial assay

2.4.1. Well diffusion method

The well diffusion method was applied to screen preliminary antibacterial activity of methanol extracts (Perez *et al.*, 1990). Using a sterile cotton swab bacterial suspensions (1.5×10^8 CFU/ml adjusted to 0.5 McFarland turbidity standard) were inoculated onto the Mueller-Hinton agar (Merck, Germany) plates. Four wells of 8 mm diameter were punched into the agar plates using a sterile well cutter. Three wells were filled with 50μl each of the extracts dissolved in DMSO (50mg/ml). The fourth well was filled with

50µl Ciprofloxacin (10µg/ml), which served as the standard drug. *E. coli* (ATCC 25922) and *S. aureus* (ATCC29213) were used as quality control strains. The plates were allowed on the bench for 50min for prediffusion of the extracts and incubated overnight at 37̊C. The experiment was carried out in triplicates and the mean zones of inhibition were regarded as antibacterial activity. All results are expressed as mean ± standard deviation.

2.4.2. Broth microdilution method

Minimum Inhibitory and Bactericidal Concentrations (MIC and MBC) were evaluated according to Clinical and Laboratory Standards Institute (CLSI) guidelines. Different concentrations of the extracts were prepared as follows: 100, 50, 25, 12.5, 6.25, 3.12, 1.56 and 0.78 mg/ml. The initial concentration of ciprofloxacin in the first well was 500 µg/ml. The experiment was carried out in triplicate. The isolates containing MBC values 4 µg/ml or more were regarded to be resistant to ciprofloxacin (Chaudhry *et al.,* 1999).

3. Results and discussion

In well diffusion assay, the extract of *Stachys schtschegleevii* was most active against *S. saprophyticus* (19.36 ± 0.32 mm) while for other isolates the inhibitory zones of extract ranged from 10.6-18 mm, approximately. *S. striata* extract exhibited less inhibitory zones on gram-negative isolates (about 8.8-10.23 mm) when compared to another extract (Table 1).

The methanol extracts of *Schrophularia striata* and *Stachys schtschegleevii* exhibited both high bacteriostatic and bactericidal activities (Table 1). In comparison to *Schrophularia striata* extract, *Stachys schtschegleevii* extract showed the greatest antibacterial effect on *E. coli* and *Enterobacter dissolvens* among gram-negative uropathogens (MIC range 1.56-6.25 mg/ml). Bacteriostatic property of *Stachys schtschegleevii* extract against gram-negative bacteria was significant. The extract of *Schrophularia striata* inhibited the growth of *S. agalactiae* and *Staphylococcus* spp. rather than other isolates (MIC values 0.39-3.12 mg/ml). According to results, *S. saprophyticus* was the most sensitive isolate towards both extracts. The higher MIC values of *Schrophularia striata* extract (6.25-12.5 mg/ml) were found to inhibit the growth of *E. faecalis* and gram-negative isolates. The highest MIC value for ciprofloxacin was 256 µg/ml against *E. coli*. All the clinical isolates were resistant to ciprofloxacin (MBC ≥ 4 µg/ml).

Our results are partially in agreement with previous ones which have proved the antibacterial effects of *Schrophularia striata* and *Stachys schtschegleevii* (Abichandani *et al.,* 2010; Mikaili*et al.,* 2011). The antibacterial property of *Stachys schtschegleevii* extract obtained from the leaves and stems has been known. The methanol extract was the most potent among the extracts and the most active against ampicillin-resistant *E. coli* (MIC =1.56 mg/ml), (Abichandani *et al.,* 2010). In our study *Stachys schtschegleevii* extract showed the greatest antibacterial effect on *E.coli* and *Enterobacter dissolvens* (MIC range 1.56-6.25 mg/ml), so this plant extract might be used to treat UTIs.

In another study, the bioactivity of the oil of *Stachys schtschegleevii* considered by Sonboli *et al.* (2005) indicated moderate effect on gram-positive bacteria. *S. aureus* was the most sensitive. Whereas gram-negative bacteria, except for *E. coli* were resistant at the concentrations of the oil used (15ml/disc). Similarly, in another study on the antibacterial activity of four Stachys species from Iran, methanol extracts were found to be more active against gram-positive bacteria (Saeedi *et al.,* 2008). Antimicrobial activity of Stachys species can be attributed to presence of monoterpenes such α-pinene as destroys the cellular integrity of gram-positive bacteria, but gram-negative ones are more resistant (Andrew *et al.,* 1980).

In a research, the antibacterial activity of leaf extract of *Schrophularia striara* was assessed against *E. coli* using microdilution method. In contrast with our study, the MIC and MBC values towards *E. coli* ranged between 32.1 µg/ml and 39 µg/ml (Bahrami and Valadi, 2010). In our study, MIC and MBC of *Schropularia striata* extract on *E. coli* were 6.25 and 12.5 mg/ml, respectively. The extract of *Schrophularia striata* inhibited the growth of *S. agalactiae* and *Staphylococcus* spp. rather than other isolates (MIC values 0.39-3.12 mg/ml). The extract to concentration of 0.39 mg/ml had greatest inhibition of growth against *S. saprophyticus*. The highest concentration of used extract was 12.5 mg/ml against *Klebsiella pneumoniae, Proteus mirabilis and Enterobacter dissolvens*.

Table 1. Antibacterial activity of *Schrophularia striata* and *Stachys schtschegleevii* extracts.

M.O	*S. schtschegleevii* extract			*S. striata* extract			CP
	IZ (mm)	MIC (mg/ml)	MBC	IZ (mm)	MIC (mg/ml)	MBC	MIC (µg/ml)
E.c1	12.7 ± 0.45	1.56	3.12	9.26 ± 0.25	6.25	12.5	256
K.p	10.6 ± 0.11	12.5	50	8.8 ± 0.55	12.5	25	128
P.m	11.26 ± 0.25	12.5	25	10.23 ±0.25	12.5	25	8
E.d	14.6 ± 0.3	6.25	12.5	9.61 ± 0.36	12.5	25	64
E.c2	10.4 ± 0.1	3.12	6.25	10.21 ± 1.24	6.25	12.5	0.008
S.sa	19.36 ± 0.32	1.56	3.12	16.2 ± 0.52	0.39	0.78	4
E.f	15.16 ± 0.2	6.25	12.5	11.9 ± 0.52	6.25	6.25	16
S.a	18 ± 0.88	3.12	6.25	14.23 ± 0.15	0.78	3.12	NA
S.au	15.53 ± 1.47	3.12	6.25	16.34 ± 0.65	3.12	6.25	0.31

M.O: Microorganism; *E.c1: E. coli; K.p: Klebsiellapneumoniae; P.m: Proteus mirabilis; E.d: Enterobacterdissolvens; E.c2: E.coli* (ATCC 25922); *S.s: Staphylococcus saprophyticus; E.f: Enterococcus faecalis; S.a: Streptococcus agalactiae; S.au: Staphylococcus aureus* (ATCC 29213); IZ: inhibition zone (mean ± SD). The experiment was carried out in triplicate. CP: Ciprofloxacin; NA: Not applicable.

The study on antibacterial activity of the methanol extract of root and aerial part of *Schrophularia striata* was evaluated against *S. aureus*, *E. coli* and *Bacillus cereus* using disc diffusion method. The most effective one was methanolic extract of root against *B. cereus* (inhibition zone = 21 mm), (Safavi *et al.*, 2012). Other species of the genus Scrophularia have also been shown to have antibacterial activity (Ahmad *et al.*, 2012a; Tasdemir *et al.*, 2008; Stavri *et al.*, 2006).

Since *Schrophularia striata* and *Stachys schtschegleevii* appear to be most promising, bioassay-guided fractionation which can elucidate their active antibacterial compounds. The antimicrobial activity of *Stachys schtschegleevii* is in relation to the presence of polar compounds, e.g. flavonoids and phenylethanoid glycosides (caffeic acid derivatives), (Saeedi *et al.*, 2008). Moreover the studies on Scrophularia genus have shown flavonoids and terpenoids, e.g., caryophyllene, phytol, linalool which are common and responsible for various pharmacological activities in this genus (Pasdaran *et al.*, 2013). Other studies reveal that the components of both Stachys and Scrophularia genera are responsible for their therapeutic effects, particularly in bacterial infections and inflammation (Azadmehr *et al.*, 2013; Valiyari *et al.*, 2012). The studies indicate that *E. coli* is still the most common cause of UTIs in Iran (Ranjbar *et al.*, 2009). In addition, coagulase negative *Staphylococcus* spp. are prevalent cause of UTI among gram-positive bacteria (Huebner and Goldmann, 1999). Our study results support traditional uses of these medicinal plants in the treatment of UTIs. As UTIs being a major part of the nosocomial infections, these herbal extracts may treatment acute infection caused by some of the test isolates.

4. Conclusion

In this study, the antibacterial effect of *Stachys schtschegleevii* and *Scrophularia striata* extracts were determined on some of prevalent uropathogens. On considering antibacterial activity of both the extracts, *Stachys schtschegleevii* extract was found to exhibit more activity against gram-negative uropathogens than *Schrophularia striata* extract while the *Schrophularia striata* extract inhibited the growth of *S. agalactiae* and *Staphylococcus* spp to the large extent. These Iranian native plants can be used as an antiseptic agent to eliminate bacterial uropathogens.

5. Acknowledgement

The authors are thankful to Faculty of Medical Sciences, Shahrood Branch, Azad University for providing the facilities carry out the present research work.

6. References

Abichandani, M., Nahar, L., Singh, P., Chitnis, R., Nazemiyeh, H., Delazar, A., Sarker, S.D. 2010. Antibacterial and free-radical-scavenging properties of *Stachys schtschegleevii* (Lamiaceae). *Archives of Biological Science,* 62: 941-945.

Ahmad, M., Muhammad, N., Mehjabeen, Jahan, N., Alam, S.M., Ahmad, M., Obaidullah. 2012a. Biological screening of *Scrophularia nodosa* extract and its fractions. *Pakistan Journal of Pharmaceutical Sciences,* 25: 307-313.

Ahmad, M., Muhammad, N., Mehjabeen, Jahan, N., Ahmad, M., Obaidullah, Qureshi, M., Jan, S.U. 2012b. Spasmolytic effects of *Scrophularia nodosa* extract on isolated rabbit intestine. *Pakistan Journal of Pharmaceutical Sciences,* 25: 267-275.

Amin, M., Mehdinejad, M., Pourdangchi, Z. 2011. Study of bacteria isolated from Urinary Tract Infections and determination of their susceptibility to antibiotics. *Jundishapour Journal of Microbiology,* 2: 118-123.

Amiri, H, Lari, Y.H, Esmaeili, A, Samsamnia, F, Eghbali, D., Viskarami, G. 2011. Essential oil composition and anatomical study of *Scrophularia striata* Boiss. *Iranian Journal of Medicinal and Aromatic Plants,* 27: 271-278.

Andrews, R.E., Parks, L.W. and Spence, K.D. 1980. Some effects of Douglas fir terpenes on certain microorganisms. *Applied Environmental Microbiology,* 40: 301-304.

Azadmehr, A., Hajiaghaee, R., Zohal, M.A and Maliji, G. 2013. Protective effects of *Scrophularia striata* in Ovalbumin-induced mice asthma model. *DARU Journal of Pharmaceutical Sciences,* 21(1):56.

Bahrami, A.M., Valadi, A. 2010. Effects of *Scrophulari astriata* ethanolic leaves extracts on *Staphylococcus aureus*. *International Journal of Pharmacology,* 6: 431-434.

Baron, E.J, Finegold S.M. 1990. *Bailey and Scotts Diagnostic Microbiology.* 8th ed., St. Louis, C.V. Mosbey Co.

Bhandari, S.P.S., Roy, A., Agrawal, P.K. 1996. Scrokoelziside A, a triterpene glycoside from *Scrophulariakoelzii*. *Phytochemistry,*41:879-882.

Boros, C.A., Stermitz, F.R. 1990.Iridoids. An updated review. Part I. *Journal of Natural Products,* 53:1055-1147.

Beyene, G., Tsegaye, W. 2011. Bacterial uropathogens in Urinary Tract Infection and antibiotic susceptibility pattern in Jimma university specialized hospital, southwest Ethiopia. *Ethiopian Journal of Health Sciences,* 21: 14.1-146.

Chaudhry, N.A., Flynn, H.W.J., Murray, T.G., Tabandeh, H., Mello, M.O.J., Miller, D. 1999. Emerging ciprofloxacin-resistant *Pseudomonas aeruginosa*. *American Journal of Ophtalmology,* 128:509-510.

Cheesbrough, M. 2002. District laboratory practice in tropical countries, vol. 2. E.C.B.S edition. Cambridge University Press. pp 97-182.

Diaz, A.M., Abad, M.J., Fernandez, L., Silvan, A.M., Desantos, J., Bermejo, P. 2004. Phenylpropanoid glycosides from *Schrophularia scordonia*: In vitro anti-inflammatory activity. *Life Sciences,*74:2515-2526.

Fernandez, M.A., Garcia, M.D., Sachz, M.T. 1996. Antibacterial activity of phenolic acids fraction of *Scrophularia furtescens* and *Scrophularia sambucifolia*. *Journal of Ethnopharmacology,* 53: 11-14.

Garcia, M.D., Ahumada, M.C., Saenz, M.T. 1998. Cytostatic activity of some phenolic acids of *Scrophularia frutescens* L. var. frutescens. *Zeitschrift Naturforschung,* 53:1093-1095.

Germplasm Resources Information Network (GRIN), 2011. UnitedStates Department of Agriculture, Agriculture Research Service, Beltsville Area, USA. Available on Internet at: http://www.ars-grin.gov/cgi-bin/npgs/html/splist.pl?11000.

Huebner, J., Goldmann, D.A. 1999. Coagulase-negative staphylococci: role as pathogens. *Annual Review of Medicine,* 50: 223-236.

Kamat, U.S., Fereirra, A., Amonkar, D., Motghare, D.D. andKulkarni, M.S. 2009. Epidemiology of hospital acquired Urinary Tract Infections in a medical college hospital in Goa. *Indian Journal of Urology,* 25: 76-80.

Loi, M.C., Maxia, L., Maxia, A. 2005. Ethno-botanical comparison between the villages of Escolca and Lotzorai (Saridinia, Italy). *Journal of Herbs, Spices & Medicinal plants,* 11:67-84.

Mikaili, P., Jazani, N.H., Shayegh, J., Haghighi, N., Aghamohammadi, N., Zartoshti, M. 2011. The aerial parts of *Stachys schtschegleevii Sosn.* as hydroalcoholic extract has antibacterial activity on multi-drug resistant isolates in comparison to ciprofloxacin. *Journal of American Science,* 7:754-759.

Miyase, T., Mimatsu, A. 1999. Acetylated iridoid and phenylethanoid glycosides from the aerial parts of *Scrophularianodosa. Journal of Natural Products,* 62: 1079-1084.

Monsef-Esfahani, H.R., Hajiaghaee, R., Shahverdi, A.R. 2010. Flavonoids, cininamic acid and phenylpropanoid from aerial parts of *Scrophulariastriata. Pharmaceutical Biology,* 48: 333-336.

Mozaffarian, V. 1996. *A dictionary of Iranian plant names,* Farhang Moaser Press.pp 522.

Nazemiyeh, H., Shoeb, M., Movahhedin, N., Kumarasamy, Y., Talebpour, M., Delazar, A., Nahar, L., Sarker, SD. 2006. Phenolic compounds and their glycosides from*Stachys schtschegleevii* (Lamiaceae). *Biochemical Systematics and Ecology,* 34:721-723.

Norouzi-Arasi, H., Yavari, I. andAlibabaeii, M. 2004. Chemical constituents of the essential oil of *Stachys schtschegleevii Sosn.* from Iran. *Journalof Essential Oil Research,* 16:231-232.

Pasdaran, A., Nahar, L., Asnaashari, S., Sarker, S.D., Delazar, A. 2013. GC-MS analysis, free-radical-scavenging and insecticidal activities of essential oil of *Scrophularia oxysepala* Boiss. *Pharmaceutical Sciences,* 19:1-5.

Perez, C., Pauli, M., Bazerque, P. 1990. An antibacterial assay by agar well diffusion method. *Acta Biochimica et Medicine Experimental,* 15:113-115.

Ranjbar, R., Haghi-Ashtiani, M., Jafari, N.J., Abedini, M. 2009. The prevalence and antimicrobial susceptibility of bacterial uropathogens isolated from pediatric patients. *Iranian Journal of Public Health,* 38: 134-138.

Rechinger, K.H. 1982. *Stachys* L. In: Rechinger KH (Ed) Flora Iranica, Akademische Druck Verlags Antalt Graz, Austria, pp. 354-396.

Rezazadeh, S., Kebryaeezadeh, A., Pirali-Hamedani, M., Shafiee, A. andIsfahani, S.G. 2005. Anti-inflammatory and analgesic activity of methanolic extracts of aerial parts of *Stachys schtschegleevii Sosn., Stachys balansae* Boiss. and *Kotschy ex* Boiss. in rats. *DARU Journal of Pharmaceutical Sciences,* 13:165-169.

Saeedi, M., Morteza-Semnani, K., Mahdavi, M.R., Rahimi, F. 2008. Antimicrobial studies on extract of four species of Stachys. *Indian Journal of Pharmaceutical Sciences,* 70: 403-406.

Safavi, F., Meighani, H., Ebrahimi, P., Hafez, G.S. 2012. Antioxidant and antibacterial activity of *Scrophulariastriata. Researchin Pharmaceutical Sciences,* 7, S: 852.

Sonboli, A., Salehi, P., Ebrahimi, S.N. 2005. Essential oil composition and antibacterial activity of the leaves of *Stachys schtschegleevii* from Iran. *Chemistryof Natural Compounds,* 41:171-174.

Stavri, M., Mathew, K.T., Gibbons, S. 2006. Antimicrobial constituents of *Scrophulariadeserti. Phytochemistry,* 67:1530-1533.

Stevenson, P.C., Simmonds, M.S., Sampson, J., Houghton, P.J., Grice, P. 2002. Wound healing activity of acylatediridoid glycosides from *Scrophularianodosa. Phytotherapy Research,* 16: 33-35.

Tasdemir, D., Burn, R., Franzbla, S.G., Sezgin, Y., Calis, L. 2008. Evaluation of antiprotozoal and antimycobacterial activities of the resin glycosides and the other methabolities of *Scrophularia cryptophila. Phytomedicine,* 15: 209-215.

Valiyari, S., Baradaran, B., Delazar, A., Pasdaran A., Zare, F. 2012. Dichloromethane and methanol extracts of *Scrophularia oxysepala* induces apoptosis in MCF-7 human breast cancer cells. *Advance Pharmaceutical Bulletin,* 2: 223-231.

Antibacterial activities of *Stachys lavandulifolia* Vahl. extract against eight bacteria

Ziba Fooladvand*, Bahman Fazeli-nasab

Center of Agricultural Biotechnology and Center of Agricultural Research, University of Zabol, Zabol, Iran;

***Email:** *zibafooladvand83@gmail.com**

ARTICLE INFO

***Topic:** Ethnopharmacology*

Key words:

- ✓ Stachys lavandulifolia
- ✓ *Extract plant*
- ✓ *Antibacterial activity*
- ✓ *Human pathogenic*

ABSTRACT

Background & Aim: Interest in alternative medicine and plant-derived medications that affect the "mind" is growing. *Stachys lavandulifolia Vahl* subsp. *lavandulifolia* (Lamiaceae) is widely used in south Anatolia as herbal tea. It is used for the treatment of gastrointestinal and respiratory disorders. The aim of the present study was to investigate the effects of the hydro-alcoholic extract of *Stachys lavanduifolia* Vahl against eight bacteria.

Experimental: The present study was done to determine the antimicrobial activity and minimum inhibitory concentration (MIC) of extract *Stachys lavandulifolia* against human pathogenic bacteria. The antimicrobial effect of ethanolic extracts of *Stachys lavandulifolia* was determined using a deep-well broth micro dilution method on commercially available bacterial strains.

Results: The result indicated that the MICs were observed ranges from 25 to 100 ppm for antibacterial activity of the extract from *S. lavandulifolia* against eight bacteria. The least MIC value was observed against *P. mirabilis* and *E. faecalis.*

Recommended applications/industries: It suggests that the extract from *Stachys lavanduifolia* might be a promising approach for developing new anti-bacterial drugs.

1. Introduction

The genus *Stachys* (Lamiaceae) includes about 200 to 300 species in the world In Iran, 34 species of this genus are present among which, 13 are endemic (Mozaffarian, 1996). *Stachys* species are traditionally used in different conditions: headache, neuralgia, nervous conditions, as tonic at dyspepsia and for treating wounds and skin inflammation as astringent and antidiarrheal (Grieve, 1971). In pharmacological studies, *Stachys* species showed variety of effects, including: anti-inflammatory (Khanavi *et al.,* 2005), antibacterial (Skaltsa *et al*., 1999; Skaltsa *et al*., 2003) anti-nephritic (Hayashi *et al*., 1994), and anxiolitic (Rabbani *et al*., 2003).

Investigators reported that the extracts or constituents of plants belonging to the genus *Stachys* exert significant anti-inflammatory, antitoxic (Zinchenko *et al*., 1981), antihepatitis (Savchenko, *et al*., 1978), antibacterial (Skaltsa *et al*., 1999), anti-anoxia (Yamahara *et al*., 1990) and anti-nephritic (Hayashi *et al*., 1994) effects. As active principals phenylethanoid glycosides (Nishimura *et al.,* 1991; Miyase *et al.*, 1996) triterpenoids, steroids (Ross *et al.,* 1975; Yamahara *et al.,* 1990), and flavonoids (Zinchenko and Farm, 1970; EL-Ansari *et al.,* 1991) were identified in the genus *Stachys*. The present study was done to determine the inhibitory concentrations of *Stachys lavandulifolia* Vahl extracted against pathogenic bacteria.

2. Materials and methods

2.1. Preparation extracts

Plant material was dried at 35 °C for three days. After drying, the material was ground within industrial grinder. Sample was submerged in 100 ml of 96% ethanol and left to macerate for seven days, after maceration the plant material was filtered and 100 ml 96% ethanol was added to the water extracts to allow faster solvent removal. The solvent was evaporated to complete dryness using a standard Buchi rotary-evaporator. The resulting dry extracts were re-suspended in 5 ml distilled water. In order to determine the real concentration of each extract, 1 ml of previous homogenization of the respective extracts was removed and again completely oven-dried and then weighed to determine amount of extract per ml of final solution. The remaining extract was used for MIC assays.

2.2. Agar disk diffusion assay

The susceptibility of all antibiotics was done using disc diffusion method on Muller-Hinton agar as recommended by CLSI (2012). The procedure followed is briefly described here. *Streptococcus pyogenes* ATCC® 19615™, *Streptococcus pneumoniae* ATCC 49619, *S. saprophyticus* ATCC®1535, *Hafnia alvei* ATCC 51873, *Acinetobacter.* *baumannii* ATCC 19606, *Enterococcus faecalis* ATCC 29212, *Proteus mirabilis* ATCC 35659, and *Serratia marcescens* ATCC 274 plates were grown overnight on blood agar. Nutrient agar and colony suspension was prepared using the sterile saline water equivalent to a 0.5 McFarland standard. Suspension (100 µl) was spread over the media plate and antibiotic disc was transferred aseptically on the surface of inoculated media plate. Isolated plates were tested with different antibiotics and their concentration shown in parenthesis viz. ceftazidim (30 µg), erythromycin (15 µg), ceftazidime (30 µg), and tetracyclin (30 µg).

2.3. Antimicrobial assays

Streptococcus *pyogenes* ATCC® 19615™, *Streptococcus pneumoniae* ATCC 49619, *Staphylococcus saprophyticus* ATCC®15305, *Hafnia alvei* ATCC 51873, *Acinetobacte baumannii* ATCC 19606, *Enterococcus faecalis* ATCC 29212, *Proteus mirabilis* ATCC 35659, and *Serratia marcescens* ATCC 274 were used and was sub-cultured on Nutrient agar (Oxoid) and stored at 4 °C. Following the initial incubation, the organisms were suspended in 10 ml of physiological saline solution and optical density readings were compared to a 0.5 McFarland standard. For the MIC determination, bacterial solutions of 5×10^5 colony-forming units (cfu/ml) were employed.

Tablel. Antimicrobial activity of the extract and Standard antibiotics

Bacterial	MIC extract plant(ppm)	Antibiotic resistance
S. pyogenes	100	-
S. pneumoniae	100	E, CE, CF
H. alvei	100	E, TE
S. saprophyticus	100	E, CF, TE
A. baumannii	100	CE, TE
E. faecalis	25	E, CE
P. mirabilis	25	E, TE
S. marcescens	100	CE

E: Erythromycin, CE: Cefixime, CF: Ceftazidime, TE: Tetracycline

The antibacterial activity of the plant extract was determined using sterile 2 ml 96-well plates (Wiegand *et al.*, 2008). The 12 wells of each row were filled with 0.5 ml sterilized Mueller Hinton agar. Sequentially, wells 2–11 received an additional 0.5 ml of a mixture of culture medium and plant extract serially diluted to create a concentration sequence from 0.512 ml to 0.008 ml. The deep-wells were incubated for 24 h at 37 °C. The resulting turbidity was observed. After 24 h, MIC was determined to be where growth was no longer visible by assessment of turbidity by optical density readings at 600 nm with a Beckman DU-70 UV-Vis Spectrophotometer. At least three repetitions were run for each assay. The levels of MIC was observed ranges from 25 to 100 ppm.

3. Results and discussion

The selection of plant material for this study was based on ethno-botanical data on the traditional use of the plants in treatment of bacterial diseases, and conditions classified by the traditional healers as "infection" and "inflammation," the latter characterized by reddening (e.g. in wounds), or internal afflictions causing gastric discomfort. The plant species was initially tested in simple agar-bioassays, which included plants that are used or other purposes by the local population (Bussmann *et al.*, 2007; Bussmann *et al.*, 2008; Bussmann *et al.*, 2009).

Table 1 shows the antibacterial activity of *Stachys lavandulifolia* Vahl against *P. mirabilis* and *E. faecalis*. The MIC concentrations ranged from 25 to 100 ppm. The very high values in many species indicate only a very limited antibacterial efficacy. Recent findings indicate that some natural phenolic compounds found in plants have an anti-biofouling effect on biofilm formation by Gram-negative bacteria (Jagani *et al.*, 2009). There has been no large scale systematic investigation into the relationship between bacterial inhibition and total phenolic content of spices and herbs. The anti-biofouling activities of 14 selected phenol and natural phenolic compounds were tested against *Pseudomonas aeruginosa*, using a micro titer-plate (Shan *et al.*, 2005). Anti-*Candida* activity of ethanolic extracts of endemic medicinal herbs against *Candida albicans* has been studied (Rohi *et al.*, 2012). A study by Mahzooni-kachapi et al. (2012), the *S. lavandulifolia* Vahl oil at that concentration showed moderate activity against the two tested microorganism, but gram-negative microorganism, *E. coli*, was more sensitive to oil than other one. Whereas activity detected against the examined Gram-positive microorganism, *S. aureus*, was found to be less sensitive to the oil (Mahzooni-kachapi *et al.*, 2012). Essential oils from 13 plants indicated anti-*Candida* activity; one of them is *Stachys byzantina*. The extracts of *Stachys byzantina*, *S. inflata*, *S. lavandulifolia* and *S. laxa* exhibited concentration-dependent activity against Gram-positive microorganisms (Duarte *et al.*, 2005). Kursat et al. (2009) reported that the extract of *S. lavandifolia* did not show any antimicrobial activity against *B. megaterium*, and *Trichophyton* spp. while the extract showed antibacterial activity against *P. aeruginosa, K. pneumoniae, S. aureus, C. albicans, C. globrata* and *Epidermophyton* sp.

4. Conclusion

The high concentration of active constituents in *S. lavandulifolia Vahl.* revealed antimicrobial activity in this study and in the previous reports on other Stachys species.Simple agar assays alone are not reliable for determin-ing the efficacy of plants used in traditional medicine. The present study however confirms that simple laboratory methods are indeed well suited for the initial assessment of the efficacy of traditionally used medicinal plants in inhibiting bacterial growth. A comparison to the traditional uses also indicated that local knowledge can provide im-portant leads for the development of new drugs: Our hy-potheses that plants traditionally used as antibacterials do have a much higher incidence of efficacy than other me-dicinally used species, and that plants used for cleansing baths are more likely to have antibacterial properties than other species used for ritual purposes could be verified. An efficacy analysis of these mixtures, as well as assays to evaluate the toxicity of single species as well as mixtures would be an interest-ing comparative study.

5. References

Bussmann, R., Sharon, D., Castro, M., Cardenas, R., Chait, G., Regalado, S., Del, T. C., Malca, G. and Perez AF, G. A. 2009. Phyto-chemical analysis of peruvian medicinal plants. *Arnaldoa*, 16(1):105-110.

Bussmann, R., Sharon, D., Diaz, D., Cardenas, R., Chait, G., Castro, M., Regalado, S., Del Toro, C., Malca., GG, P. A. and Glenn, A. 2011. Antibacterial activity of medicinal plant species in Northern Peru. *Ethnobotany Research and Applications,* 9:067-096.

Bussmann, R., Sharon, D. and Lopez, A. 2007. Blending traditional and western medicine: medicinal plant use among patients at Clinica Anticona in El Porvenir, Peru. *Ethnobotany Research & Applications* , 5:185-199.

Bussmann, R., Sharon, D., Perez, F., Díaz, D., Ford, T., Rasheed, T. and Silva, R. 2008. Antibacterial activity of Northern-Peruvian medicinal plants - a low cost laboratory approach to assess biological activity. *Arnaldoa* , 16(1):93-103.

Duarte, M., Figueira, G., Sartoratto, A., Rehder, V. and Delarmelina, C. 2005. Anti-*Candida* activity of Brazilian medicinal plants. *Journal Ethnopharmacology*, 97(2):305-11

EL-Ansari, M., Barron, D., Abdalla, M., Saleh, N., LE, Q. J. 1991. Flavonoid constituents of *Stachys aegyptica*. *Phytochemistry*, 30(4): 1169–1173.

Grieve, M. 1971. A Modern Herbal. *Publications, Inc.*

Hayashi, K., Nagamatsu, T., Ito, M., Hattori, T. and Suzuki, Y. 1994. Acteoside, a component of Stachys sieboldii MIQ, may be a promising antinephritic agent (1): Effects of acteoside on crescentic-type anti-GBM nephritis in rats. *The Japanese Journal of Pharmacology*, 65: (2) 143-151

Hayashi, K., Nagamatsu, T., Ito, M. Hattori, T. and Suzuki, Y. 1994. Acteoside, a component of *Stachys sieboldii* MIQ, may be a promising antinephritic agent (2): Effects of acteoside on leukocyte accumulation in the glomeruli of nephritic rats. *The Japanese Journal of Pharmacology,* 66(1):47-52.

Jagani, S., Chelikani, R. and Kim, D. 2009. Effects of phenol and natural phenolic compounds on biofilm formation by *Pseudomonas aeruginosa*. *Biofouling: The Journal of Bioadhesion and Biofilm Research*, 25 (4): 321-324

Khanavi, M., sharifzadeh, M., Hadjiakhoondi, A. and Shafiee, A. 2005. Phytochemical investigation and anti-inflammatory activity of aerial parts of *Stachys byzanthina* C. Koch. *Journal Ethnopharmaco*logy, 97(3):463-8.

Kursat, M., Erecevit, P., Kirbag, S. and Civelek, S. 2009. Antimicrobial activity of some medicinal plants from turkey. . *E-Journal of New World Sciences Academy*, 4 (2): 42-47.

Mahzooni-kachapi, S., Mahdavi, M., Roozbeh-nasira'ei, L., Akbarzadeh, M., Rezazadeh, F. and Motavalizadehkakhky, A. 2012. Antimicrobial activity and chemical composition of essential oils of *Stachys lavandulifolia* Vahl. from Mazandaran , Iran. *Journal of Medicinal Plants Research*, 6(24), pp. 4149-4158

Miyase, T., Yamamoto, R. and Ueno, A. 1996. Phenylethanoid glycosides from *Stachys officinalis*. Phytochemistry, 43(2):475-9.

Mozaffarian, V. 1996. *A Dictionary of Iranian Plant Names*. Farahang Moaser,.

Nishimura, H., Sasaki, H., Inagaki, N., Chin, M. and Mitsuhashi, H. 1991. nine phenethyl alcohol glycosides from Stachys sieboldii. *Phytochemistr y.,*30(3):965-9.

Rabbani, M., Sajjadi, S. and Zarei, H. 2003. Anxiolytic effects of *Stachys lavandulifolia* Vahl on the elevated plus-maze model of anxiety in mice. *Journal Ethnopharmacology,* 89(2-3):271-276.

Rohi Boroujeni, H., Ghasemi Pirbalouti, A., Hamedi, B., Abdizadeh, R. and Malekpoor, F. 2012. Anti-Candida activity of ethanolic extracts of Iranian endemic medicinal herbs against *Candida albicans*. *Journal of Medicinal Plants Research, 6*(12): 2448-2452.

Ross , S.T. and Zinchenko, F.L. 1975. Study of triterpenoids and steroids of *Stachys palustris*. *Farmatsevtychnyi Zhurnal (Kiev)*, 30: 91–92.

Savchenko, V. and Khvorostinka, V. 1978. Effects of a preparation from Stachys inflata on the course of experimental hepatitis in rats. *Farmatsevtychnyi Zhurnal (Kiev)* ,(4): 50-53

Shan, B., Cai, Y. Z., Sun, M. and Corke, H. 2005. Antioxidant capacity of 26 spice extracts and characterization of their phenolic constituents. *Journal Agricultural Food Chem*istry, 53 (20), pp 7749–7759

Skaltsa, H., Demetzos, C. Lazari, D. and Sokovic, M. 2003. Essential oil analysis and antimicrobial activity of eight *Stachysspecies* from Greece. *Phytochemistry*, 64(3):743-52.

Skaltsa, H., Lazari, D. Chinou, I. and Loukis, A. 1999. Composition & antibacterial activity of the essential oils of *Stachys eandica* & *S. chrysantha* from southern Greece. *Planta Medica,* 65(3): 255-256.

Wiegand, L., Hilpert, K. and Hancock, R. 2008. Agar and broth dilution methods to determine the minimal inhibitory concentration (MIC) of antimicrobial substances. *Nature Protocols*, 3(2):163-75.

Yamahara, J., Kitani, T., Kobayashi, H., Kawahara, Y. and Yakugaku, Z. 1990. Studies on Stachys sieboldii MIQ. II. Anti-anoxia action and the active constituents. *Yakugaku Zasshi,* 110(12):932-5

Yamamoto, R., Miyase, T. and Ueno, A. 1994. Stachyssaponins I-VIII, new oleanane-type triterpene saponins from *Stachys riederi* Chamisso. Chemical & Pharmaceutical Bulletin (tokyo), 42(6): 1291-1296.

Zinchenko, T. V. 1970. Flavonoid glycosides of Stachys neglecta. *Farmatsevtychnyi Zhurnal (Kiev),* 25(4):81-2.

Zinchenko, T.V., Voitenko, G.N. and Lipkan, G.N. 1981. Anti-inflammatory, antitoxic, and hypoazotemic effect of a *Stachys recta* preparation, stachyrene. *Farmakol Toksikol,* 44(2):191-4.

Effect of *Ferulago angulata* sub. *carduchorum* on total serum antioxidant activity and some of the humoral immune responses in broiler chicks

Reza Govahi, Gholamreza Ghalamkari*, Majid Toghyani, Shahin Eghbal Saied, Mohammad Mohammadrezaei, Mahdi Shahryari, Alireza Dehghani Abari

Department of Animal Science, Khorasgan Branch, Islamic Azad University, Isfahan, Iran;
***Email:** *gh.ghalamkari@gmail.com**

ARTICLE INFO

Topic: *Pharmacology & Ethnoveterinary*

Key words:

- ✓ Ferulago angulata
- ✓ *Antioxidant Activity*
- ✓ *Immune Responses*
- ✓ *Vitamin E*
- ✓ *Broiler Chick*

ABSTRACT

Background & Aim: *Ferulago angulata* sub. *carduchorum* (locally name: Chavir or Chavil) is an important medicinal plant in Iran. The powder of aerial parts of this plant contains variety of components with different therapeutical effects such as antioxidant activities (AOA). This study was conducted to investigate the effect of dietary supplementation powder of aerial parts of this plant on total activities of serum antioxidant and some of the humoral immune responses in broiler chicks.

Experimental: Three hundred of 16 days-old commercial chicks (Ross 308) were randomly allocated to six treatments with five replicates. The dietary treatments consisted of the basal diet as control (A), 100 ppm (150 IU) of vitamin E (B), 70 g / 100 kg Flavofosfolipol (C), 0.3% (D), 0.6% (E), and 1% (F) of the powder of the aerial parts of this plant added to the basal diet. At 25 days, from each treatment of experiment, two chicks were randomly selected and sheep red blood cell (SRBC) was injected through their wings veins. At 30 days, blood samples (ten sample of per treatment) for the test of antibody measurement produced against SRBC, the influenza virus and Newcastle were prepared. Moreover, with the blood extension and numbering of Hetrophil and Lymphocyte calculated and hetrophil to lymphocyte ratio were estimated. At 42 days, blood samples (ten samples per treatment) were taken for measuring total activities of serum antioxidant.

Results & Discussion: Results indicated that supplementing of 0.6% of *F. angulata* significantly increased total activities of serum antioxidant compared to control birds ($p \leq 0.05$). There is no significant difference among the treatments of experiment in the number of Hetrophil, Lymphocyte their ratio and the antibody against the virus of Newcastle and SRBC. However, this antibody against the influenza virus at the treatment of 3 g/kg *F. angulata* in comparison to control treatment was more.

Recommended applications/industries: Use of *F. angulata* in broiler diet could be increase total serum antioxidant activity and improve humoral immunity.

1. Introduction

The use of antibiotic growth promoters (AGP) to improve animal performance has been a usual practice for more than half century. After 2005, in the Europe Union the use of all such antibiotics was banned by regulatory measures (Isabel *et al.*, 2009). This is because of the potential risks associated with their use and development of resistant strains of bacteria, mainly in humans. There are various products for replacing AGP, such as medicine herbs. There is sufficient evidence to show that potential herbs are effective for enhancement of the immune system and increasing antioxidant activity for poultry (Ghalamkari *et al.*, 2011). *Ferulago angulata* subsp. *carduchorum*, belonging to the family Apiaceae, is an important medicinal plant of Iran. *Ferulago* species are used in folk medicine for their sedative, tonic, digestive and anti-parasitic effects (Yesilbag *et al.,* 2011). In addition, the antibacterial, antifungal, and anti-oxidant effects of this plant have been reported (Ghasempour *et al.*, 2007; Yesilbag *et al.*, 2011). The main constituents of this plant are monoterpens and among, α-pinene, bornyl acetate and *cis*-ocimene (Dorman *et al.*, 2000) and β- pinene (Homann *et al.*, 1999; Lopez *et al.*, 1994; Billany *et al.*, 1995) have the most antioxidant activity. The mechanism of these compounds is to damage the membrane of lipoprotein cell bacteria that is lead to leaking and decreasing of cytoplasm compound (Hosseini Mansob *et al.*, 2011). On the other hand, the antioxidant compounds, with adding of some parts to free radicals to deactivate these poisonous materials. Moreover, the herb has the compounds with antibacterial activity, such as α- terpineol, terpenen-4-ol (Cosentino *et al.*, 1999), α-pinene, β-pinene, and *ρ*-cymene have anti-fungous (Adam *et al.*, 1998; Lis-Balchin *et al.*, 1998). Antibacterial and antifungal activities of the plant are also presented on both positive -Gram like *Staphylococcus* and negative-Gram like *E. coli*, and fungi like *C. albicans* (Ghasempour *et al.*, 2007). The chemical composition of *F. angulata* such as β-hydroxy-13-epi-manoyloxide, α-pinene, 2,5-dimethoxy-*p*-cymene, *p*-cymene, methyl carvacrol, transchrysanthenyl, transchrysanthenyl acetate, γ-terpinene, (*Z*)-β ocimene, α-pinene, myrcene, terpinolene, 2,4,5-trimethylbenzaldehyde, and α-phellandrene was reported by Taran et al. (2010) and, Ghasempour et al. (2007). Since there have not been any study on the effects of antioxidant activity and humoral immunize of *F. angulata* in broiler chicks ROOS (308), this study was conducted to investigate the effect of powder of aerial parts of this plant on total activities of serum antioxidant and immune system function of broiler chicks.

2. Materials and Methods

2.1. Bird, diets and management

The aerial parts of *Ferulago angulata* were collected from Shahoo Mountain western Iran, dried in shed and added to broiler diet as a powder. In present research, 360 one-day old broiler chicks (Ross-308) randomly allocated into six treatments, each with free replicates with 12 broiler chickens. Vitamin E, Flavofosfolipol, and the aerial parts of *F. angulata* were supplemented to no additive added basal diet. Six treatments were as follows:

a) Basal diet (control)
b) Basal diet + 100 mg / kg (150 IU) Vitamin E;
c) Basal diet + 70 g Flavofosfolipol / 100 kg diet;
d) Basal diet + 0.3 kg *F. angulata* / 100 kg diet;
e) Basal diet + 0.6 kg *F. angulata* / 100 kg diet;
f) Basal diet +1 kg *F. angulata* / 100 kg diet;

The trial comprised three 2-weeks periods. The birds were fed a starter diet from days 1-14, a grower diet from days 14-28 and finisher from days 28-42 (Table 1). The diets were formulated to meet the requirements of broilers as recommended by the Catalog Ross (Ross Co., 2007). The dried aerial parts of *F. angulata* were added at the expense of powder. The birds were allowed to free access to feed and water during the 42-d grow out period. The lighting cycle was 23 h/d maintained. The ambient temperature in experimental house was maintained at 32 °C during the first week and gradually decreased by 3 °C in the second and third week, and then fixed at 22 °C.

2.2. Total activities of serum antioxidant

At 42 days from each repetition of treatments, two chicks were randomly selected, and the blood samples were taken by cylinder 2.5 ml from wings vein. The blood samples of serum were prepared by centrifuge for Fenton type reaction. AOA was measured by the spectrophotometry method. In summary, standard solution of Fe–EDTA complex reacts with hydrogen peroxide by a Fenton type reaction, leading to the formation of hydroxyl radicals. These reactive oxygen species degrade benzoate, resulting in the release of TBARS. Antioxidants from the added sample of broiler serum cause suppression of the production of TBARS. This reaction can be measured by spectrophotometer and the inhibition of color development defined as the AOA (Ghalamkari *et al.*, 2011).

2.3. Calculation of Hetrophil to lymphocyte ratio

At 30 days from each repetition of experiment, two chicks were randomly selected and the blood samples were taken from wings vein. Blood extensions samples were prepared and colored based on Gimsa method (Thrall *et al.*, 2004). One hundred white blood cells for each sample with the separation of Heterophil and lymphocyte were counted, and the Heterophil to lymphocyte ratio was calculated and then registered. Then data gained were analyzed statistically.

2.4. The measurement of the anti-body produced against SRBC

At 25 days from each treatment of experiment, two chicks were randomly selected and then 1 ml SRBC 1% was injected through the wings veins. At 30 days, taking blood process was performed from the wings veins of the same chicks for determining of antibody against SRBC by the method of Hemaglutination (HA) method. Then the blood samples were placed in centrifuge 1500 T/m for 15 min. Their serums were separated, and kept in the temperature of - 20 °C for experiment. Then from the average of each repetition, was under the analysis and survey statistics.

2.5. The measurement of the anti-body produced against Newcastle and Influenza virus

At 30 days from each treatment of experiment, two chicks were randomly selected and taking blood through the wings vein was performed. After separation of serum from blood samples, the measurement of special antibody produced against Newcastle and Influenza vaccine were measured separately by the Hemaglutination inhibition (HI) method.

2.6. The measurement of Lymphatic organs weight

At the end of the experiment (at 42 days), two chicks that their average weight was about the average of their group, were randomly selected (10 chicks from each treatment), and their carcasses were examined. For each bird, the weight of effective glands in immune system of the chicks (Bursa of fabricius and spleen) was measured. In final, the data was calculated in percent of body weight and analyzed statistically.

2.7. Statistical analysis

Data subjected to one–way analysis of variance using SAS statistical package (version 6.08, 1989). Significant effect of dietary treatments was compared with Least Significant Difference Test (LSD) with $p < 0.05$.

3. Results and Discussion

3.1. Total activities of serum antioxidant

The AOA of serum in broiler chicks under six g *F. angulata* / kg treatment significantly ($p \leq 0.05$) increased than those control and antibiotic treatments (Table 2). But, there was no significant difference between *F. angulata* treatment and vitamin E treatment.

Table 2. The effect of dietary inclusion of feed additives on AOA (mmol/lit) of serum in broiler chicks.

Treatments	AOA
Control	0.45^{b}[¶]
Vitamin E	0.54^{ab}
Flavofosfolipol	0.35^{b}
0.3% *F. angulata*	0.40^{b}
0.6% *F. angulata*	0.67^{a}
1% *F. angulata*	0.56^{ab}
SEM	±0.03

[¶] Mean values followed by the same letters in the column do not differ according to LSD test.

3.2. Heterophil and Lymphocyte ratio

There was no significant difference among the treatments ($p > 0.05$) (Table 3). However, the least numbers of Heterophil among treatments were belonged to the control treatment, and the most numbers of Lymphocyte were belonged to 3 and 6 g/kg of *F. angulata*. In addition, the least Heterophil to Lymphocyte ratio was belonged to 3 g/kg *F. angulata* treatment, and the most were belonged to antibiotic treatment ($p > 0.05$).

3.3. The measurement of antibody produced against Newcastle, Influenza (HI) and SRBC (HA)

The measurement of antibody produced against the Influenza virus in the chicks of treatment 3 g/kg *F. angulata* in comparison to other groups of treatments was significant ($p \leq 0.05$) (Table 4). No significant effect on the antibody against Newcastle virus and, SRBC also were seen ($p > 0.05$). However, the most measurement of the antibody produced against the Newcastle virus was observed in the chicks diet with 3 g/kg *F. angulata* and the vitamin E treatment ($p > 0.05$). The measurement of the antibody produced against SRBC was not affected by treatment experiment significantly ($p > 0.05$). It is clear that the most measurement of the antibody produced against SRBC, in the treatment 6 g/kg *F. angulate* (Table 5).The least measurement of antibody produced was belonged to the treatment of 3 g/kg *F. angulata* ($p > 0.05$).

*3.4. Weight comparison of Lymph*atic organs

Treatments had no significant effect on weight average of Lymphatic organs at 42 days (Table 5). At 42 days, the maximum weight of fabricius bursa was in control group and in treatment that received 6 g/kg *F. angulate*. The minimum weight of fabricius bursa belonged to treatment of vitamin E. In addition, among the treatments, the maximum weight average of Bursa of fabricius was for 6 g/kg *F. angulata*, and the minimum weight of that was for 3 g/kg *F. angulata*. Moreover, there was no significant difference between the weights of spleen at 42 days in different treatments experiments. The maximum of spleen weight is for antibiotic treatment, and the minimum of that, is for the treatment of 10 g/kg *F. angulata*. The maximum of spleen weight in chicks of 3 g/kg *F. angulata* and the minimum of that is for 10 g/kg *F. angulata*.

Since there was no experiment on the effect of this plant on the total serum antioxidant activity and immune responses in broiler chickens, the effects of other plants that are similar to *F. angulata* were chosen and discussed. The maximum total serum antioxidant activity belonged to the treatment of 6 g/kg dietary and had significant effect to decreasing oxidation of tissues specially lipid tissues (Table 2).

The active ingredients of a medicinal plant are mainly its phenolic compound that is also an important antioxidant (Huda-Faujan *et al.*, 2009; Khanavi *et al.*, 2009). The phenolic compounds are generic term for multiple aromatic groups including mainly flavonoids, phenols acid, isoflavonoids, and anthocyanins. These ingredients are naturally produced during a plant's growth metabolic process, the active substances with antioxidant function such as scavenging reactive oxygen species, free radicals or non-free radical reactive oxygen species production from body metabolism (Rath *et al.*, 2006).

Vossen et al. (2009) clarified that the chicks, under the test of oxidative plasma, have more antioxidant properties in serum when they applied *Rosmarinces officinalis* in their diet. They reported that the chicks, which got 500 g/kg oil of the herb, had less meat cholesterol oxidation in comparison to control treatment ($p \leq 0.05$). In contrast, Roofchaee et al. (2011) in their experiment showed that adding oregano essential oil level 300, 600, and 1200 mg/kg dietary, had no significant effect on the serum antioxidant activity.

Botsoglou et al. (2002) claim that high concentration of unsaturated fatty acids in poultry meat increases susceptibility of chicken meat lipids to oxidative deterioration during storage. In this study, it seems that the antioxidant activity of *F. angulata* due to the presence of phenolic components having off group these components act as hydrogen donors to the peroxy radicals produced during the first step in lipid oxidation thus retarding the hydroxy peroxide formation (Farag *et al.*, 1989).

F. angulata treatments had no significant effect on the titer of produced antibody against Newcastle virus and sheep red blood cell (SBRC) (Table 5). However, the treatments of *F. angulata* had significant effect on the titer of produced antibody against Newcastle virus. In this way, AL-ankari et al. (2004) reported the titer of produced antibody against Newcastle antigene in the chicks fed by mint was higher. They also suggested the herb could stimulate immune system and improve the responses of immune system against Newcastle virus.

Results of a study by Mathivanan and Kalaiarasi (2007) showed that the titer of produced antibody against SRBC, in the dietary completed by herbs in comparison to the dietary with antibiotics of Virginiamycin was increased. Kabir et al. (2004) and Ramarao et al. (2004) concluded that increasing antibody in the herbal treatments in comparison to control and dietaries is due to hypertrophy and hyperplasia of lymphatic organs in herbal treatments.

Table 1. The ingredient and chemical composition of basal starter, grower and finisher diets

Ingredients	Starter	Grower	Finisher
Corn	55.18	57.94	62.4
Soybean meal	39.2	36.4	32.4
Oil	1.32	2.1	2
DCP	1.66	1.4	1.3
$Caco_3$	1.29	1.12	1
Vitamin-Premix[1]	0.25	0.25	0.25
Mineral -Premix[2]	0.25	0.25	0.25
NaCl	0.35	0.3	0.25
DL-Methionine	0.31	0.2	0.15
L-Lysine	0.19	0.04	-
Calculated composition (mg/kg)			
M. energy (kcal/kg)	2830	2900	3000
Crude protein(%)	21.8	20.7	19
Calcium(%)	0.98	0.84	0.81
Av. phosphorus(%)	0.46	0.42	0.39
Meth.+ cysteine(%)	0.96	0.87	0.76
Lysine (%)	1.33	1.77	1.0

[1]To provide the following per kg of diet: Vit A 10,000 IU, vitamin D3 2000 IU, vitamin E 5 IU, vitamin K 2 mg, riboflavin 4. 20 mg; vitamin B12 0.01 mg; pantothenic acid 5 mg; nicotinic acid 20 mg; folic acid 0.5 mg.

[2]To provide the following per kg of diet: choline 3 mg; Mg 56 mg; Fe 20 mg; Cu, 10 mg; Zn 50 mg; Co 125 mg; Iodine 0.8 mg.

Table 3. The effect of dietary inclusion of feed additives on Heterophil, Lymphocyte and their ratio at 42 days

Treatment	H/L	Lymphocyte%	Heterophil%
Control	0.47	72	32
Vitamin E	0.52	70	35
Flavofosfolipol	0.66	65	38
F. angulata 3g/Kg	0.45	76	34
F. angulata 6g/Kg	0.46	76	35
F. angulata 10g/Kg	0.51	75	37
SEM	0.03	1.54	1.4

Table 4. The effect of dietary inclusion of feed additives on the antibody produced against Newcastel, Influenzae Virus and SRBC of chicks at 30 days

Treatment	The measurement of the antibody produced against SRBC	The measurement of the antibody produced against Influenza Virus	The measurement of the antibody produced against Newcastle Virus
Control	6.6	4.8 ^{b}	5.0
Vitamin E	6.2	6.7 ^{a}	5.2
flavofosfolipol	5.6	6.2 ^{ab}	4.6
F. angulata 3 gr/kg	5.4	7.2 ^{a}	5.0
F. angulata 6 gr/kg	5.8	3.3 ^{c}	4.2
F. angulata 10 gr/kg	5.7	4.8 ^{b}	4.3
SEM	0.17	0.27	0.13

Followed by the same letters in the column do not differ according to LSD test ($p \leq 0.05$).

Table 5. The effect of dietary inclusion of feed additives on weight average of lymphatic organs at 42 days

Treatment	Spleen	Bursa of fabricius
Control	0.115	0.18
Vitamine E	0.115	0.15
Flavofosfolipol	0.126	0.16
F. angulata 3g/kg	0.116	0.16
F. angulata 6g/kg	0.113	0.18
F. angulata 10g/kg	0.112	0.17
SEM	0.004	0.005

AbdEl – Moteal et al. (2008) in their experiments preformed on brown laying hens observed that adding eucalyptus leaves powder to the dietary, decreased hetrophil to Lymphocyte ratio significantly. In birds, the heterophil are phagocytic cells whose main is protection against invading microorganisms, whereas primary functions of Lymphocyte is cell mediated and humoral immunity. The H/L ratio is a recognized measure of stress in birds (Davison *et al.*, 1983; Gross *et al.*, 1983; Maxwell *et al.*, 1993) that has become a valuable tool in stress research especially when combined with the convenience and repeatability of automated blood cell count. As it is clear from the results of the comparison of the weight averages related to Lymphotic organs (Bursa of Fabricius and spleen) experiment treatments (Table 5), had no significant effect on the weight of these organs, and the maximum weight of Bursa Fabricius in the chicks fed by control treatment and treatment of 6 g/kg *F. angulata* was observed. The maximum spleen weight was for the chicks of 3 g/kg treatment.

4. Conclusion

According to this result, the treatment of 6 g/kg *F. angulata* has increased the total serum antioxidant activity in broilers and has proper effects on the function of their immune system. In addition, it could be improving meat oxidative stability but a further research is necessary.

5. References

Abd El – Motaal, A.M., Ahmed, A.M.H., Bahakaim, A.S.A, Fathi, M.M., 2008. Productive performance and immune competence of commercial laying hens given diets supplemented with Eucalyptus. *International Journal of Poultry Science.*, 7 (5): 445-449.

Al-Ankari, A.S., Zaki, M.M., Sultan, S.I., 2004. Use of habek mint (*Mentha longifolia*) in broiler chicken diets. *International Journal Poultry Science.*, 3(10): 629-634.

Botsoglou, N.A., Florou-Paneri, P., Christaki, E., Fletouris, D.J., Spais, A.B., 2002. Effect of dietary oregano essential oil on performance of chickens and on iron-induced lipid oxidation of breast, thigh and abdominal fat tissues. *British Poultry Science.*, 43: 223-230.

Cosention, S., Tuberoso, S.I., Pisano, B., 1999. In vitro antimicrobial activity and chemical composition of Sardinian *Thymus* essential oils. *Letters in Applied Microbiology*, 29: 130-135.

Davison, T.F., Rowell, L.G., Rea J., 1983. Effects of dietary corticosterone on peripheral blood lymphocyte and granulocytes populations in immature domestic fowl. *Research in Veterinary Science.*, 34: 236-239.

Farag, R.S., Badei, A.Z.M.A., Hewedi, F.M., El-Baroty, G.S.A., 1989. Antioxidant activity of some spice essential oils on linoleic acid oxidation in aqueous media. *Journal American Oil Chemical Society.*, 66: 792-799.

Ghalamkari, G., Landy, N., Toghiani, M., Modaresi, M., Ghalamkari, Z., 2011. Efficiency of *Echinacea purpurea* on total antioxidant activity in serum of broiler chicks. *The 9th International Conference on Food Engineering and Biotechnology*, Bangkok, Thailand.

Ghasempour, H.R., Shirinpour, E., Heidari, H., 2007. The constituents of essential oils of *Ferulago angulata* (Schlecht) Boiss at two different habitats, Nevakoh and Shahoo, Zagross Mountain, Western Iran. *Iranian Journal of Science and Technology.*, Transaction A, 31(A3).

Gross, W.B., Siegel, P.B., 1983. Evaluation of the heterophil / lymphocyte ratio as a measure of stress in chickens. *Avian Disease.*, 27: 972-979.

Hosseni Mansob, N., Nezhady, M.M., 2011. The effect of using thyme, garlic and nettle on performance, carcass quality and blood parameters. *Annale of Biological Research.*, 4: 315-320.

Huda-Faujan, N., Noriham, A., Norrakiah, A.S., Babji, A.S., 2009. Antioxidant activity of plants methanolic extracts containing phenolic compounds. *African Journal of Biotechnology.*, 8: 484-489.

Isabel, B., Santos, Y., 2009. Effects of dietary organic acid and essential oils on growth performance and carcass characteristics of broiler chickens. *Journal Apply Poultry Research.*, 18: 472-476.

Kabir, S.M.L., Rahman, M.M., Rahman, M.B., Ahmad, S.U., 2004. The dynamics of probiotics on growth performance and immune response in broilers. *International Journal Poultry Science.*, 3: 361-364.

Khanavi, M., Hajimahmoodi, M., Cheraghi-Niroomand, M., Kargar, Z., Ajani, Y., Hadjiakhoondi, A., Oveisi, M.R., 2009. Comparison of the antioxidant activity and total phenolic contents in some *Stachys* species. *African Journal of Biotechnology.*, 8: 1143-1147.

Lis–Balchin, M., Deans, G., Stanley., Eaglesham, E., 1998. Relationship between bioactivity and chemical composition of commercial essential oils. *Journal Flavour and Fragrance.,* 13: 98-104.

Lopez-Bote, C.J., Gray, J.I., Gomma, E.A., Flegal, C.J., 2010. Effect of dietary administration of oil extracts from rosemary and sage on lipid oxidation in broiler meat. *British Poultry Science.*, 39: 235-240.

Mathivanan, R., Kalaiarasi, K., 2007. Panchagavya and *Andrographis panculata* as alternatives to antibiotic growth promoters on haematological, serum biochemical parameters and immune status of broilers. *Journal Poultry Science.*, 44: 2. 198-204.

Maxwell, M.H., 1993. Avian blood leukocyte responses to stress. *World's Poultry Science Journal.*, 49: 34-43.

Ramarao, S.V., Reddy, M.R., Raju, M.V.L.N., Panda, A.K. 2004. Growth, nutrient utilization and immune competence in broiler chicken fed probiotic, gut acidifier and antibacterial compounds. *Indian Journal Poultry Science.,* 39: 125-130.

Rath, N.C., Huff, W.E., Huff, G.R., 2006. Effects of humic acid on broiler chickens. *Poultry Science.*, 85: 410-414.

Roofchaee, A., Irani, M., Ebrahimzadeh, M.A., Akbari, M.R., 2011. Effect of dietary oregano (*Origanum vulgare* L.) essential oil on growth performance, cecal microflora and serum antioxidant activity of broiler chickens. *African Journal of Biotechnology.*, 10: 6177-6183.

Ross Company., 2007. Ross 308 broiler Performance Objectives, Alabama, USA: Aviagen, page, 24.

SAS Institute., 2008. SAS User's guide version 9.02 review edition, Cary NC: SAS Institute Inc, 176

Taran, M., Ghasempour, H.R., Shirinpour, E., 2010. Antimicrobial activity of essential oils of *Ferulago angulata* subsp. *Carduchorum. Jundishapur Journal of Microbiology.*, 3(1): 10-14.

Thrall, M.A., 2004. *Veterinary Hemotalogy and Clinical Chemistry*. Lippincott Williams & Wilkins, pp.10.

Vossen, E., Ntawubizi, M., Ntawubizi, K., Raes, K., Smet, G., Uyghebaert, S., Arnouts, S., De Smet., 2011. Effect of dietary antioxidant supplementation on the oxidative status of plasma in broilers. *Journal of Animal Physiology and Animal Nutrition.*, 95: 198–205.

Yesilbag, D., Eren, M., Agel, H., Kovanlikaya, A., Kovanlikaya, F., 2011. Effects of dietary rosemary, rosemary volatile oil and vitamin E on broiler performance, meat quality and serum sod activity. *British Poultry Science.*, 52: 472-482.

Permissions

All chapters in this book were first published in JHD, by Islamic Azad University, Shahrekord Branch; hereby published with permission under the Creative Commons Attribution License or equivalent. Every chapter published in this book has been scrutinized by our experts. Their significance has been extensively debated. The topics covered herein carry significant findings which will fuel the growth of the discipline. They may even be implemented as practical applications or may be referred to as a beginning point for another development.

The contributors of this book come from diverse backgrounds, making this book a truly international effort. This book will bring forth new frontiers with its revolutionizing research information and detailed analysis of the nascent developments around the world.

We would like to thank all the contributing authors for lending their expertise to make the book truly unique. They have played a crucial role in the development of this book. Without their invaluable contributions this book wouldn't have been possible. They have made vital efforts to compile up to date information on the varied aspects of this subject to make this book a valuable addition to the collectionof many professionals and students.

This book was conceptualized with the vision of imparting up-to-date information and advanced data in this field. To ensure the same, a matchless editorial board was set up. Every individual on the board went through rigorous rounds of assessment to prove their worth. After which they invested a large part of their time researching and compiling the most relevant data for our readers.

The editorial board has been involved in producing this book since its inception. They have spent rigorous hours researching and exploring the diverse topics which have resulted in the successful publishing of this book. They have passed on their knowledge of decades through this book. To expedite this challenging task, the publisher supported the team at every step. A small team of assistant editors was also appointed to further simplify the editing procedure and attain best results for the readers.

Apart from the editorial board, the designing team has also invested a significant amount of their time in understanding the subject and creating the most relevant covers. They scrutinized every image to scout for the most suitable representation of the subject and create an appropriate cover for the book.

The publishing team has been an ardent support to the editorial, designing and production team. Their endless efforts to recruit the best for this project, has resulted in the accomplishment of this book. They are a veteran in the field of academics and their pool of knowledge is as vast as their experience in printing. Their expertise and guidance has proved useful at every step. Their uncompromising quality standards have made this book an exceptional effort. Their encouragement from time to time has been an inspiration for everyone.

The publisher and the editorial board hope that this book will prove to be a valuable piece of knowledge for researchers, students, practitioners and scholars across the globe.

List of Contributors

Oshi, M.A.M, Abdelkareem, A.M and Eltohami, M.SH
Department of Pharmaceutical Technology, Faculty of Pharmacy, Omdurman Islamic University, Omdurman, Sudan

Eltohami
Department of Pharmacognosy, Faculty of Pharmacy, Omdur

Jude Efiom Okokon and Bawo Michael
Department of Pharmacology and Toxicology Faculty of Pharmacy, University of Uyo, Uyo, Nigeria

Saadat Moshkelani
Department of Surgery, Faculty of Specialized Veterinary Sciences, Tehran Science and Research Branch, Islamic Azad University, Tehran, Iran

Mohamad Javaheri-Koupaei
Young Researchers and Elite Club, Shahrekord Branch, Islamic Azad University, Shahrekord, Iran

Hassan Momtaz
Faculty of Veterinary Medicine, Shahrekord Branch, Islamic Azad University, Shahrekord, Iran

Emad Khalilzadeh, Reza Hazrati and Gholamreza Vafaei Saiah
Division of Physiology, Department of Basic Science, Faculty of Veterinary Medicine, University of Tabriz, Tabriz, Iran

Mohammad Momen Heravi, Shahla Daneshmehr and Ali Morsali
Department of Chemistry, Mashhad Branch, Islamic Azad University, Mashhad, Iran

Jude E. Okokon
Department of Pharmacology and Toxicology, Faculty of Pharmacy, University of Uyo,Uyo, Nigeria

Koofreh Davis
Department of Physiology, Faculty of Basic Medical Sciences, University of Uyo, Uyo, Nigeria

Azare
Department of Biological Sciences, University of Abuja, Nigeria

Malek Taher Maghsoodlou, Javad Mottaghipisheh and Nahid Rahneshan
Department of Chemistry, University of Sistan and Baluchestan, Zahedan, Iran

Jafar Valizadeh
Department of Biology, University of Sistan and Baluchestan, Zahedan, Iran

Maedeh Rezghi and Jinous Asgarpanah
Department of Pharmacognosy, Faculty of Pharmacy, Pharmaceutical Sciences Branch, Islamic Azad University, Tehran - Iran (IAUPS)

Seyyed Reza Hoseinidoust
Department of Microbiology, Faculty of Pharmacy, Pharmaceutical Sciences Branch, Islamic Azad University, Tehran - Iran (IAUPS)

Salar Hafez Ghoran
Department of Chemistry, Faculty of Sciences, Golestan University, Gorgan 4913815739, Iran

Boshra Azadi
Phytochemistry Department, Faculty of Medicinal Chemistry, Pharmaceutical Sciences Branch, Islamic Azad University, Tehran, Iran

Hussain Hidayat
UoN Chair of Oman's Medicinal plants and Marine Natural products, University of Nizwa, Nizwa, Sultanate of Oman

Forough Talazadeh and Mansoor Mayahi
Department of Clinical Sciences, Faculty of Veterinary Medicine Shahid Chamran University of Ahvaz- Iran

Hossein Najafzade Varzi and Hadis Norouzizade
Department of Basic Sciences, Faculty of Veterinary Medicine Shahid Chamran University of Ahvaz- Iran

Louis U. Amazu
Department of Pharmacology and Therapeutics, College of Medicine, Evans Enwerem University, Orlu Campus, Imo State

Lucky L. Nwidu
Department of Pharmacology and Toxicology, Faculty of Pharmacy, Niger Delta University, Wilberforce Island, Bayelsa State

Alaleh Nikooie and Amir Pouya Ghandehari Yazdi
Department of Food Science and Technology, Shahrekord Branch, Islamic Azad University, Sharekord, Iran

Mina Shamsaei
Department of Food Science and Technology, Khorasgan Branch, Islamic Azad University, Isfahan, Iran

Leila Sedaghat Boroujeni
Department of Food Science and Technology, Science and Research Branch of Tehran, Islamic Azad University, Tehran, Iran

Ali Azizi and Maryam Pirbodaghi
Department of Horticultural Sciences, Faculty of Agriculture, Bu-Ali Sina University, Hamedan, Iran

Mahtab Esfahanizadeh Hoseinpoor
Young Researcher and Elit Club, Isfahan (khorasgan) Branch, Islamic Azad University, Isfahan, Iran

Forough Mortazaeinezhad
Department of Horticultural Sciences, Isfahan (khorasgan) Branch, Islamic Azad University, Isfahan, Iran

Hamidreza Ardalani
Department of Horticultural Sciences, Science and Research Branch, Islamic Azad University, Tehran, Iran

Mohammad Hojjatoleslamy, Fatemeh Raisi and Masoumeh Asadi
Department of Food Science and Technology, Faculty of Agriculture, Islamic Azad University, Shahrekord Branch, Shahrekord, Iran

Mehran Mohammadian
Laboratory of Vice-chancellor for Drug and Food Organization, Shahrekord, Iran

Narges Samanian
Department of Food Engineering, Ferdowsi University, Mashhad, Iran

Shahrbanoo Alami Rostami
Department of Biology, Islamic Azad Univercity, Gomishan center, Gorgan Branch, Gorgan Iran

Maryam Rafieirad
Department of Biology, faculty of Sciences, Islamic Azad University, Izeh branch, Izeh-Iran

Sonia Johri, Nasir Khan, Sarita Tiwari and Lovie Shakyawar
Department of Life Sciences, ITM University, Gwalior

Fatemeh Sadeghi Samani and Hossein Sazegar
Department of biology, Faculty of Basic Sciences, Shahrekord Branch, Islamic Azad University, Sahrekord, Iran

Abdollah Ghasemi Pirbalouti
Department of Medicinal Plants, Shahrekord Branch, Islamic Azad University, Shahrekord, Iran

Koofreh Davies
Department of physiology, Faculty of basic medical sciences, University of Uyo, Uyo, Nigeria

Bassey S Antia
Department of chemistry, University of Uyo, Uyo, Nigeria

Leila Firoozian
Falavarjan Branch, Islamic Azad University, Isfahan, Iran

Leila Amjad
Department of Biology, Falavarjan Branch, Islamic Azad University, Isfahan, Iran

Monir Doudi
Department of Microbiology, Falavarjan Branch, Islamic Azad University, Isfahan, Iran

Emeje Martins, Isimi Christianah, Izuka Amaka, and Olayemi Olubunmi
National Institute for Pharmaceutical Research & Development (NIPRD), Abuja, Nigeria

Yaser Rahimian
Department of Animal Science, Shahrekord Branch, Islamic Azad University, Shahrekord, Iran
Extension Agent, Agriculture Organization of Jihad, Chaharmahal and Bakhtiari Province, Shahrekord, Iran

Farshid Kheiri
Department of Animal Science, Shahrekord Branch, Islamic Azad University, Shahrekord, Iran

Mohammad Alavi
Department of Herbal Plant Science, Shahrekord Branch, Islamic Azad University, Shahrekord, Iran

Mehran Aboozar
Department of Animal Science, Abhar Branch, Islamic Azad University, Abhar, Iran

Omotuyi Idowu Olaposi
Center for Bio-computing and Drug Development, Adekunle Ajasin University Akungba Ondo State, Nigeria

Ovuakporie-Uvo Oghale and Idu MacDonald
Department of Plant Biology and Biotechnology, University of Benin, Benin City, P.M.B. 1154. Edo State, Nigeria

Kumar Ravendra, Prakash Om and Pant Anil K
Department of Chemistry, College of Basic Sciences and Humanities, G.B. Pant University of Agriculture & Technology, Pantnagar, U.S. Nagar, Uttarakhand, India

Kumar Mahesh
Department of Vet. Epidemiology and Preventive Medicine, College of Veterinary & Animal Sciences. G.B. Pant University of Agriculture & Technology, Pantnagar, U.S. Nagar, Uttarakhand, India

Isidorov Valary A and Szczepaniak Lech
Institute of Chemistry, Białystok University, Division of Environmental Chemistry, UL. Hurtowa 1,15-399, Białystok, Poland

Zahra Dehbashi and Forough Forghani
Department of Obstetrics' & Gynecology, Faculty of Medicine, Zabol University of Medical Science, Zabol, Iran

Seyed Kazem Sabbagh
Department of Biology, Faculty of Science, Yazd University, Yazd, Iran

Saeideh Saeidi
Laboratory expert of Microbiology, Institute of Plant Biotechnology, University of Zabol, Zabol, Iran

Somayeh Azami and Bijan Fahimi
Department of Laboratory Sciences, Faculty of Medical Sciences, Shahrood Branch, Islamic Azad University, Shahrood, Iran

Mehdi Bagheri
Research Committee, Semnan University of Medical Sciences, Semnan, Iran

Shabnam Mohsenzadeh
International Jolfa Branch, Islamic Azad University, Jolfa, Iran

Ziba Fooladvand and Bahman Fazeli-nasab
Center of Agricultural Biotechnology and Center of Agricultural Research, University of Zabol, Zabol, Iran

Reza Govahi, Gholamreza Ghalamkari, Majid Toghyani, Shahin Eghbal Saied, Mohammad Mohammadrezaei, Mahdi Shahryari and Alireza Dehghani Abari
Department of Animal Science, Khorasgan Branch, Islamic Azad University, Isfahan, Iran

Index